Imperial County

Lars Borges

Texts by William T. Vollmann and Enno Kaufhold

KEHRER

Imperial County
Giving a Face to a Place

Enno Kaufhold

America—the United States of America, to be precise—is the ultimate land of photography. Although photographic technology originated on the old continent of Europe, it was in America that more favorable external conditions enabled this new visual medium to develop more quickly. The American intelligentsia with their European roots were well-versed in European cultural and art historical traditions. But they were much less reserved than their European counterparts when it came to the emerging technology of photography. For it was through photographs that they discovered their own country as it was settled from east to west. Photography could provide a reliable representation of their immense nation—according to prevailing notions of photographic objectivity. Photography was also used early on to document times of historic upheaval, such as the American Civil War in the early 1860s. Afterwards, photographers following the expansion of the western frontier gave Americans views of the newly settled areas with their spectacular natural landscapes.

This specifically American tradition was continued in the images that were taken across the nation by photographers working for the Farm Security Administration (FSA) during the Depression in the 1930s. Walker Evans and Dorothea Lange were among the best known such photographers, who helped establish the genre of social documentary photography, which was marked by increasingly existential and dramatic images due to the rampant poverty in rural areas. The image of America changed with Swiss-born photographer Robert Frank, who traveled with his camera through America from 1955 to 1957 on a Guggenheim Fellowship, and in 1959 published the resulting pictures in a book that would be celebrated as a seminal work of modern documentary photography: *The Americans*. Through the eyes of a foreigner, Frank saw the American people and less their landscapes and cities. And in contrast to the more affirmative images that dominated popular media at the time, Frank's view was decidedly more confrontational. His insistence on the subjective, which included the critical, explains why his book was initially met with vehement disapproval—a fact that is gladly overlooked today. His images reveal nothing of the glorifying national self-image of the American way of life. A positive assessment of Frank's *Americans* would occur only some years later, when the next generation of photographers sought to identify the forefathers of their purposeful work. These included the likes of Lee Friedlander, Garry Winogrand, William Eggleston, Joel Sternfeld, Joel Meyerowitz,

Stephen Shore, Mitch Epstein, Jeff Mermelstein, and in more recent years Alex Soth. Their extensive output has significantly contributed to the image of America and its people, reaching well beyond America's borders. Judging by his international success, the Danish photographer Jakob Holdt should also not be left off the list. In the 1970s, Holdt hitchhiked across America and focused his lens on its dark side, especially racial discrimination. Shot with an automatic camera, his amateur-like photographs document the extensive reports he made of his experiences, and in this combination, convey a very authentic portrait of society.

It is against this backdrop that we can regard the photographic work of Lars Borges. Although the well-known photographers of bygone days were never naive in their work, today's well-trained photographers tend to be much more informed about the work of their photo-historical predecessors. And so it is with Lars Borges, whose pictures of America reveal his familiarity not only with his photographic forebears, but also the road movie genre. The work of filmmaker Terrence Malick has also had a particular influence on him. Parallel to his work in commercial photography, Borges resolutely pursues his own independent projects as well. It was by chance that he came upon the subject of Imperial County. En route to Los Angeles, he looked out of the airplane window to glimpse a vast swath of green adorning the middle of a desert landscape. This aroused his interest, prompting a spontaneous visit to this southernmost region of both California and the USA, so he could have a look and get a picture—literally—of its characteristics. It's a place with a relatively short history and an extremely hot climate, which seems to exist in apparent contradiction to its flourishing agricultural economy. And despite yielding enormous profits, the region is accompanied by a high poverty rate. Following an initial short stay, Borges proceeded to visit Imperial County several times, seeking out personal contact with the local men and women. Only after establishing a certain familiarity with them did he make use of his rather unassuming, albeit professional digital camera. The result is a remarkable photographic portrait, and "portrait" in the broadest sense, for his work comprises pictures of people as well as local landmarks and landscapes.

"Landscape" is an important keyword in this respect, for it describes a fundamental element of the visual world. In the long history of art, the traditional landscape has been based on the horizon as we experience it on a daily basis, making the landscape format inextricably bound to its subject matter. Conversely, images of people walking and standing are usually represented in the upright portrait format. Lars Borges consistently depicts his motifs—including his portraits of people—in the landscape format. This allows him to include more of the people's surroundings. The people enter into a variety of relationships with their environment, interacting with one other both in the photographs, and all the more so in reality. The connection they have is profound, one that might even reach into their DNA. According to what is referred to as milieu theory, the specific characteristics of a region are inscribed over several generations into the external and internal characteristics of the people living there. (One of the main proponents of milieu theory in the late 19th century was the influential French critic and historian Hippolyte Taine.) Given Lars Borges's decidedly person-oriented perspective, which can also be surmised from the sheer number of his portraits, we can ask to what extent his subjects' external features might be directly linked to Imperial County. Considering the historic fact that this region was first settled at the beginning of the 20th century, there are no generations-long genealogies that might help to define a regional typology. This can be seen in the photographs, which show a wide variety of ethnicities and their intermingling, with a strong emphasis on Latin Americans and African Americans. They do, however, point to immigration trends of the past decades, especially from nearby Mexico. At the same time, the faces in his pictures disclose an unfettered familiarity with the photographer. This speaks for the empathy with which Borges encountered these people, and for his special ability and talent to intuitively connect with people and gain their trust. The result is a sense of unforced naturalness.

After photographers like Frank, Winogrand, and Friedlander, who worked with black and white film in the classical manner of concerned photography, we have become accustomed to seeing America in color, beginning with William Eggleston's iconic color photographs of everyday life. Today, black and white photography maintains an aura of nostalgia, in the sense of old fashioned. For Lars Borges, it was clear from the outset that he would use color as an important aesthetic component of his visual understanding. Just as clear was his decision to work exclusively with available light. That applies to the motifs that were taken in glaring daylight as well as at dusk, and also for those images taken with the existing electrical light in both indoor and outdoor situations. Given Lars Borges's—technically speaking—precise depictions, the likes of which are often described as being documentary in style, it would be helpful to consider their content and form. Photographers such as Stephen Shore, Joel Meyerowitz, and Mitch Epstein not only established the use of color in artistic photography, they also demonstrated that the high degree of detail they achieved with their large-format photographs was not relegated to the documentary realm, but was also a matter of artistic expression. It is also in this sense that we can understand Borges's documentary-style photographs.

How many airplane passengers have—like Lars Borges—looked down from their position of comfortable height onto the striking agricultural landscape of Imperial County? It seems that he is one of the few, if not the only one, who developed a long-term photographic interest from this chance sighting. With his perspective of the United States, Borges continues in the photographic tradition of those mentioned above, and categorically avoids anything that might be considered a tourist attraction. Today we often read and hear that, since everything in the world has already been photographed, it no longer makes sense to produce more images. Just how far this is from the truth convincingly demonstrated in the work of Lars Borges. Calexico, El Centro, Slab City, Holtville, Heber, Hot Springs, Orita, Ocotillo Mountains, East Jesus, Niland, Glamis, Imperial, Greeson Wash, Dixieland, Seeley, Brawley, Salton City, Mount Signal, Wilsie, Bombay Beach, Tortuga, Fuller, Calipatria—it's a long list of places that hardly a soul outside of Imperial County has ever heard of. Borges's photographs have now given them a face—from the ground, as well as from the air. Aerial photographs along with perspectives from elevated positions count among the tried and true means of photography, when the aim is to provide the viewer with an overview at a glance. In this case, they provide an immediate idea of what comprises Imperial County both ecologically and economically. What we see is a modern agricultural economy with largescale cultivation of fruits and vegetables, and an equally effective livestock industry. Uniform green patches of farmland and the neat alignment of livestock facilities are the visual manifestations of this optimized efficiency. Unmistakable in this desert region is the crucial importance of water, which stems from the Colorado River, and which by necessity precedes all life. Without water, nothing would thrive, neither plant nor animal, and only in its presence could humans settle here in the first place. The people portrayed in the context of these production processes allow us to guess how few workers are needed by these large, streamlined companies. Next to this, everyday life comes all the more sharply into view, and with it a sense of normality in the most diverse places. We see members of simple social circles as well as societal leaders such as the mayor. They are all depicted as individuals; in their totality, however, down to the details of their clothing and their individual gestures, they embody Imperial County and show us its version of the American way of life.

The insights into Imperial County that these photographs give us enable us to experience the present-day continuation of 19th-century frontier photography, which placed nature's vast panoramas at its heart. Just as those photographs provided those who did not set off for the American west with a visual impression of the unknown, so do these photographs by Lars Borges give us a view of the American southwest today—far removed from the typical travel guide destinations compiled for foreign tourists. And it may well be that these photographs will open the eyes of Americans as well, when they see—possibly for the first time—the origin of the fruit, vegetables, and meat that they buy in their local supermarkets and enjoy on their plates at home every day. Although they cannot entirely erase the disconnect between the production and consumption of food, these images do bring us visually closer to both the origin of certain everyday items, and the unique characteristics of their region of origin. With their compelling visuality, the photographs of Lars Borges thus succeed in expanding our overall awareness of the world, the United States of America, and especially Imperial County.

Imperial County
Eine Region bekommt ein Gesicht

Enno Kaufhold

Amerika, die Vereinigten Staaten von Amerika, um genauer zu sein, ist das Land der Fotografie schlechthin. Die Erfindungen der fotografischen Technik hatten zwar auf dem alten Kontinent Europa ihren Ursprung, für die weitere und schnellere Entwicklung dieses neuen technischen Bildverfahrens bestanden aber in Amerika die besseren äußeren Bedingungen. Die führenden gesellschaftlichen Kreise hatten in ihrer Mehrzahl europäische Wurzeln, auch im Wissen um die kultur- und kunstgeschichtlichen Traditionen, gleichwohl betrachteten sie die technisch erzeugten Bilder mit weniger Vorbehalten, als das in Europa der Fall war. Denn sie lernten ihr Land, das sie von der Ost- wie von der Westküste aus besiedelten, in wesentlichen Teilen durch die neuen fotografischen Bilder kennen. Diese gaben ihnen, nach damaligem Verständnis, womit vor allem die ungemein frappierende Abbildtreue gemeint ist, eine verlässliche Vorstellung von ihrem riesigen Land. Das galt selbst für so markante historische Einschnitte wie den Sezessionskrieg in den frühen 1860er-Jahren. Danach öffneten die im Zuge der weiteren Besiedelung des Westens tätig gewordenen Fotografen, die Frontierfotografen, den Amerikanern den Blick auf die neu erschlossenen Gebiete mit ihren spektakulären Naturarealen.

Diese spezifisch amerikanische Tradition fand in den landesweit aufgenommenen Bildern der Fotografen und Fotografinnen der Farm Security Administration (FSA), während der Depression in den 1930er-Jahren seine Fortsetzung. Genannt seien Walker Evans oder Dorothea Lange als bekannteste Exponenten. Damit gingen die Vorstellungen des Dokumentarismus einher, allerdings aufgrund der in den Landregionen grassierenden Armut mit wesentlich existenzielleren und dramatischeren Motiven. Erst mit dem Schweizer Robert Frank, der von 1955 bis 1957 mit einem Guggenheim-Stipendium durch Amerika reiste und der dann 1959 das heute als Inkunabel der Fotografie gefeierte Buch *The Americans* herausgab, änderte sich die Wahrnehmung des Landes. Aus dem Blickwinkel eines Ausländers sah Frank die Amerikaner, weniger die Landschaften und die Städte, und das im Unterschied zu den vorherrschenden affirmativen Bildauffassungen auf höchst subjektive Weise. Dieses Insistieren auf dem Subjektivem, und das schließt die kritische Sicht ein, erklärt, warum sein Buch zunächst, was heute gerne übersehen wird, vehement kritisiert wurde. Seine Bilder ließen nichts von dem glorifizierenden nationalen Selbstverständnis des American Way of Life erkennen. Eine positive Würdigung von Franks Fotografien sollte erst Jahre später einsetzen, als die nachwachsende

Fotografengeneration nach Vorläufern für ihr engagiertes Arbeiten suchte. Genannt seien Lee Friedlander, Garry Winogrand, William Eggleston, Joel Sternfeld, Joel Meyerowitz, Stephen Shore, Mitch Epstein, Jeff Mermelstein und in jüngeren Jahren Alex Soth. Die umfangreichen Arbeiten dieser Fotografen haben erheblich zu dem Bild beigetragen, das außerhalb der amerikanischen Grenzen von Amerika und seinen Menschen existiert. Gemessen an seinem internationalen Erfolg darf der Däne Jakob Holdt nicht ungenannt bleiben, der in den frühen 1970er-Jahren durch Amerika getrampt ist und dessen thematischer Schwerpunkt auf den Schattenseiten Amerikas und da im Besonderen der Rassendiskriminierung lag (in Deutschland erstmals 1978 veröffentlicht). Seine amateurhaft mit einer automatischen Kamera fotografierten Bilder illustrierten seine umfangreichen Erlebnisberichte und vermittelten in dieser Kombination ein sehr authentisches Gesellschaftsporträt.

Vor diesem Hintergrund ist die aktuelle fotografische Arbeit von Lars Borges zu sehen. Wenngleich die namhaften Fotografinnen und Fotografen vergangener Tage zu keiner Zeit naiv an ihre Arbeiten gingen, was die Kenntnis der Bilder der vorausgegangenen Generationen betrifft, kennen sich die heute in der Regel gut ausgebildeten Fotografen besser mit den fotohistorischen Vorläufern aus. Das trifft uneingeschränkt auf Lars Borges zu. Mit Blick auf sein Amerikabild sind ihm neben den Vorläufern in der Fotografie nicht weniger die einschlägigen Roadmovies vertraut. Im Besonderen hat ihn der Filmemacher Terrence Malick beeinflusst. Ausgehend von seiner kommerziellen Fotografie verfolgt er zielstrebig seine für ihn wichtigen freien Arbeiten. Auf das Thema Imperial County kam er, als er beim Anflug auf Los Angeles aus dem Fenster die riesigen, schon durch ihr formales Ornament ins Auge fallenden Grünflächen inmitten einer Wüstenlandschaft zu Gesicht bekam. Das weckte sein Interesse und bewog ihn spontan, in diese südlichste Region Kaliforniens und mithin der USA zu fahren, um sich dort umzusehen und sich im wortwörtlichen Sinn ein Bild von den Eigenheiten dieser Region zu machen. Einer Region mit relativ kurzer Vergangenheit, einem extrem heißen Klima und einer damit im scheinbaren Widerspruch stehenden florierenden Agrarwirtschaft, der trotz ihrer enormen Gewinne eine hohe Armutsrate gegenübersteht. Nach einem ersten Kennenlernen reiste Lars Borges in der Folge mehrmals ins Imperial County und suchte vor Ort gezielt persönliche Kontakte zu den dort lebenden Frauen und Männern. Erst nachdem sich jeweils eine gewisse Vertrautheit eingestellt hatte, setzte er seine eher unauffällige, aber dennoch professionelle Digitalkamera ein. Entstanden ist in der Summe ein bemerkenswertes fotografisches Porträt, Porträt im weitesten Sinn, denn seine Arbeit schließt Bilder von Personen ebenso ein wie von lokalen Auffälligkeiten und Landschaftspanoramen.

„Landschaft" ist insofern ein wichtiges Stichwort, weil damit Grundsätzliches der Bilderwelt berührt wird. Das traditionelle Landschaftsbild bevorzugt seit kunstgeschichtlichen Urzeiten in Anlehnung an den Horizont, wie wir ihn täglich erleben und wie er demzufolge diesem Sujet eigen ist, das Querformat, während das Bildnis dem aufrecht gehenden und stehenden Menschen entsprechend traditionell als Hochformat auftritt. Lars Borges hat seine Motive für diese Arbeit durchgehend im Querformat fotografiert, einschließlich der Porträts. Auf diese Weise kommt mehr von dem Umfeld, in dem sich die Personen befinden, mit ins Bild. Die Personen und das Ambiente gehen eine wie auch immer geartete Beziehung ein, sie interagieren miteinander im Bild, aber – und auf einer höheren Bedeutungsebene liegend – mehr noch in der Realität. Denn es stellt sich eine Verbindung ein, die nach Auffassung der Milieutheorie bis ins Genetische reicht. Danach übertragen sich die spezifischen Eigenheiten eines Landstriches im Verlaufe vieler Generationen auf die äußeren wie inneren Charakteristika der dort lebenden Menschen (einer der Mitbegründer und Haupttheoretiker der modernen Milieutheorie war in der zweiten Hälfte des 19. Jahrhunderts der Franzose Hippolyte Taine). Angesichts der von Lars Borges bewusst auf die Menschen ausgerichteten Perspektive, wie sie allein schon an der reinen Menge der Porträts abzulesen ist, liegt die Frage nahe, in welchem Maße die Porträtierten äußerliche Merkmal erkennen lassen, die im unmittelbaren Zusammenhang mit dem Imperial County interpretiert werden können. Im Hinblick auf die historische Tatsache, dass diese Region erst seit Beginn des 20. Jahrhunderts besiedelt wurde, konnten sich keine über gewachsene Traditionsketten zurückreichende Genealogien und demzufolge auch noch kein landestypischer Menschenschlag herausbilden. Das kann aus den Porträts direkt abgeleitet werden, denn sie zeigen verschiedenste Ethnien und Mischethnien mit deutlichem Schwerpunkt auf Hispanos und Afroamerikaner. Als solche lassen sie den Zuzug erkennen, der während der zurückliegenden Jahrzehnte stattgefunden hat, insbesondere den aus dem nahegelegenen Mexiko. Zugleich geben die Gesichter eine wohltuende Vertrautheit mit dem Fotografen zu erkennen. Das spricht für die Empathie, mit der Lars Borges die Personen aufnimmt, und für seine besondere Fähigkeit, um nicht von Gabe zu sprechen, sich intuitiv auf Menschen einstellen zu können und deren Vertrauen zu gewinnen. Daraus resultiert die ungezwungene Natürlichkeit.

Nach Fotografen wie Frank, Winogrand und Friedlander, die noch nach klassischer Manier der Concerned Photography mit Schwarz-Weiß-Filmen arbeiteten, haben wir uns daran gewöhnt, Amerika farbig zu sehen, beginnend mit den Farbfotografien von William Eggleston. Heute haftet dem Schwarz-Weiß etwas Nostalgisches im Sinn von Old-Fashioned an. Für Lars Borges gab es von Beginn an keinen Zweifel an der Verwendung der Farbe als wichtiger ästhetischer Komponente seines Bildverständnisses. Genauso klar entschied er sich dafür, bei dieser Arbeit ausschließlich mit vorhandenem Licht, available light, wie es im Fachjargon heißt, zu arbeiten. Das trifft gleichermaßen auf die Motive zu, die bei gleißendem Tageslicht wie bei Dämmerlicht aufgenommen wurden, sowie auf diejenigen, in denen das vor Ort vorhandene elektrische Licht in Außen- wie in Innenräumen bildbestimmend wurde. Angesichts der, technisch gesprochen, präzisen Abbilder, die gerne mit dem Begriff des Dokumentarischen beschrieben werden, bedarf es einer Anmerkung zu Inhalt und Form der Bilder von Lars Borges. Fotografen wie Stephen Shore, Joel Meyerowitz oder Mitch Epstein etablierten nicht nur die Farbe in der künstlerischen Fotografie, zugleich demonstrierten sie mit ihren Großbildaufnahmen, dass die damit zu erzielende Abbildgenauigkeit nicht allein eine Sache des Dokumentarischen ist, sondern sehr wohl als künstlerischer Ausdruck gelten kann. In diesem Sinn müssen auch die von Lars Borges im dokumentarischen Stil aufgenommenen Fotografien verstanden werden.

Wie viele Flugpassagiere, so könnte die Frage lauten, haben wie Lars Borges aus ihrer komfortablen Höhenposition die auffälligen Agrarflächen des Imperial County gesehen? Wie es scheint, ist er einer der wenigen, wenn nicht sogar in seiner Konsequenz der einzige, der aus dem Sehen ein nachhaltiges fotografisches Interesse entwickelt hat. Damit nahm er eine Perspektive auf die USA ein, in der er an die genannten Vorläufer anschließt, darüber hinaus setzt er sich damit zugleich fundamental von allen eher touristischen Attraktionen ab. Angeblich, so ist immer wieder zu lesen und zu hören, sei alles, was die Welt ausmacht, bereits fotografiert worden und es mache demzufolge keinen Sinn mehr, weitere Bilder zu produzieren. Dass dem nicht so ist, demonstriert seine Arbeit auf eindrucksvolle Weise. Calexico, El Centro, Slab City, Holtville, Heber, Hot Springs, Orita, Ocotillo Mountains, East Jesus, Niland, Glamis, Imperial, Greeson Wash, Dixieland, Seeley, Brawley, Salton City, Mount Signal, Wilsie, Bombay Beach, Tortuga, Fuller, Calipatria, das ist eine lange Reihe solcher Ortsnamen, die kaum jemand außerhalb des Imperial County kennt, die jetzt dank der Fotografien ein Gesicht bekommen, am Boden, aber ebenso aus der Luft. Luftaufnahmen gehören ebenso wie Perspektiven von erhöhten Standpunkten zu den probaten Mitteln der Fotografie, wenn es darum zu tun ist, dem Betrachter auf einen Blick eine Übersicht zu bieten. In diesem Fall geben sie eine unmittelbare Vorstellung von dem, was das Imperial County ökologisch wie ökonomisch ausmacht. Zu sehen ist eine moderne, auf Effizienz ausgerichtete Agrarwirtschaft mit großflächigem Obst- und Gemüseanbau sowie einer nicht minder effektiven Viehwirtschaft. Das gleichförmige

Ornament, wie es die rechteckigen Grünflächen entstehen lassen, und die parallel gestaffelten Anlagen der Viehwirtschaft sind bildgewordene Zeichen für eben diese optimierte Wirtschaftlichkeit. Unübersehbar erschließt sich die eminente Bedeutung des Wassers in der Wüstenregion, ausgehend vom Colorado River, das allem Leben zwingend vorauszugehen hat. Denn ohne Wasser würde nichts gedeihen, keine Pflanze, kein Tier, und auch den Menschen ermöglicht es erst das Leben an diesem Ort. Die in Verbindung mit den Produktionszusammenhängen porträtierten Personen lassen ahnen, mit wie wenigen Arbeitskräften die durchrationalisierten Großbetriebe auskommen. Daneben rückt in weit größerem Maße das Alltagsleben in den Blick und damit die an den verschiedensten Orten anzutreffende Normalität. Wir sehen Repräsentanten einfachster gesellschaftlicher Kreise genauso wie die gesellschaftlich führenden Persönlichkeiten einschließlich des Bürgermeisters. Sie alle sind individuell erfasst, in ihrer Summe verkörpern sie aber bis in alle Details der Bekleidung und des jeweiligem individuellen Gestus hinein das Imperial County und zeigen den Status des dortigen American Way of Life.

Indem wir anhand der Fotografien diese Einblicke in das Imperial County bekommen, erleben wir die aktuelle Fortsetzung der Frontierfotografie des 19. Jahrhunderts, für die noch die großen Naturpanoramen im Mittelpunkt stand. Wie diese seinerzeit all denen, die sich nicht auf die Reise in den Westen des Landes gemacht haben, wenigsten eine visuelle Vorstellung des ihnen Unbekannten gaben, vermitteln uns die Fotografien von Lars Borges jetzt ein Bild des Südens, und das jenseits dessen, was die Reiseführer dem Besucher der USA als landestypische Attraktionen anpreisen. Vermutlich dürften diese Fotografien selbst vielen Amerikanern die Augen öffnen, sehen sie doch, möglicherweise zum ersten Mal, woher ihr Obst, Gemüse und Fleisch kommt, das sie tagtäglich in den Supermärkten kaufen und das sie zuhause auf den Tellern haben. Damit wird die bestehende Entfremdung nicht aufgehoben, das Wissen um die Herkunft bestimmter zum Leben gehörender Produkte erschließt sich aber visuell und wird somit ebenso bewusst wie all das, was die Eigenheiten der Herkunftsregion ausmacht. In diesem Sinn erweitern Lars Borges' Fotografien in ihrer überzeugenden Visualität unser aller Bewusstsein hinsichtlich des Gesamtbildes, das wir von unserem Globus, den USA und dem Imperial County im Speziellen haben.

The Gardens of Paradise

William T. Vollmann

What did the bodies come here for? We all know the answer. I remember how on one of my many bus rides south I was meditating on the heat and strangeness of this corner of California when the man beside me awoke, and turned toward the window like a plant toward the sun. Soon we would come to the sign which read IMPERIAL COUNTY LINE and a few minutes later we'd pass the Corvina Cafe, which would surely be as closed and dead as one of those corvina floating belly-up in the Salton Sea. The man sat gazing alertly eastward across the desert flats toward the long deep green stripe of date plantations and the dusty red and blue mountains beyond. I inferred that this landscape was his by birth or long residence. Perhaps he had been away from it for awhile. He'd told me that he was coming from a Fourth of July party at his sister's, but I'd seen the policeman standing in the loading area, watching to make sure that he boarded this bus whose disinfectant, pretending to be pine or lemon, stung the nose with its bad chemical smell. He'd slept with his chin in his hands all the way from Indio and past the tan silence of the Jewel Date Company's former factory parallel to the railroad tracks where rusty flatbed cars gave off heat. Now he sighed a little, and turned toward me as eagerly as he had strained toward the mountains. He offered me Mexican candy, praising it because it was cheap. Openhanded, gruff and husky, he longed to tell the tale of his life. He'd served twenty-four years in the Spanish army—or maybe he'd been an American soldier stationed in Spain, this fine point being occluded by his broken English and my ignorance of Spanish. At any rate, Spain had failed him, evidently by means of woman trouble. Now he was living in El Centro to be near his eighty-two-year-old father who had once been a mechanical genius but who lately did little more than putter around the air conditioner, trying to grow coolness like a vegetable and then inbreed and harvest it. When he spoke of his father, tenderness came into his voice in just the same way that the yellow flowers of the palo verde tree come briefly back even in July or August if there is rain. His father was too old to drive a car, so once our bus pulled into the El Centro station, my friend would be walking home in the hundred-and-ten-degree heat, which killed illegal aliens easily.

The ones who crossed alone were called *solos*. The ones who paid to be taken across were *pollos*—chickens. And who better to shepherd chickens through dangerous ways than a coyote? That's truly what they were called! Coyotes never eat chickens, do they? (Every day, many pollos die, a taxi driver told me with solemn exaggeration. The newspaper said that only two hundred and fifty-four illegals had died last year, to which the taxi driver replied: Liars—assassins! Two or three a day die right here! They hide the bodies under the sand so that the Border Patrol won't see.—They do die, a lifetime *pollo* later told me, but not that many.) Then there were the chicken-handlers, the *pollistas* or *polleros* whom the bigshot coyotes deputed to do the dirty work of canal-crossings and the like. Officer Murray called them "scouts."—They're pretty chicken, he said, not meaning the pun.—Like their bosses, they sometimes ran away when it was dangerous, leaving their passengers to die of thirst. For it was so very hot! When his father died, my seatmate might move away from Imperial County, on account of the heat. In his low, hoarse, not unpleasant voice, he remarked that he didn't mind sitting outside in a hundred and five degrees, but when it got up to a hundred and fifteen, then his cold beer turned into hot coffee, and it was time to go indoors. He uttered many a melancholy jest of this character. I'd already begun to think of him as the old soldier, and was almost appalled that he was my age, thirty-eight; he looked twenty years older. This working man, dark and wiry, had resisted many solar assaults, armored by no more than an upturned cap-brim, but each attack had shriveled him a little more, so that he'd eventually be desiccated to his very soul. The hot, dry sunlight instantly warms flesh to a state near burning, then cauterizes it and stains it brown. Born in Brawley, which our Greyhound soon would reach, he'd never been to the Salton Sea in his entire life. (How far was it? Half an hour's drive?) As a boy he'd been too busy in the fields, he said; after that he'd tried his luck in Spain. And now as we continued south on Highway 111 he began to explicate the crops to me, each time weighing himself down with a new story of dreary and dangerous drudgery.

Here came another date orchard to our left, with busy birds silhouetted in the palm-crests, uplifting their beaks, clicking and crying even in the heat of midday. I admired the shade and luxurious fruit of those trees, but the old soldier turned to me with a bitter smile and said that the most perilous labor of his life had been ascending toward the birds on a rickety ladder leaned against each tree in turn, with no one holding the bottom for him; his job was to tie bags around immature dates so that they'd not be lost. Little and lean, he'd scampered into the sun which burned him until he resembled the black fly with alert yellow eyes which one often finds crouching in the dusty crease of a palm's fan. Sometimes he got dizzy; sometimes the ladder slipped. His memories were stained with terror.

By the time he'd completed this relation, our Greyhound bus had drawn close to an onion field in glorious flower, and the old soldier croaked out that working in the onion fields had left him stinking of onion juice, his eyes watering day and night. After a week the onion juice was literally under his skin. (I thought of what Officer Murray had said: When you get people out of an onion field, you wanna roll your windows down.) No matter how long he bowed beneath the showerhead, scrubbing himself red, the onion smell kept oozing out of him so that he stank even to himself and coughed himself to sleep. Eventually he began to bring up blood from too much coughing.

No, I hung it up, the old soldier said. Don't wanna pick in the fields no more. I got me a ladyfriend, she about forty, forty-five years old. And every morning she drives from El Centro all the way to Yuma. There are four of them people; they share gas. Then she picks. Imagine that, a forty-five-year-old lady and still out there picking! What a tough gal! One time she brought me a cantaloupe from the field. Another time, it was a big watermelon…

And he smiled a smile of loving pride. But then his bitterness landed on him again, like flies on a sweaty face. We'd come to a place of white puffballs left behind in the dark fields. The old soldier said that they were cantaloupes—no plants, only the pale spheres sticking out. The migrant workers would turn them up later. He had been among the up-turners of cantaloupes and of so many other crops, following the harvesters on foot, gleaning up lost fruits under that hot, dusty, greyish-white sky. He began to tell me how it was, waving his withered hands as he angrily, dolefully whispered, describing the ache between the shoulderblades, the throbbing in the small of the back, the shooting pains in the arms, the hands that after gripping and lifting all day became dirt-stained baseball mitts which could no longer open or close, painfully throbbing in the bones. Beyond these agonies he remembered with all his hatred the Imperial summers, which had moved one woman on a hundred-degree Saturday evening in Indio to tell me how she had realized that this planet truly orbits a star of immense heat and brightness; whenever she stepped outside on an Imperial day, she could keep possession of only a slender slice of moments before being overpowered by stuporous confusion. Once she was safely back inside, everything on her person, every key or card, every square inch of her blouse, gave off heat. And yet the migrant workers had to spend all day outside, sometimes working for less than the legal minimum wage. The old soldier had finished with that. He could not bear it anymore.

The Imperial Valley Press stood on his side. In a section entitled "OUR OPINION: TIME FOR A CHANGE," that newspaper laid out the problem: As important as agriculture is to the county, there are limits on a community with an economy so dependent on farming, because agricultural workers do not exactly get the highest salaries… Finally, agriculture is not as strong in the Imperial Valley as it has been in years past. The Press slavered over the smoothly-named Gateway to the Americas Project, which would soon erect houses and industrial parks near the new Calexico East Port of Entry. It could create thousands of jobs. The hoped-for future of the Imperial Valley: strip malls, office parks, chain stores, Los Angelesization. Meanwhile the old soldier's ladyfriend went on fruit-picking, and in hopes of doing the same thing the *pollos* and *solos* slithered up and down the border fence.

Die Gärten des Paradieses

William T. Vollmann

Weswegen kamen die Körper hierher? Wir alle kennen die Antwort. Ich weiß noch, wie ich auf einer meiner vielen Busfahrten in den Süden über die Hitze und die Eigentümlichkeit dieses Zipfels von Kalifornien nachsann, als der Mann neben mir aufwachte und sich zum Fenster wandte wie eine Pflanze zur Sonne. Bald sollten wir zu dem Schild mit der Aufschrift IMPERIAL COUNTY LINE kommen und wenige Minuten später würden wir das Corvina Cafe passieren, das sicher so geschlossen und tot sein würde wie einer dieser Corvina-Fische, die mit dem Bauch nach oben im Saltonsee schwammen. Der Mann saß da und starrte geistesgegenwärtig über die Wüstenebene gen Osten in Richtung der langen, tiefen, grünen Streifen von Dattelplantagen und der staubigen roten und blauen Berge im Hintergrund. Ich folgerte, dass diese Landschaft von Geburt oder nach jahrelangem Aufenthalt die seine war. Vielleicht war er eine Zeitlang fort gewesen. Er komme, so hatte er mir erzählt, von einer Feier bei seiner Schwester zum Unabhängigkeitstag, doch ich hatte den Polizisten bei der Gepäckverladung gesehen, der ihn beobachtete und dafür sorgte, dass er diesen Bus mit seinem durchdringenden Desinfektionsgeruch nach angeblich Pinie oder Zitrone bestieg. Seit Indio hatte er die ganze Zeit mit dem Kinn in den Händen geschlafen, entlang der hellbraunen Stille der ehemaligen Fabrik der Jewel Date Company neben den Eisenbahnschienen, wo verrostete Flachwagen Wärme abgaben. Nun seufzte er ein wenig und drehte sich so eifrig zu mir, wie er sich zu den Bergen hin verrenkt hatte. Er bot mir mexikanische Süßigkeiten an, pries sie an, weil sie billig waren. Freigebig, ruppig und rauchig, sehnte er sich danach, die Geschichte seines Lebens zu erzählen. 24 Jahre hatte er in der spanischen Armee gedient – oder vielleicht war er als amerikanischer Soldat in Spanien stationiert gewesen, diese Nuance blieb mir wegen seines gebrochenen Englisch und meiner fehlenden Spanischkenntnisse verborgen. Jedenfalls war er von Spanien enttäuscht, anscheinend wegen Ärger mit einer Frau. Nun lebte er in El Centro, um in der Nähe seines 82-jährigen Vaters zu sein, der einst ein genialischer Mechaniker gewesen war, in letzter Zeit aber nicht viel mehr tat, als an der Klimaanlage zu schrauben und zu versuchen, die Kühle wie Gemüse heranzuziehen und dann Inzucht zu betreiben und sie zu ernten. Wenn er von seinem Vater sprach, bekam seine Stimme einen liebevollen Klang, so wie die gelben Blüten des Jerusalemsdorns für kurze Zeit noch im Juli oder August zurückkehren, wenn es Regen gibt. Sein Vater war zu alt, um Auto zu fahren, und sobald unser Bus in den Bahnhof von El Centro einbiegen würde, würde mein Freund zu

Fuß nach Hause gehen bei 43 Grad Hitze, die illegale Einwanderer leicht umbringen konnte.

Diejenigen, die alleine rüberkamen, hießen *solos*. Diejenigen, die für das Hinüberbringen bezahlten, waren *pollos*, Hühner. Und wer war besser geeignet, Hühner über gefährliche Wege zu führen, als ein Kojote? So hießen sie ganz im Ernst! Kojoten fressen nie Hühner, oder? (Jeden Tag sterben zahlreiche *pollos*, berichtete mir ein Taxifahrer mit ehrwürdiger Übertreibung. Der Zeitung zufolge waren im letzten Jahr nur 254 illegale Einwanderer gestorben, worauf der Taxifahrer entgegnete: Lügen – Mörder! Genau hier sterben jeden Tag zwei oder drei! Sie verstecken die Leichen unter dem Sand, sodass die Grenzpatrouille sie nicht findet. – Es gibt tatsächlich Tote, bestätigte mir ein lebenslanges *pollo* später, aber nicht so viele.) Daneben gab es die Hühnerschlepper, die *pollistas* oder *polleros*, die von den Alpha-Kojoten für die Drecksarbeit der Kanalüberfahrten und Ähnliches abkommandiert wurden. Officer Murray nannte sie die „Scouts". – Es sind die hübschen Hühner, sagte er, ohne sie damit als feige bezeichnen zu wollen. – Wie ihre Bosse machten sie sich manchmal, wenn es gefährlich wurde, aus dem Staub und ließen ihre Passagiere verdursten. Denn es war einfach so unendlich heiß! Nach dem Tod seines Vaters werde er vielleicht aus Imperial County wegziehen, sagte mein Sitznachbar, wegen der Hitze. In seiner tiefen, heiseren, nicht unangenehmen Stimme bemerkte er, es mache ihm nichts aus, bei 40 Grad Hitze draußen zu sitzen, aber wenn die Temperatur auf 46 Grad steige, werde sein kaltes Bier zu heißem Kaffee und es sei Zeit, ins Haus zu gehen. Melancholische Scherze dieser Art machte er viele. Ich hatte schon angefangen, ihn mir als alten Soldaten vorzustellen, und war beinahe entsetzt, dass er mein Alter war, 38; er sah 20 Jahre älter aus. Dieser arbeitende Mann, dunkel und drahtig, hatte vielen Sonnenangriffen mit nicht mehr als dem hochgeklappten Schirm seiner Kappe widerstanden, doch jeder Angriff hatte ihn ein bisschen runzliger gemacht, sodass er irgendwann bis auf die Seele ausgedörrt sein würde. Das heiße, trockene Sonnenlicht erhitzt das Fleisch fast sofort bis auf Brenntemperatur, verödet es dann und färbt es braun. In Brawley geboren – ein Ort, den unser Greyhound bald erreichen würde –, war er in seinem ganzen Leben noch nie am Saltonsee gewesen. (Wie weit war der weg? Eine halbe Stunde mit dem Auto?) Als Junge habe er immer auf dem Feld gearbeitet, dann sein Glück in Spanien versucht. Und während wir nun weiter auf dem Highway 111 in Richtung Süden fuhren, erklärte er mir die Feldfrüchte und zog sich mit jeder neuen Geschichte von grauer und gefährlicher Schinderei ein bisschen weiter nach unten.

Hier kam eine weitere Dattelplantage zu unserer Linken mit fleißigen Vögeln, die sich in den Kronen der Palmen abzeichneten, die Schnäbel aufrichteten, selbst in der Mittagssonne noch trommelten und tirilierten. Ich bewunderte den Schatten und die kostbare Frucht dieser Bäume, doch der alte Soldat drehte sich mit bitterem Lächeln zu mir um und sagte, die gefährlichste Arbeit seines Lebens sei es gewesen, auf einer wackligen, gegen den Baum gelehnten Leiter nach oben zu den Vögeln zu klettern, ohne dass unten jemand die Leiter festgehalten habe; er habe Tüten um die noch unreifen Datteln binden müssen, um sie vor Schäden zu schützen. Klein und dürr sei er in der Sonne herumgeflitzt, die ihn verbrannte, bis er der schwarzen Fliege mit den wachen gelben Augen ähnelte, die man häufig in der staubigen Falte eines Palmfächers findet. Manchmal wurde ihm schwindlig; manchmal rutschte die Leiter weg. Seine Erinnerungen waren von schrecklichen Ängsten getrübt.

Als er seine Schilderung beendet hatte, näherte sich unser Greyhound-Bus einem Zwiebelfeld in herrlicher Blüte, und der alte Soldat stieß krächzend hervor, die Arbeit auf den Zwiebelfeldern habe ihn nach Zwiebelsaft stinken lassen, seine Augen hätten Tag und Nacht getränt. Nach einer Woche sei ihm der Zwiebelsaft buchstäblich unter die Haut gegangen. (Ich musste an die Bemerkung von Officer Murray denken: Wenn Du Leute aus 'nem Zwiebelfeld kriegst, kurbel' die Fenster runter.) Er konnte sich noch so lange unter die Brause stellen, sich rot schrubben – der Zwiebelgeruch sickerte immer noch aus ihm heraus, sodass er selbst für sein eigenes Empfinden stank und sich in den Schlaf hustete. Schließlich begann er, vom vielen Husten Blut zu spucken.

Nein, ich hab's an den Nagel gehängt, sagte der alte Soldat. Ich will nicht mehr auf den Feldern pflücken. Hab mir 'ne Freundin gesucht, sie ist um die 40, 45. Und jeden Morgen fährt sie die ganze Strecke von El Centro bis nach Yuma. Sie sind zu viert, teilen sich das Benzin. Dann pflückt sie. Stell Dir das vor, eine 45-jährige Lady und pflückt noch immer! Was für ein toughes Mädel! Einmal hat sie mir eine Cantaloupe-Melone vom Feld mitgebracht. Ein anderes Mal eine große Wassermelone…

Und er lächelte ein liebevoll stolzes Lächeln. Doch dann landete die Bitterkeit wieder auf ihm, wie Fliegen auf einem verschwitzten Gesicht. Wir waren an einen Ort gelangt, an dem weiße Boviste auf den dunklen Feldern zurückgelassen worden waren. Das seien Cantaloupe-Melonen, sagte der alte Soldat, keine Pflanzen, nur die blassen Kugeln, die herausragten. Die Wanderarbeiter würden sie später umdrehen. Er habe zu den Umdrehern von Cantaloupe-Melonen und so vielen anderen Feldfrüchten gehört, sei den Erntearbeitern zu Fuß gefolgt, habe verlorene Früchte unter diesem heißen, staubigen, grauweißen Himmel aufgesammelt. Er erzählte mir, wie es war, fuchtelte mit den verrunzelten Händen, während er wütend, niedergeschlagen flüsterte, den Schmerz zwischen den Schulterblättern beschrieb, das Pochen im Kreuz, die stechenden Schmerzen in den Armen, die Hände, die nach dem Zupacken und Hochziehen den ganzen Tag zu dreckigen Baseballhandschuhen wurden und sich nicht mehr öffnen oder schließen ließen und in den Knochen schmerzhaft puckerten. Von diesen Qualen abgesehen, erinnerte er sich mit all seinem Hass an die Imperial-Sommer, die eine Frau an einem fast 38 Grad heißen Samstagabend in Indio dazu veranlasst hatten, mir zu erzählen, wie ihr klar geworden sei, dass dieser Planet wahrhaftig einen Stern von unermesslicher Hitze und Helligkeit umkreise; jedes Mal, wenn sie an einem Imperial-Tag nach draußen ginge, könne sie es nur magere Momente dort aushalten, bevor sie von dumpfer Verwirrtheit überwältigt werde. War sie erst wieder einmal sicher drinnen, gab alles an ihr, jeder Schlüssel und jede Karte, jeder Quadratzentimeter ihrer Bluse, Wärme ab. Und dennoch mussten die Wanderarbeiter den ganzen Tag draußen verbringen, manchmal für weniger als den gesetzlichen Mindestlohn. Der alte Soldat hatte damit Schluss gemacht. Er konnte es nicht mehr ertragen.

Die Imperial Valley Press war auf seiner Seite. In einer Rubrik mit dem Titel „UNSERE MEINUNG: ZEIT FÜR EINEN WECHSEL“ schilderte die Zeitung das Problem so: So wichtig die Landwirtschaft für das County auch ist, so gibt es Grenzen für eine Gemeinschaft, deren Wirtschaft derart von der Feldarbeit abhängt, weil Landarbeiter nicht gerade die höchsten Gehälter bekommen… Schließlich ist die Landwirtschaft im Imperial Valley nicht mehr so stark wie in den vergangenen Jahren. Die Zeitung konnte das unverfänglich Gateway-to-the-Americas-Projekt genannte kaum abwarten, für das bald Häuser und Industrieparks in der Nähe des neuen Calexico-Ost Zollhafens entstehen würden. Es könne Tausende neuer Jobs schaffen. Die erhoffte Zukunft des Imperial Valley: Einkaufszentren, Bürogebäude, Ladenketten, Los Angelesisierung. Unterdessen pflückte die Freundin des alten Soldaten weiter Früchte, und in der Hoffnung, dasselbe zu tun, schlängelten sich die *pollos* und *solos* den Grenzzaun hinauf und hinunter.

“Water is king, here is its kingdom.”

Imperial Press, front page, June 8, 1901

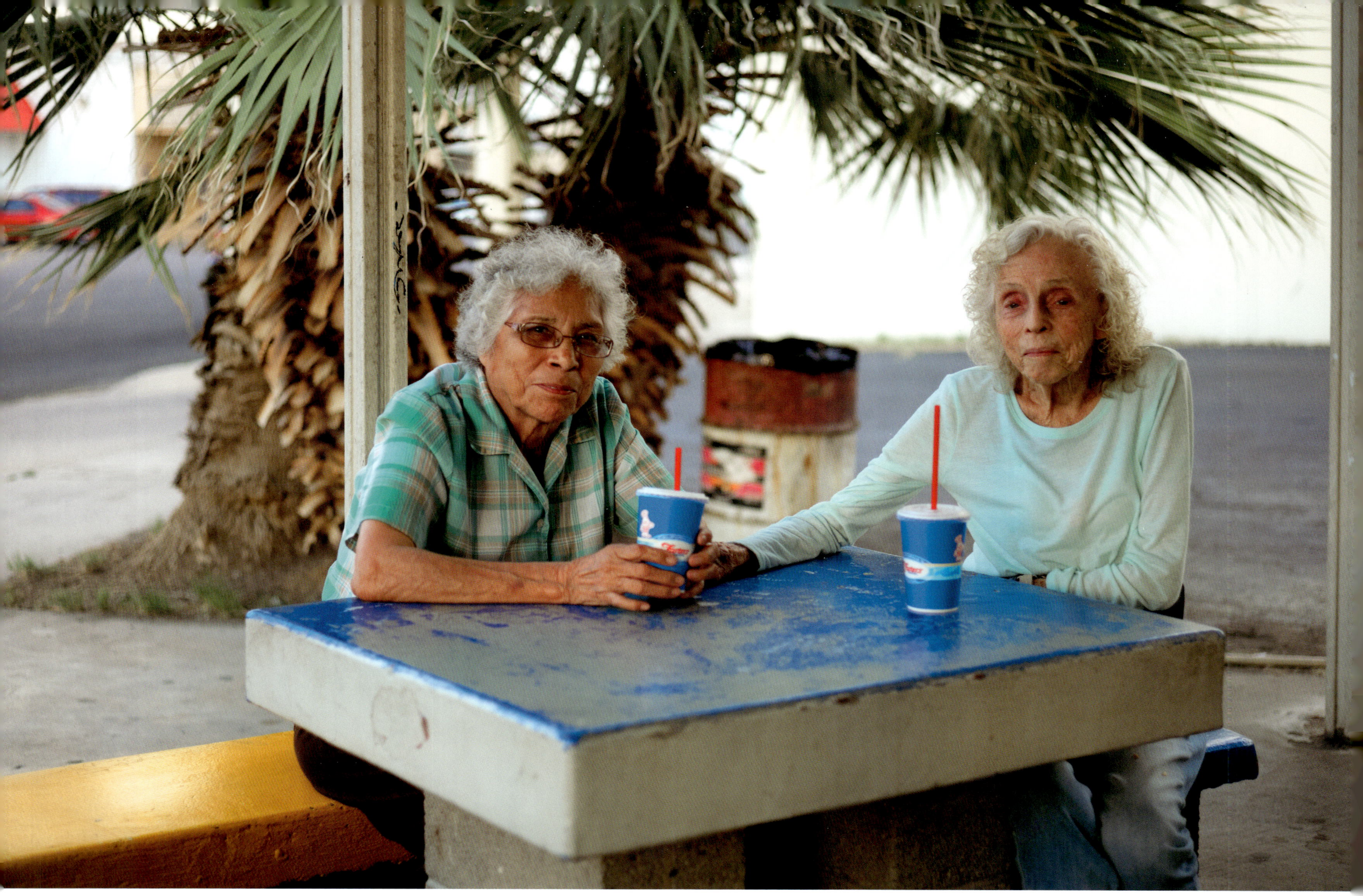

Kate and Agnes, Brawley

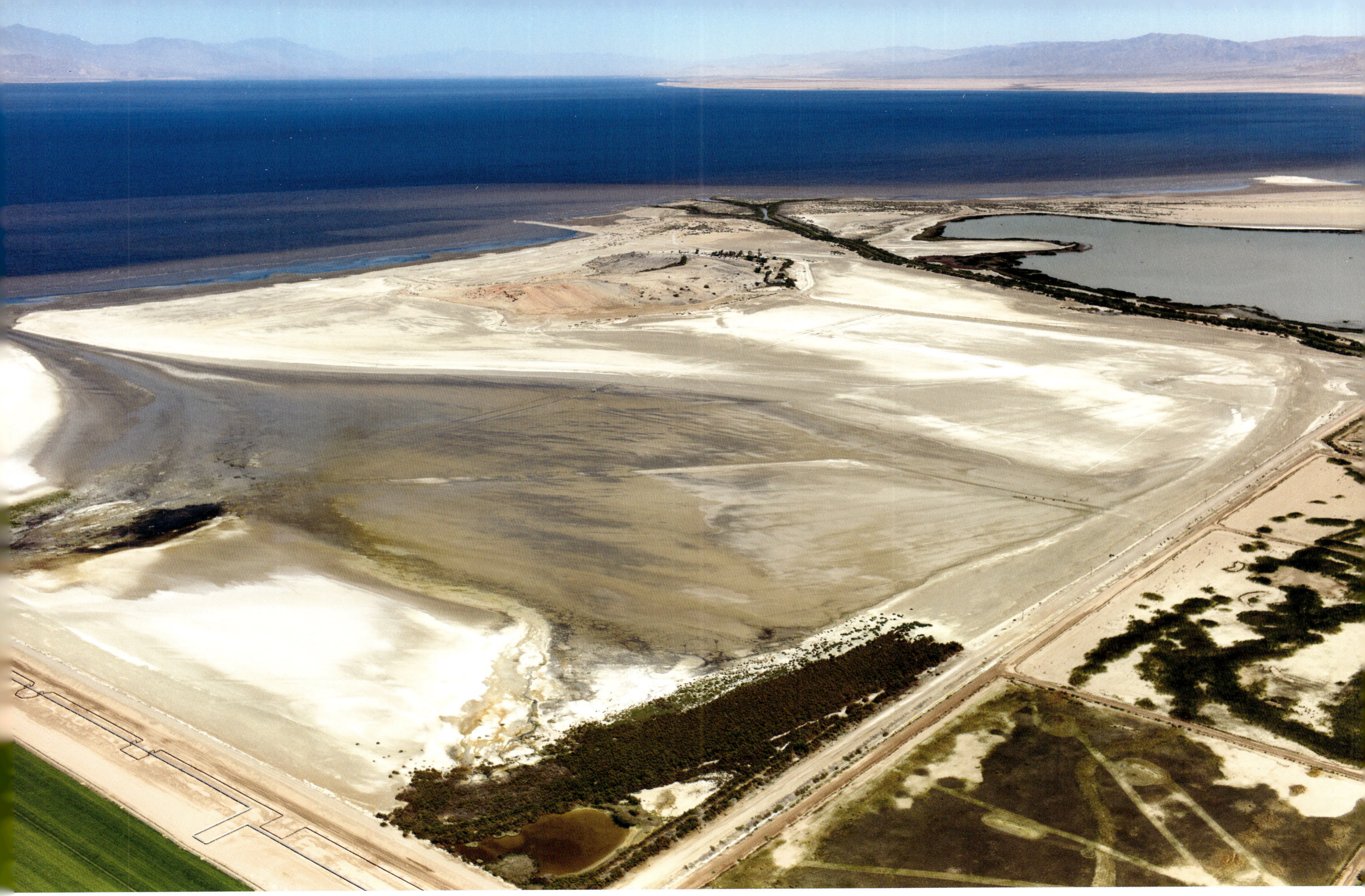

Sonny Bono Wildlife Refuge, Salton Sea

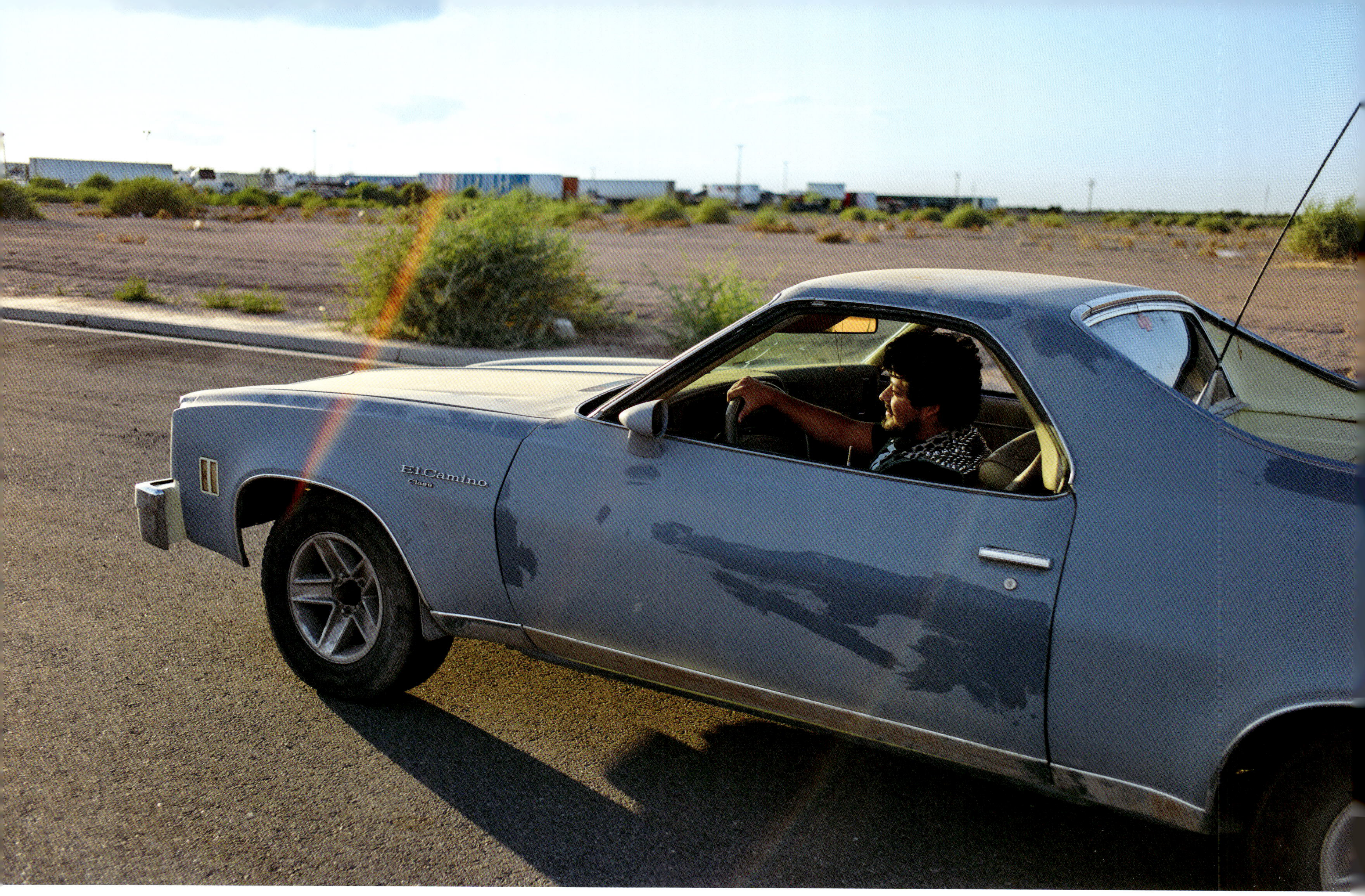

Hector Junior, Calexico

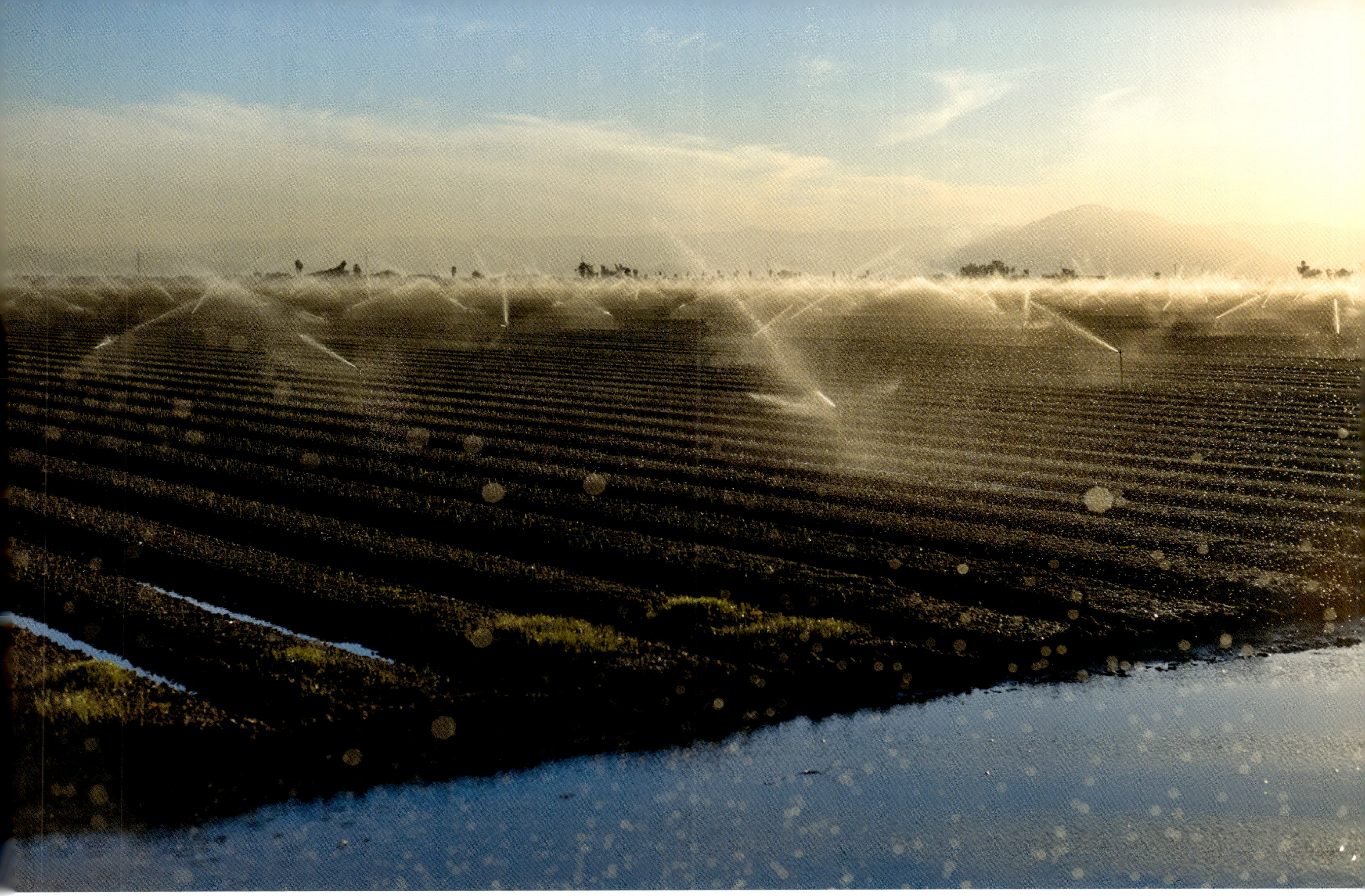

Onion field, near Seeley

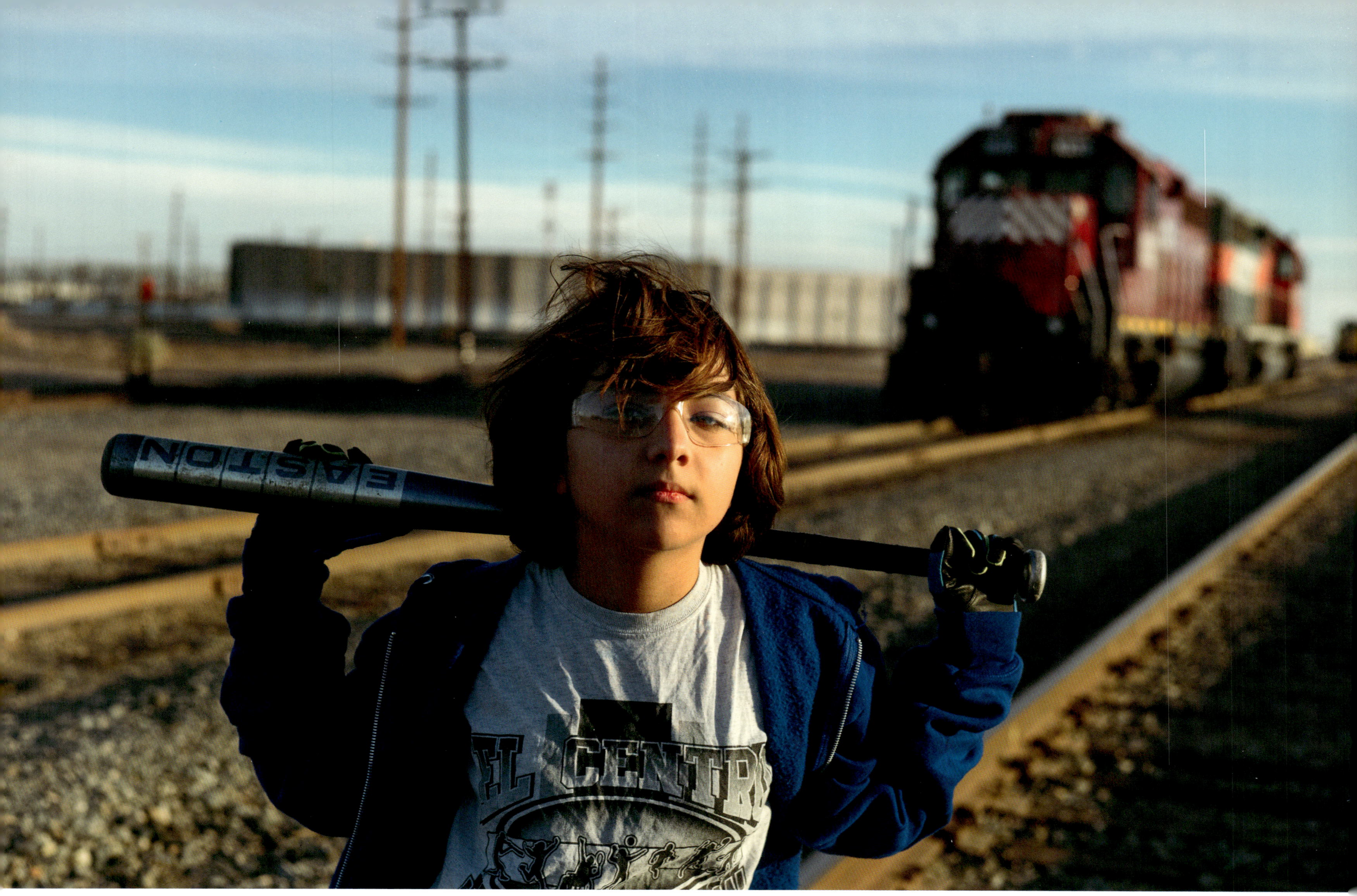

Hailey, El Centro

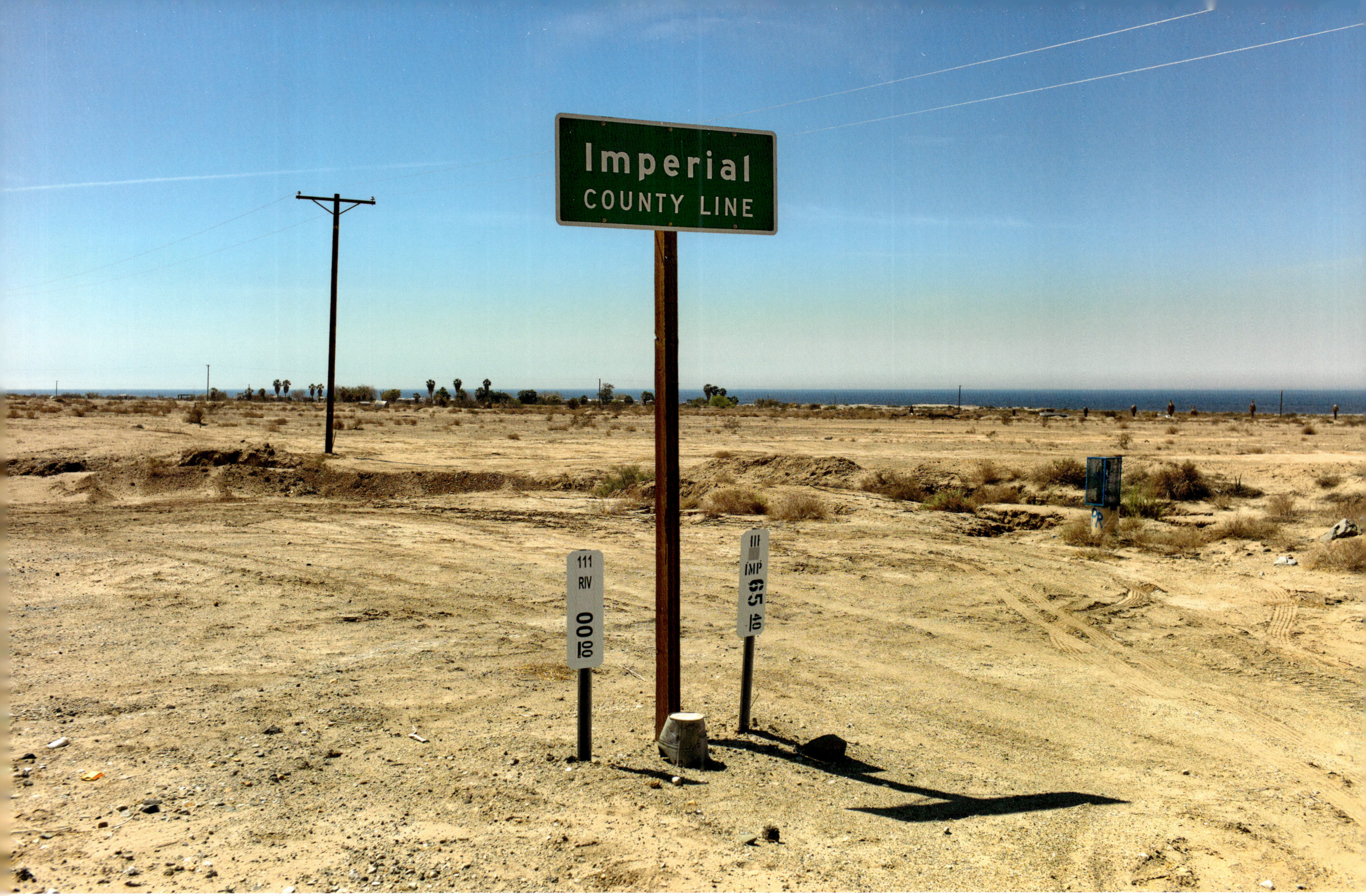

Highway 111, north of Bombay Beach

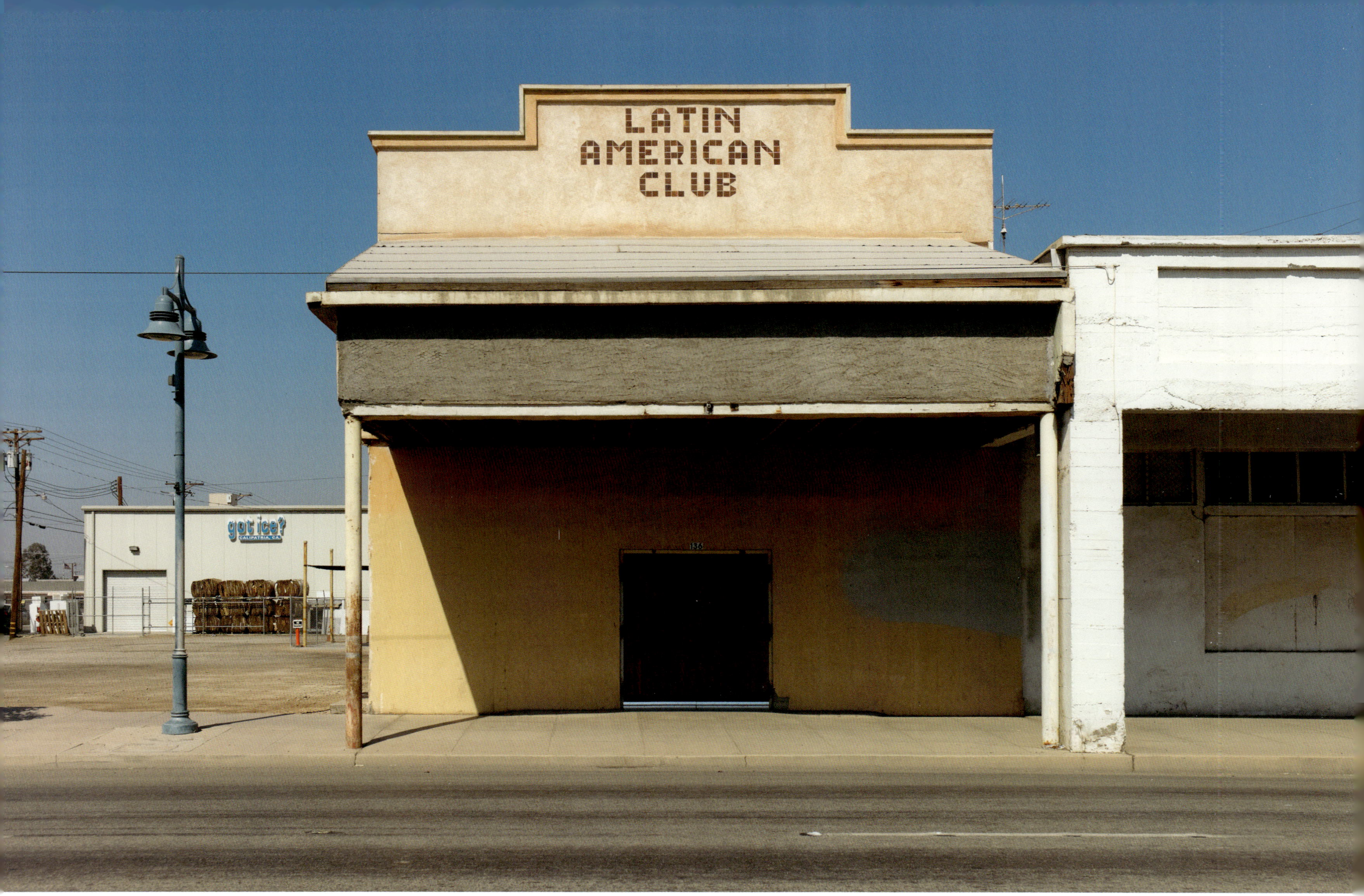

Sorensen Avenue, Calipatria

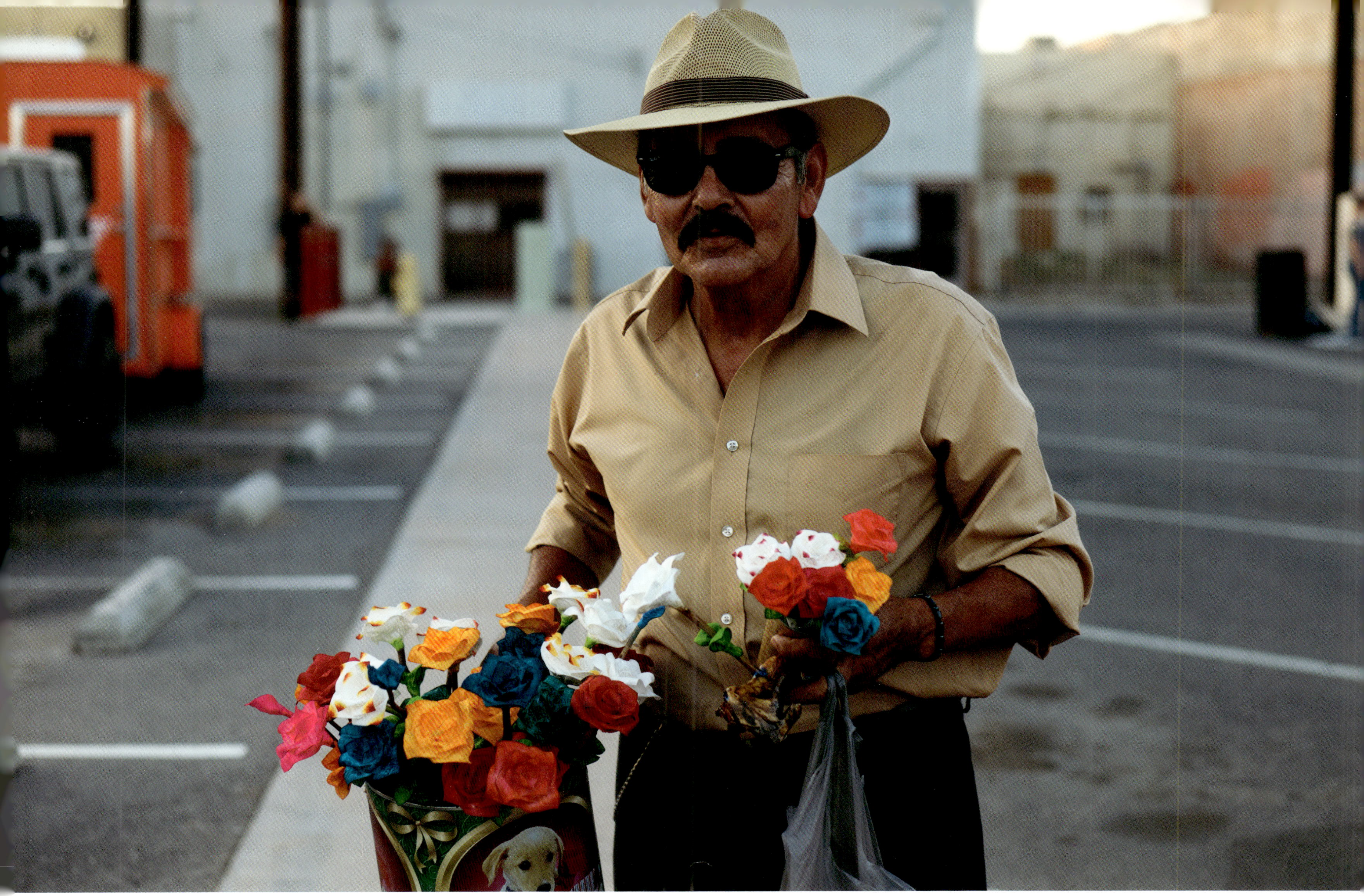

Gilbert, Brawley

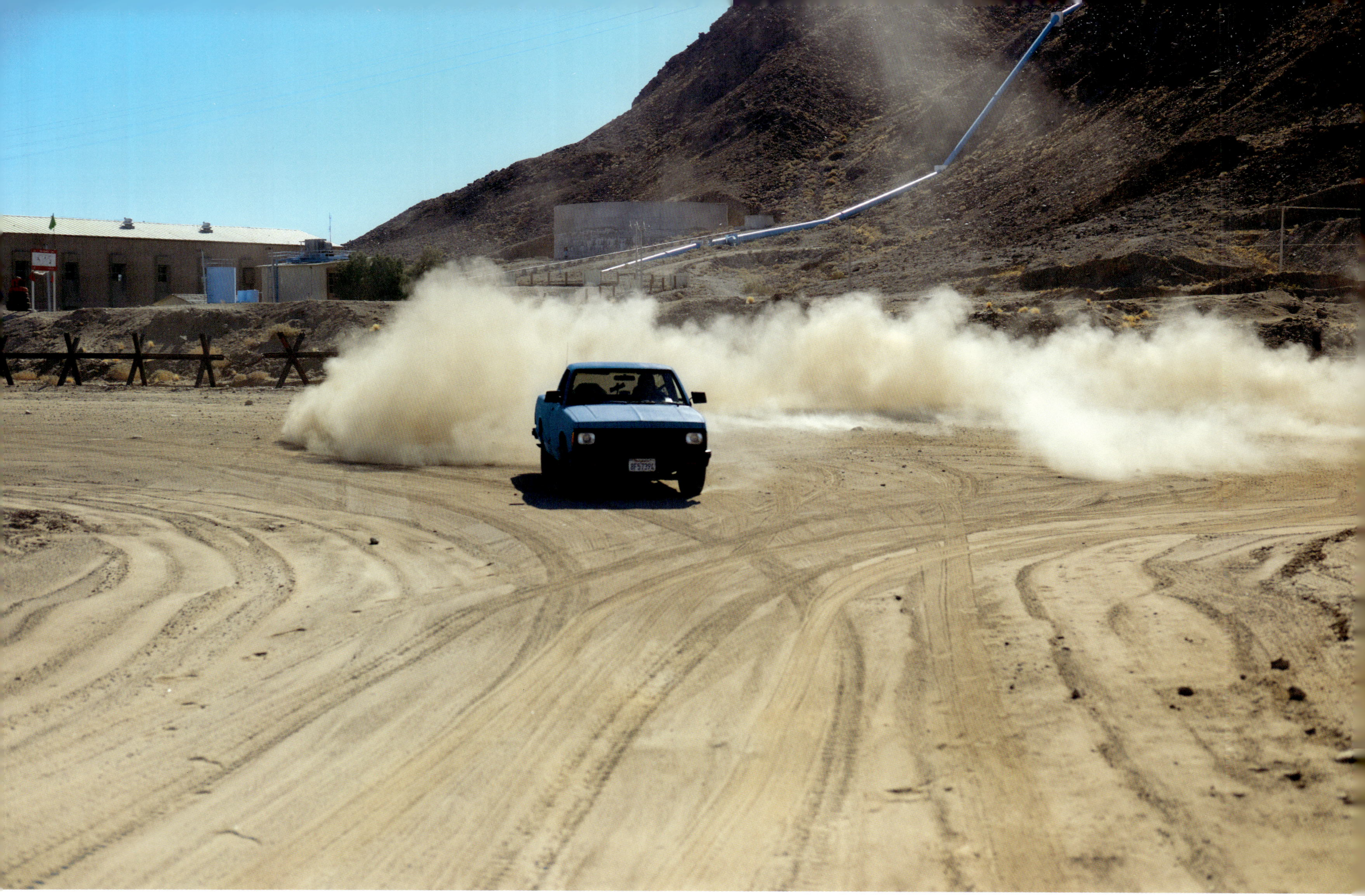

Next to La Rosita drug tunnel, Mount Signal

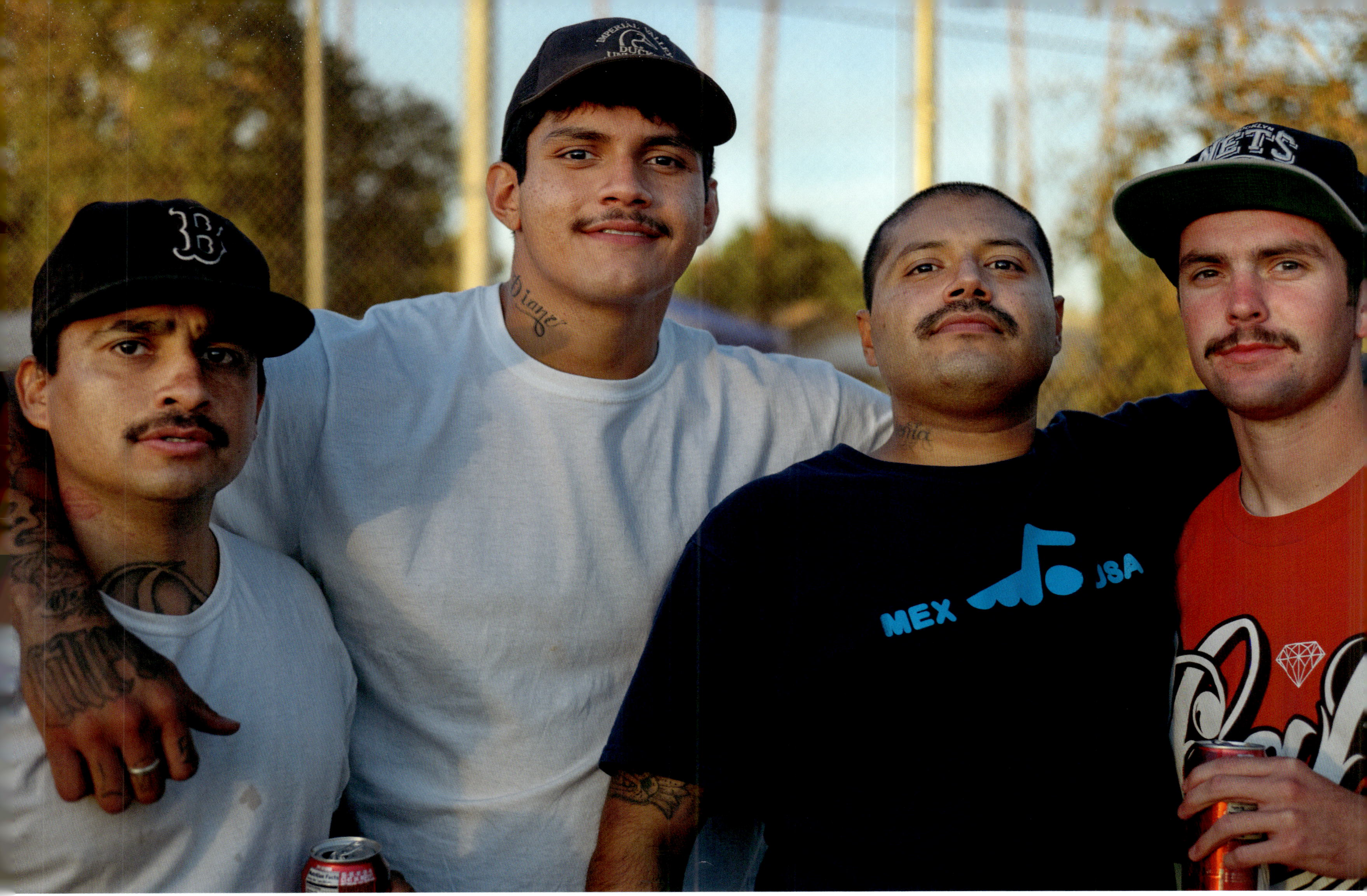

Team Jesus, Holtville

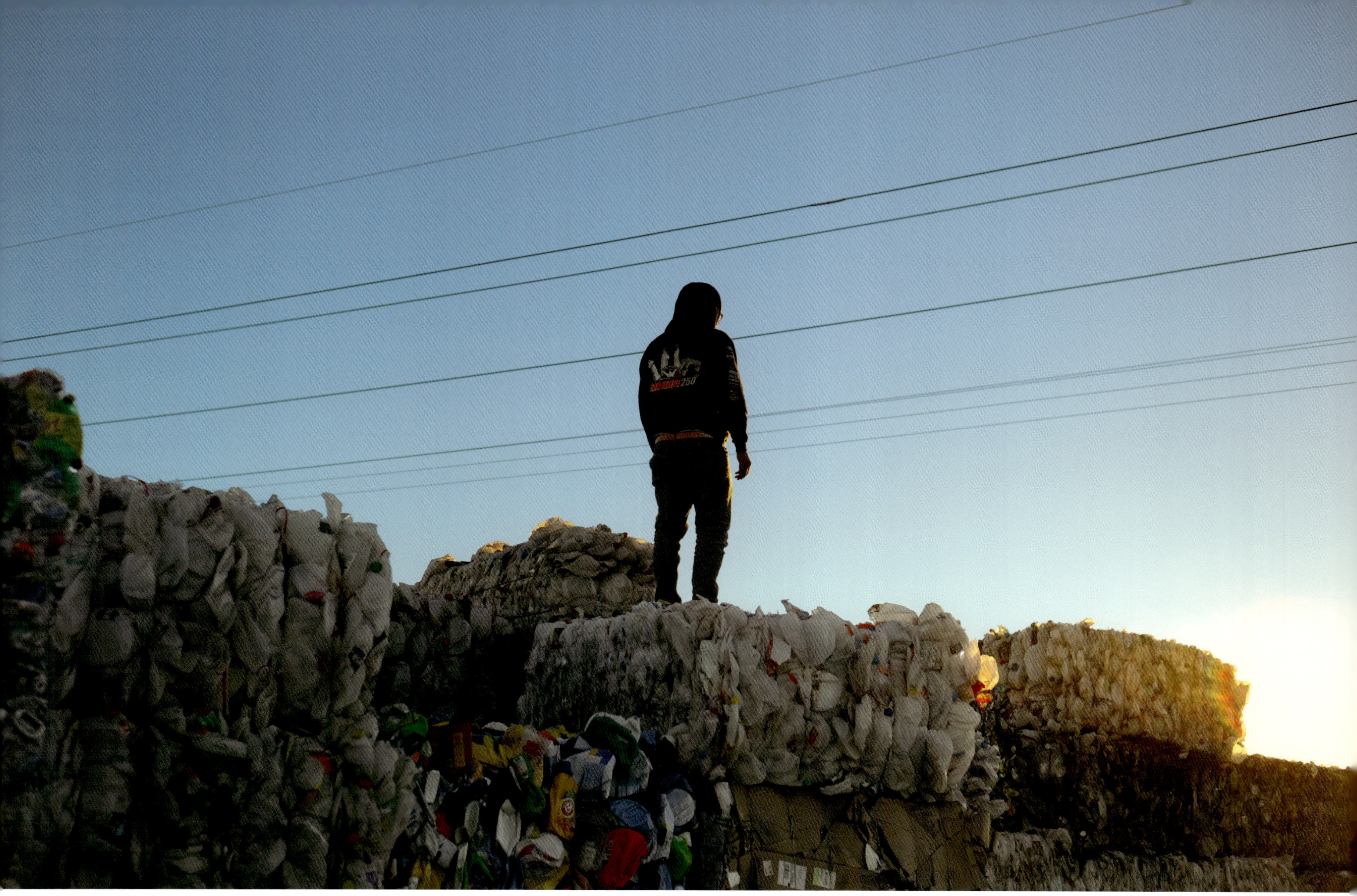

Oscar, El Centro

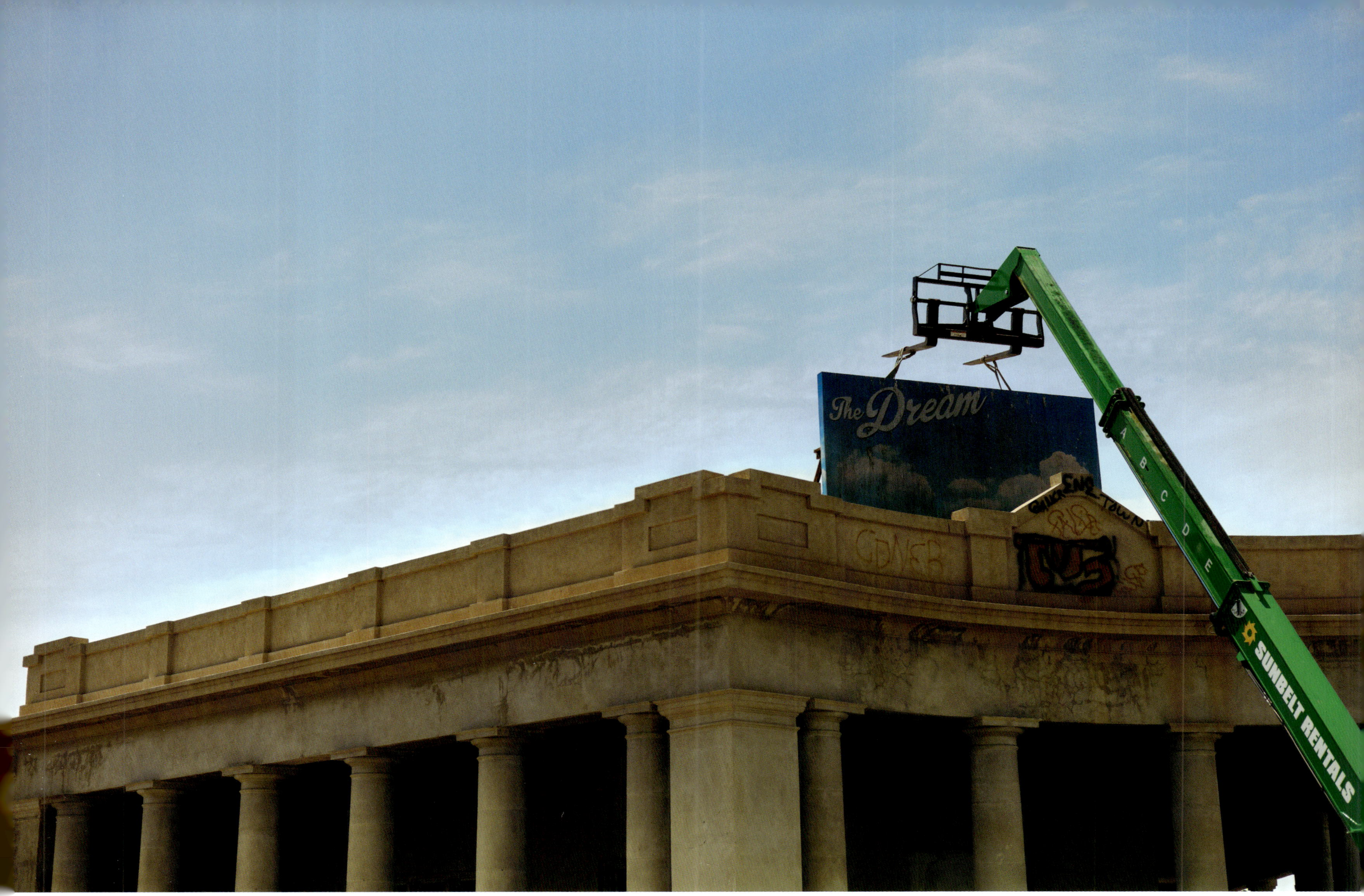

Old Commercial Building, Niland

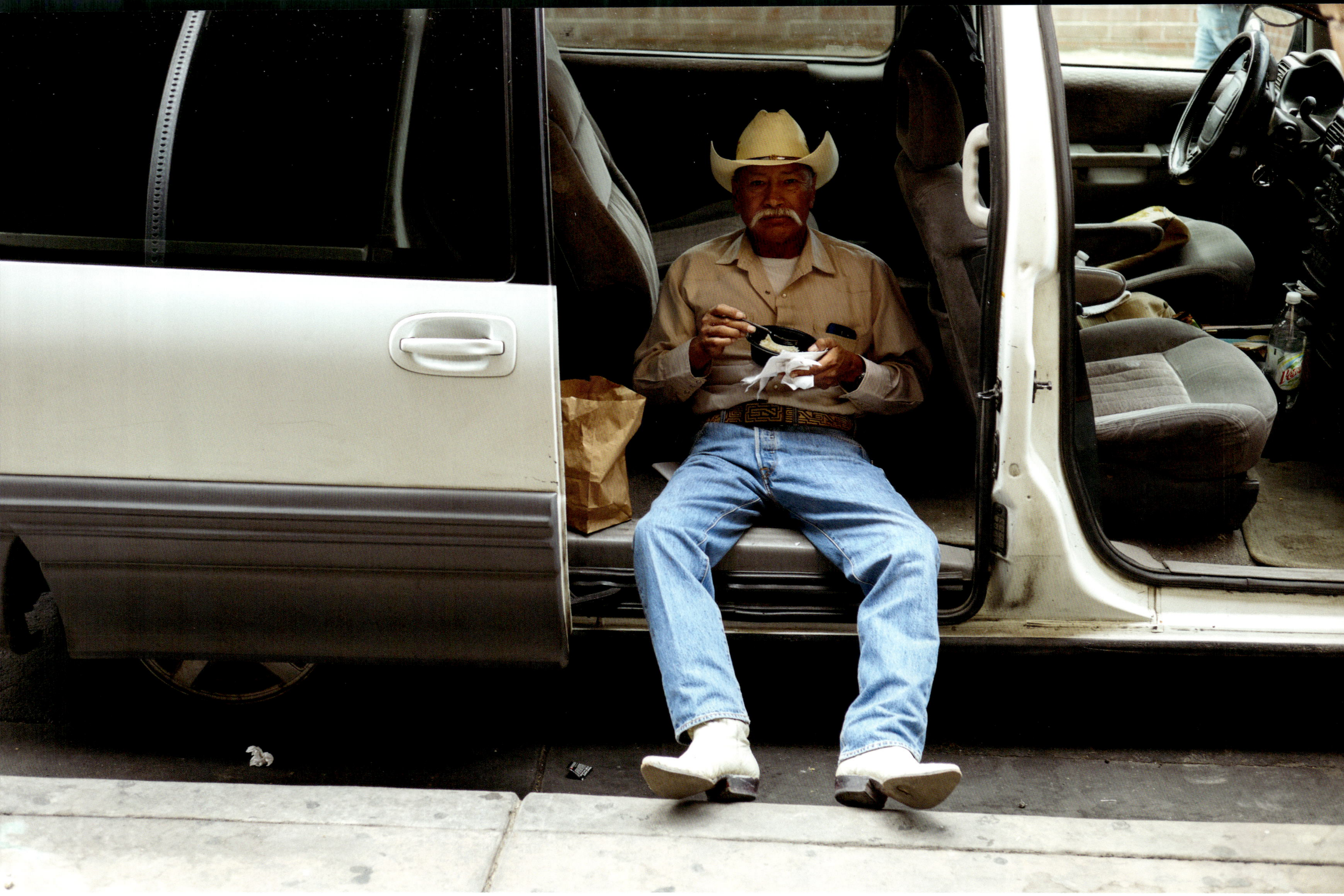

Tony in his minivan, Calexico

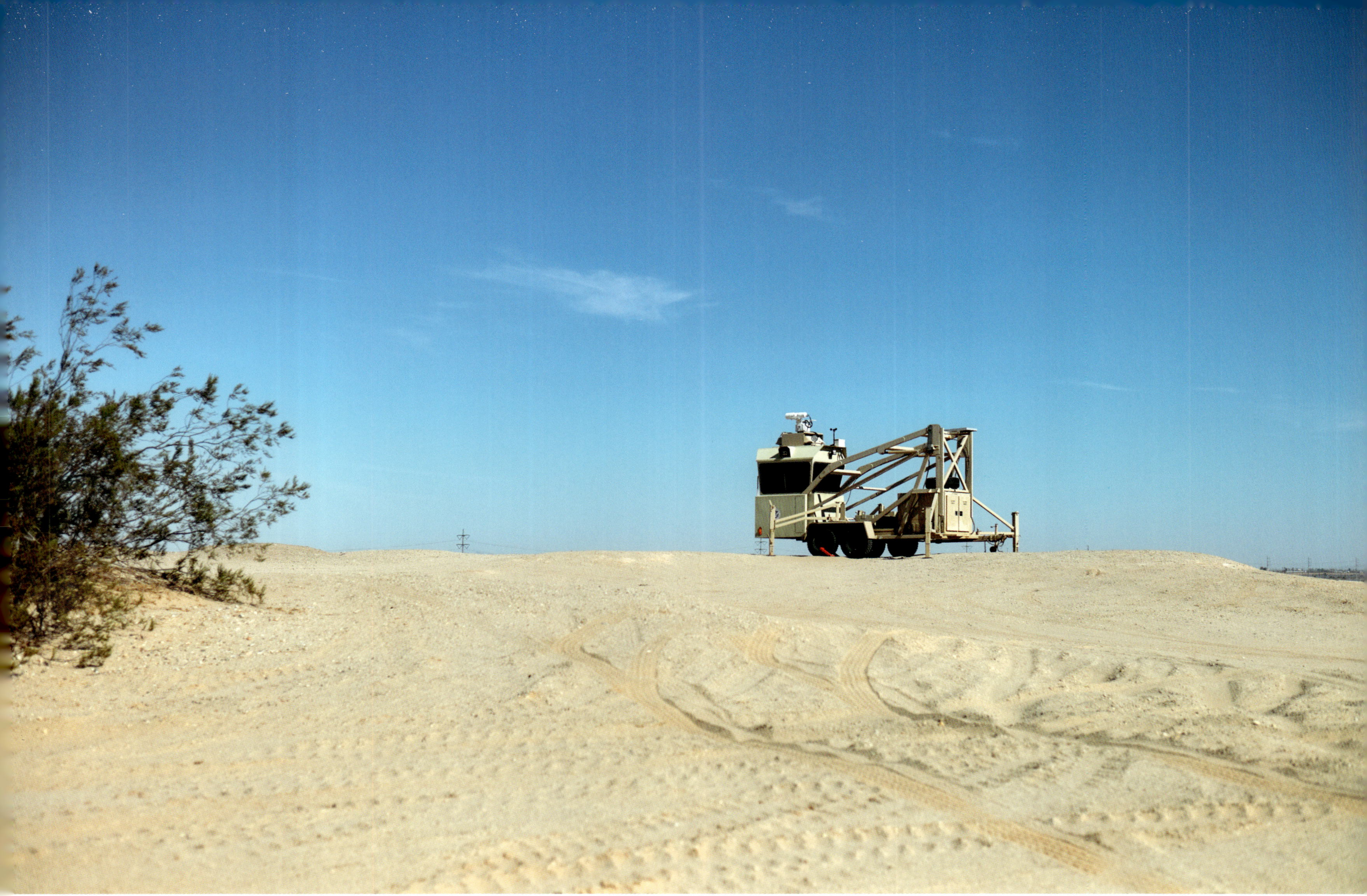

Border Patrol surveillance unit, Mount Signal area

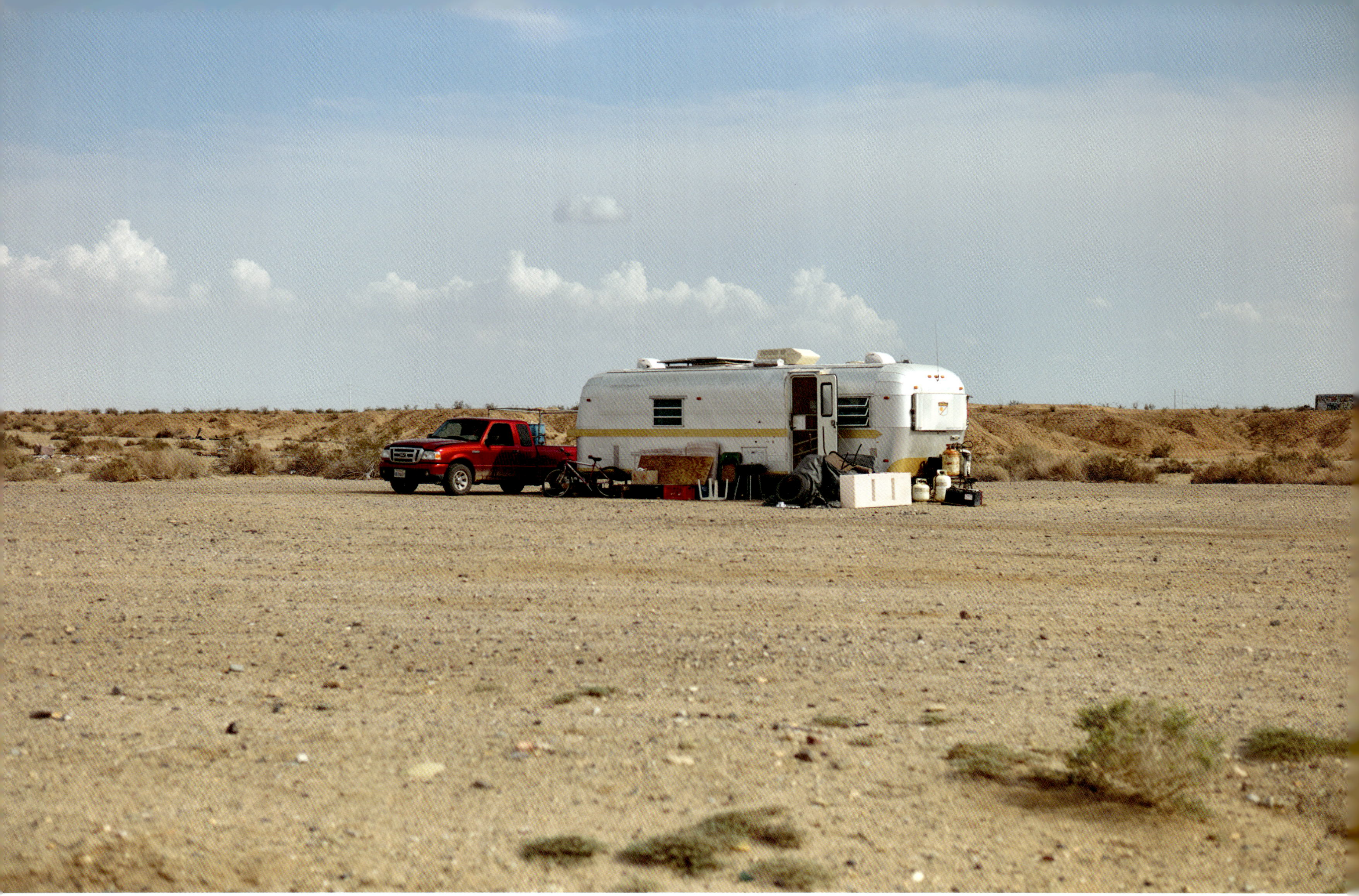

Desert home, Niland

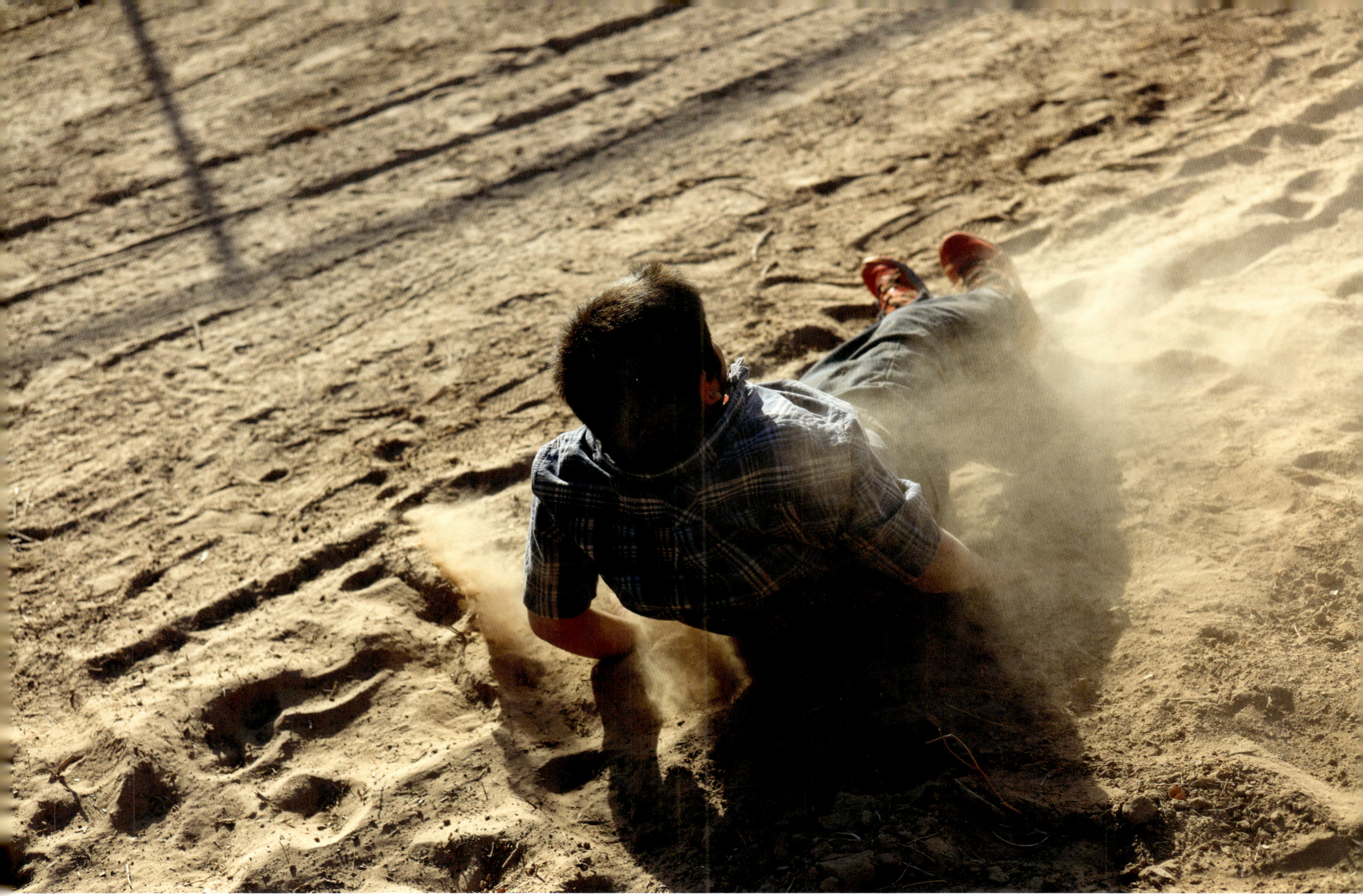

Angel, Brawley

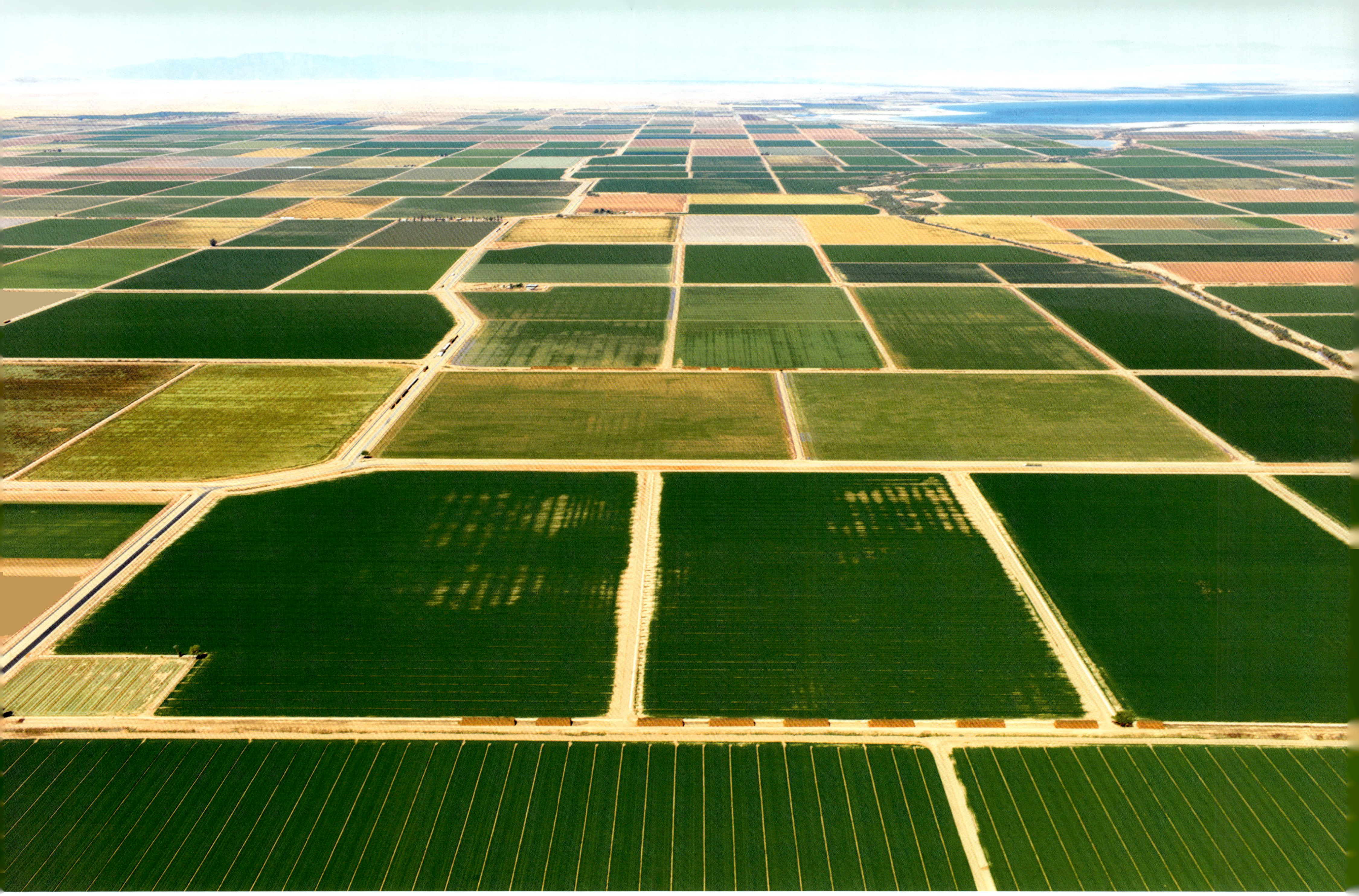

Farmland, desert and the Salton Sea, Fondo area

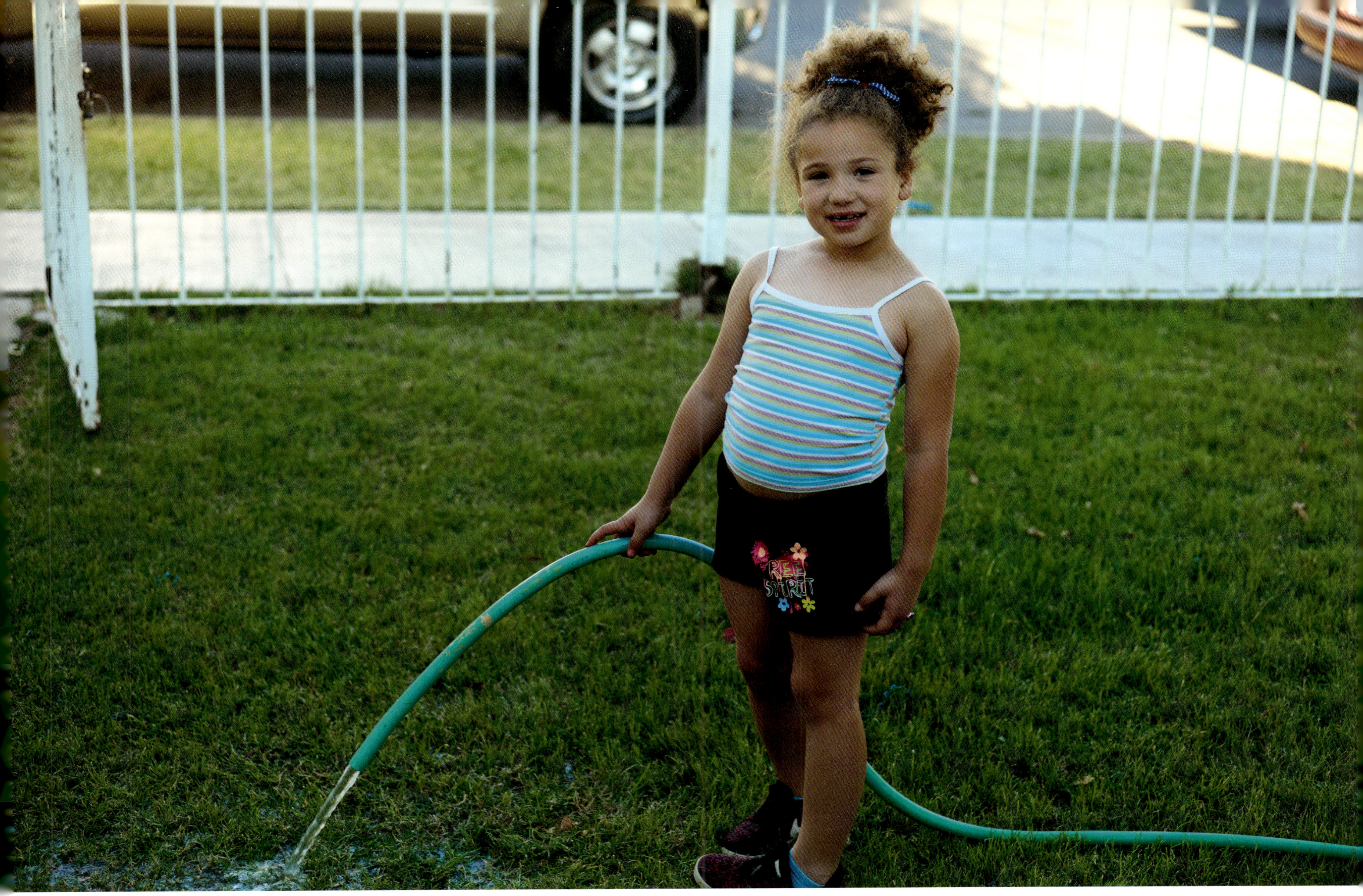

Anabell, Calexico

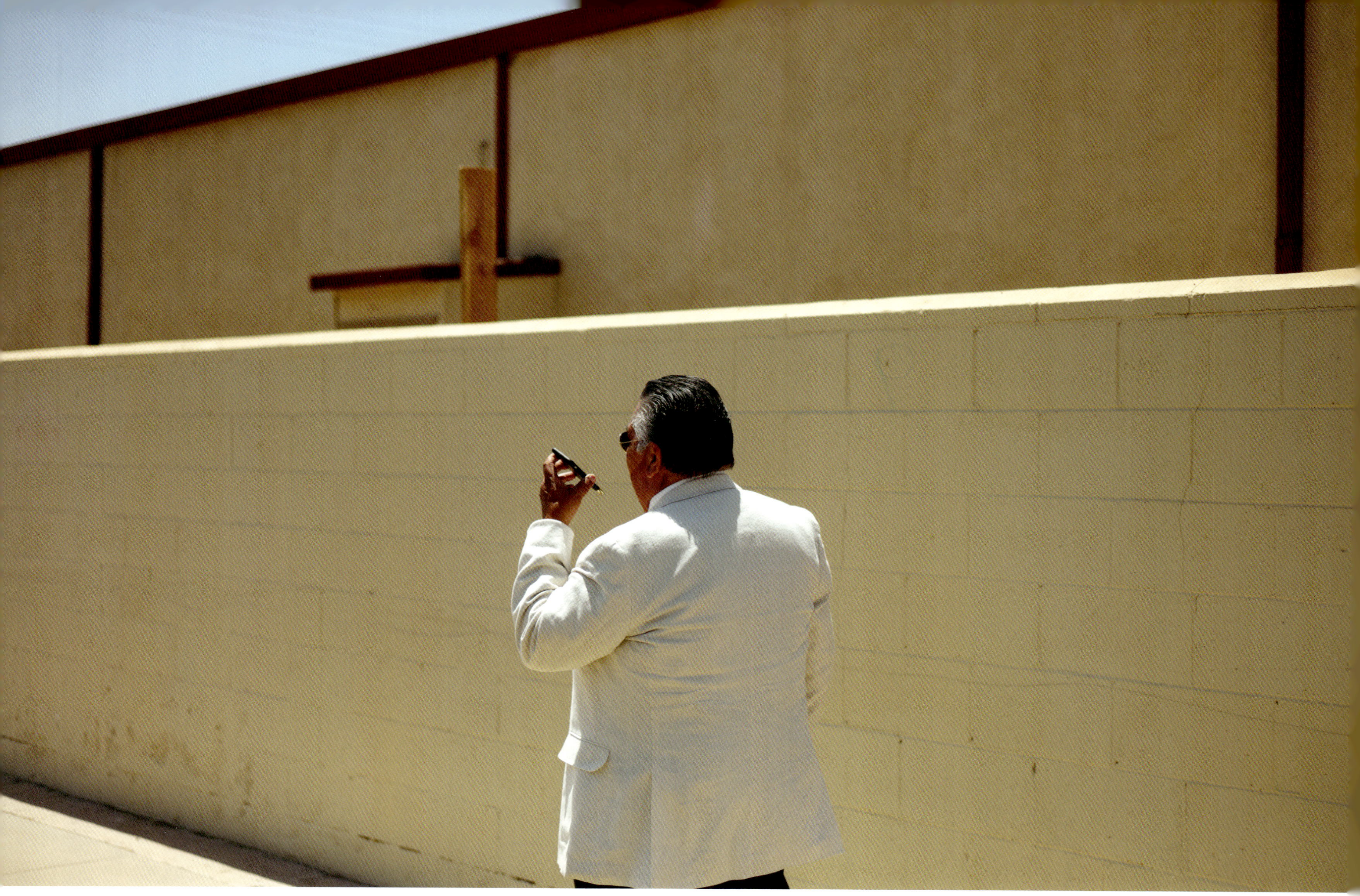

Tio, El Centro

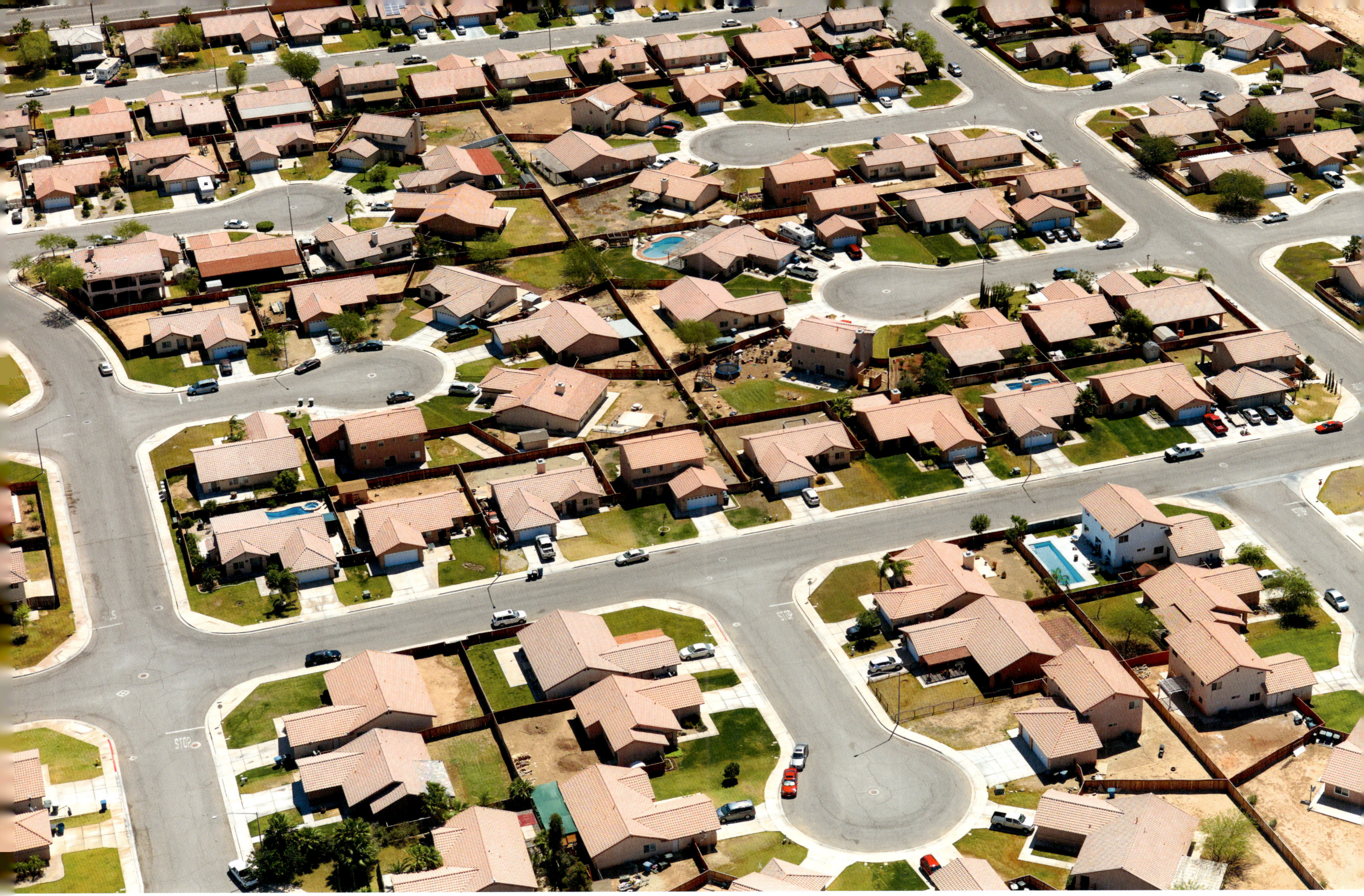

Sunset Ranch Estates, Imperial

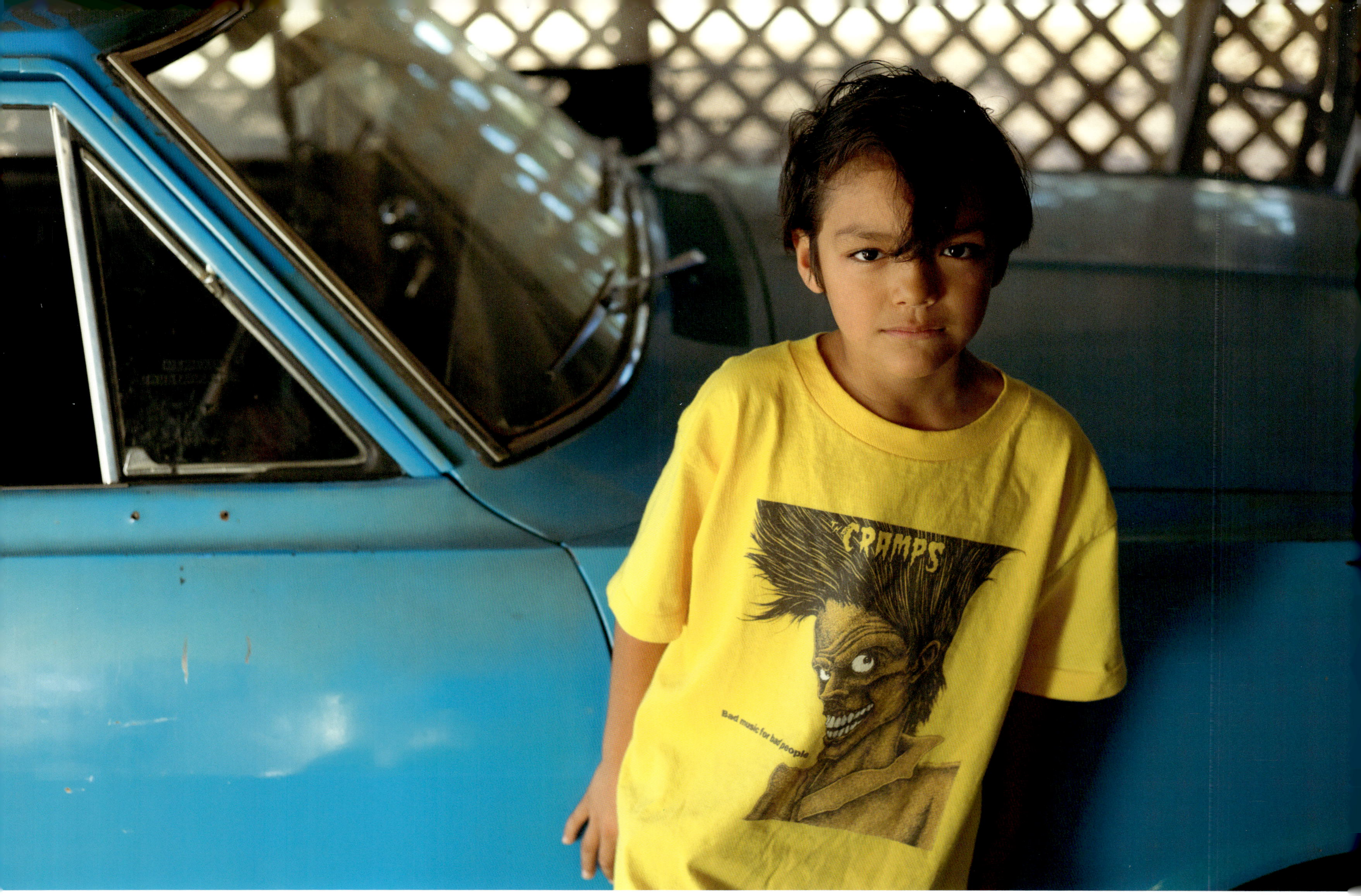

Andrew, El Centro

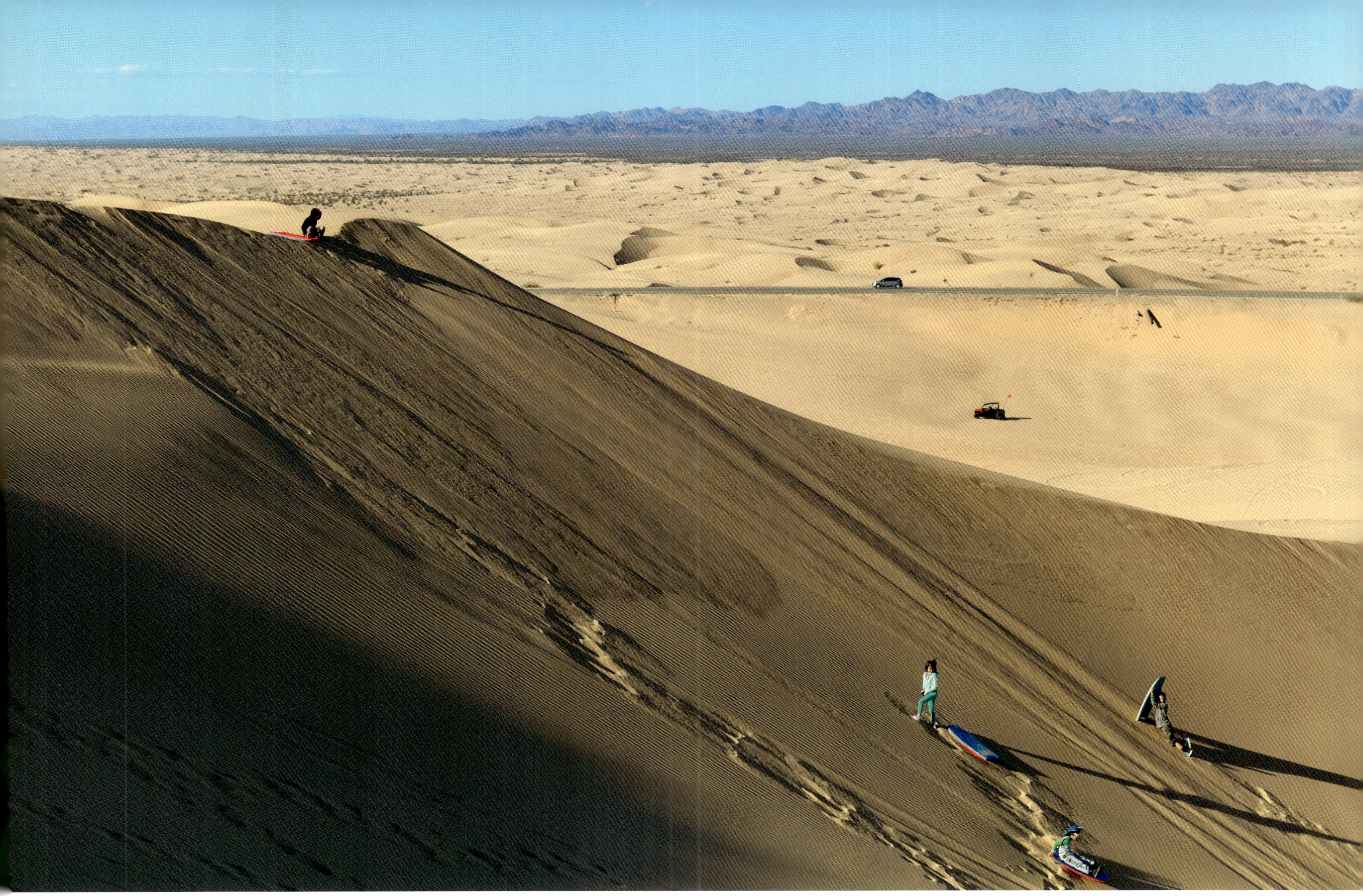

Hugh T. Osborne Lookout Park, Glamis

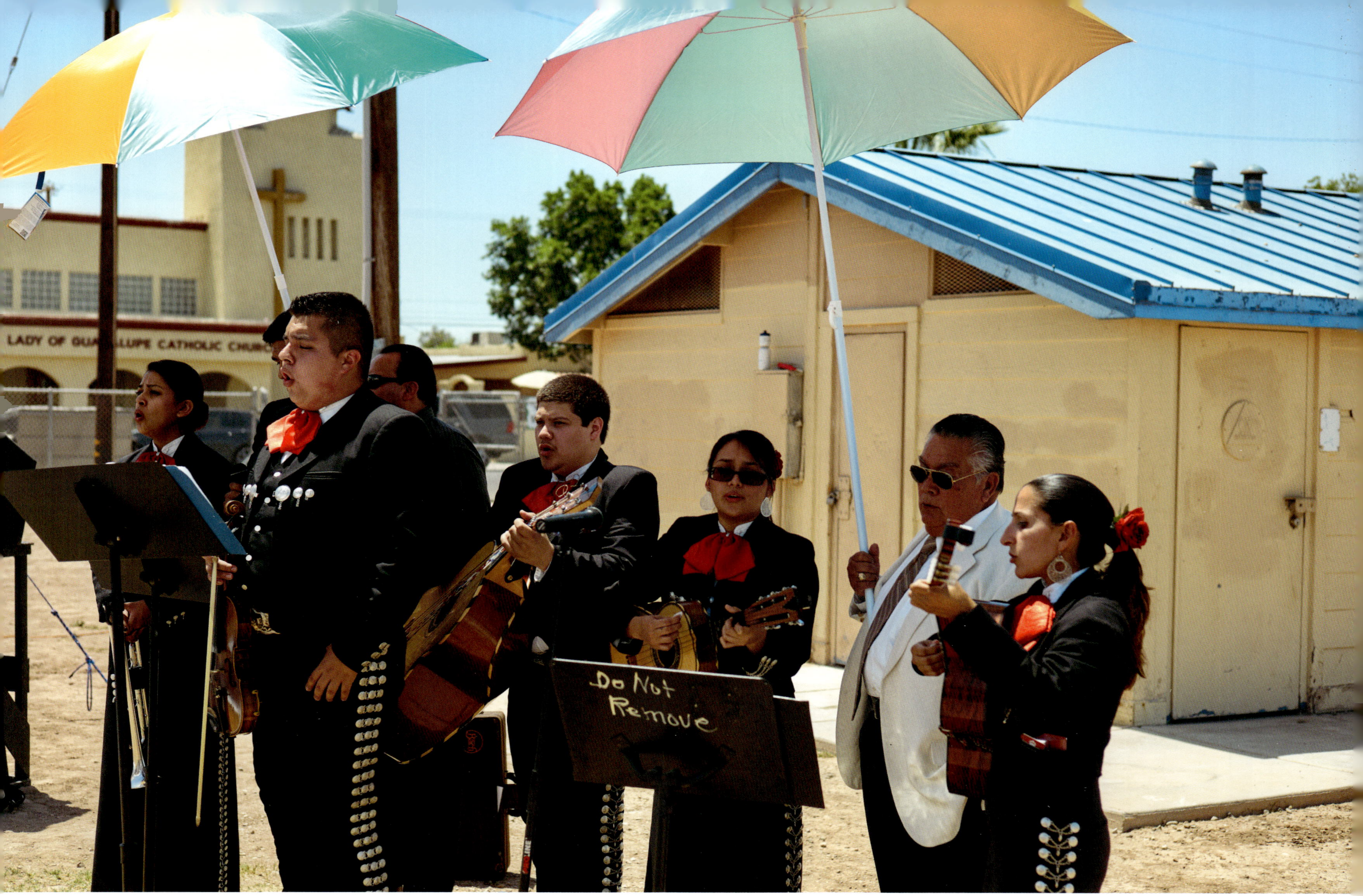

Cinco de Mayo celebration, El Centro

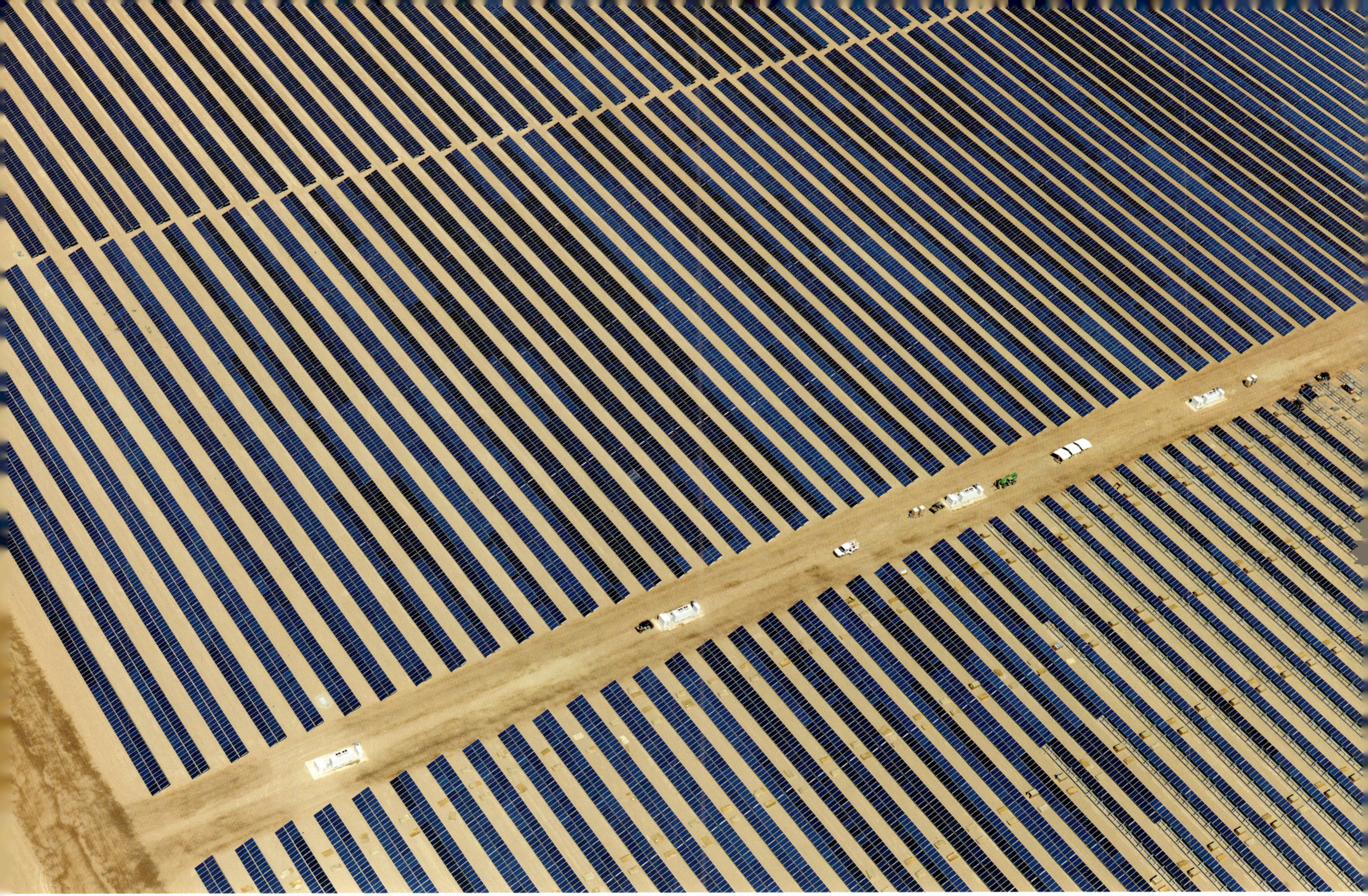

Imperial Valley Solar Company 1, Niland

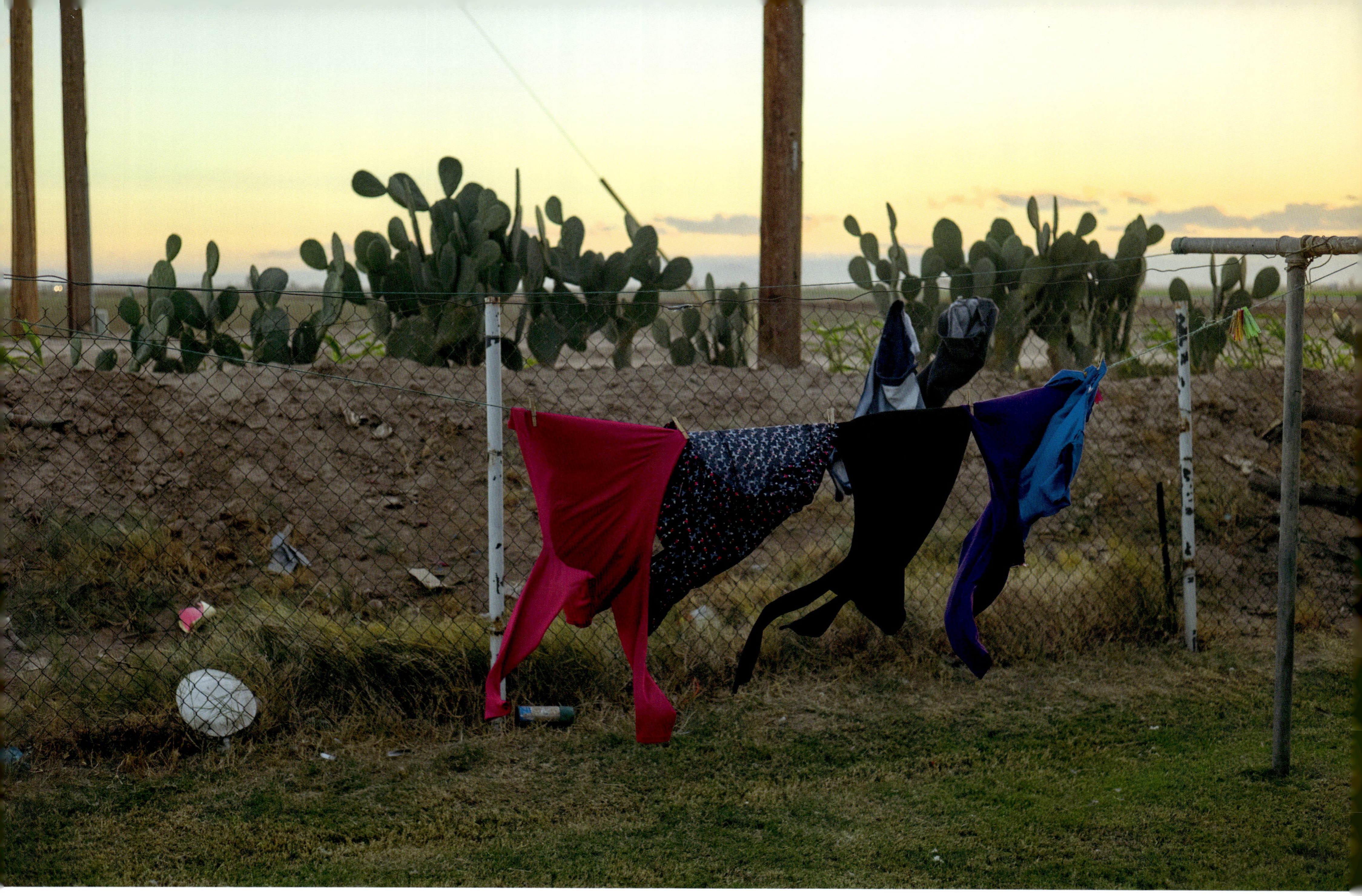

Tio Felipe's yard, Fuller

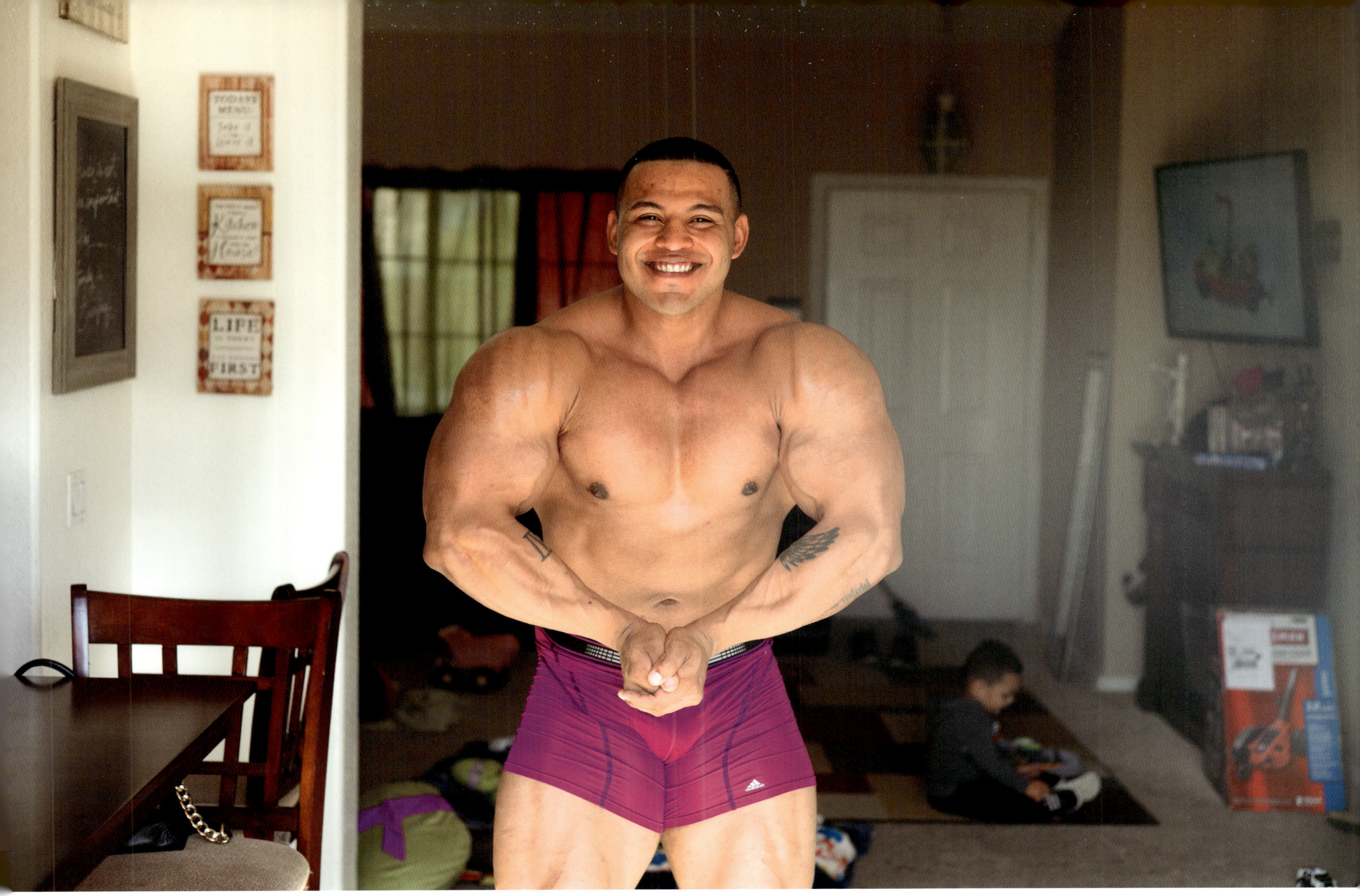

Carlos and his son, Calexico

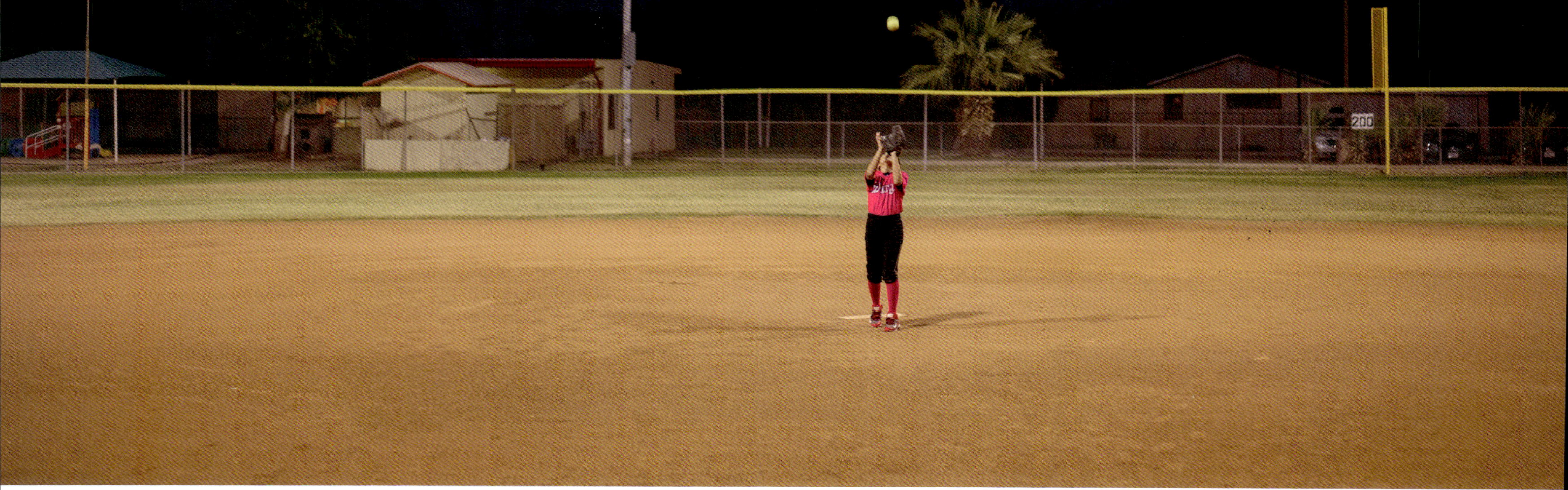

Samantha, Calexico

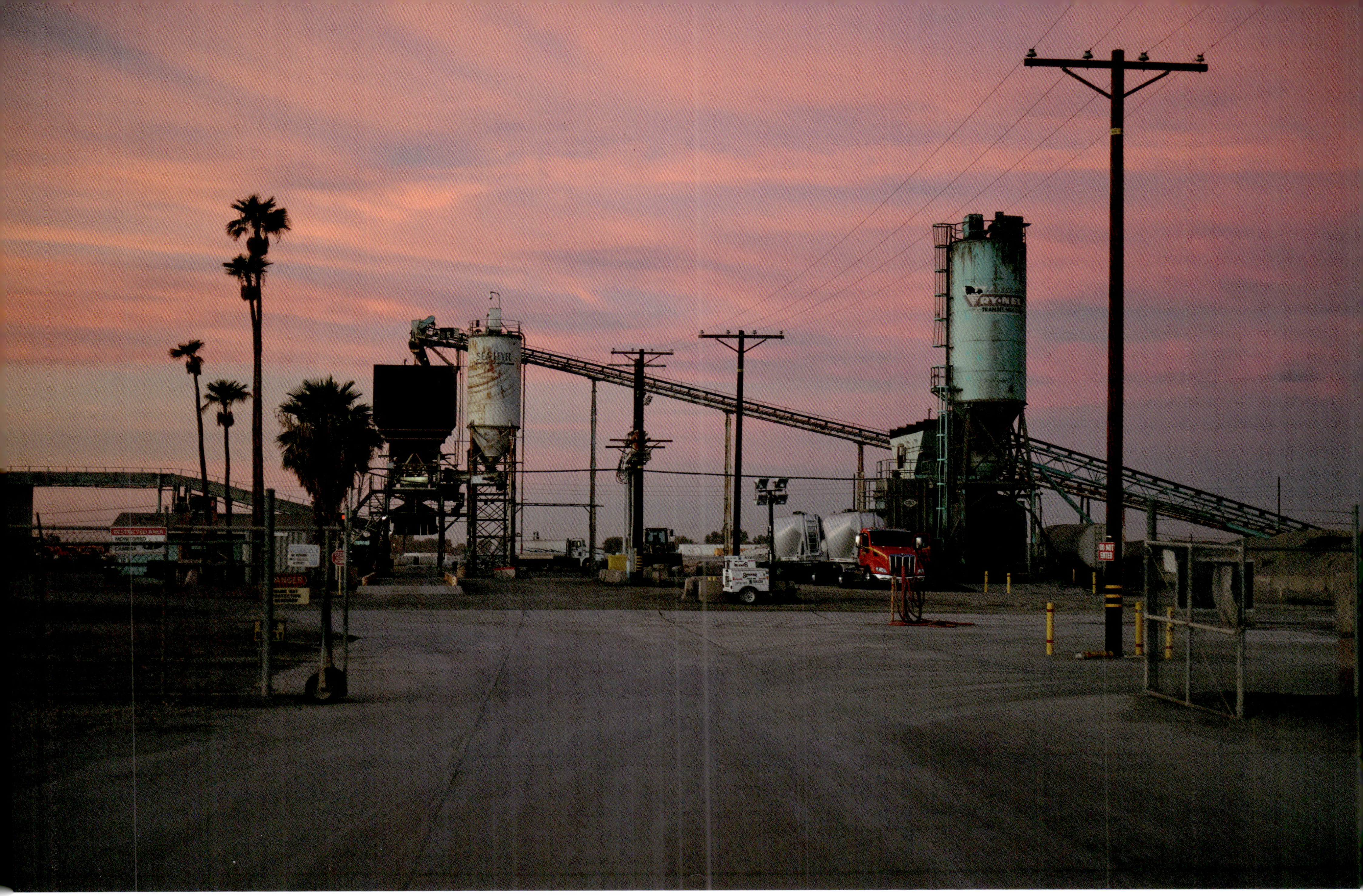

Fertilizer silos, Brawley

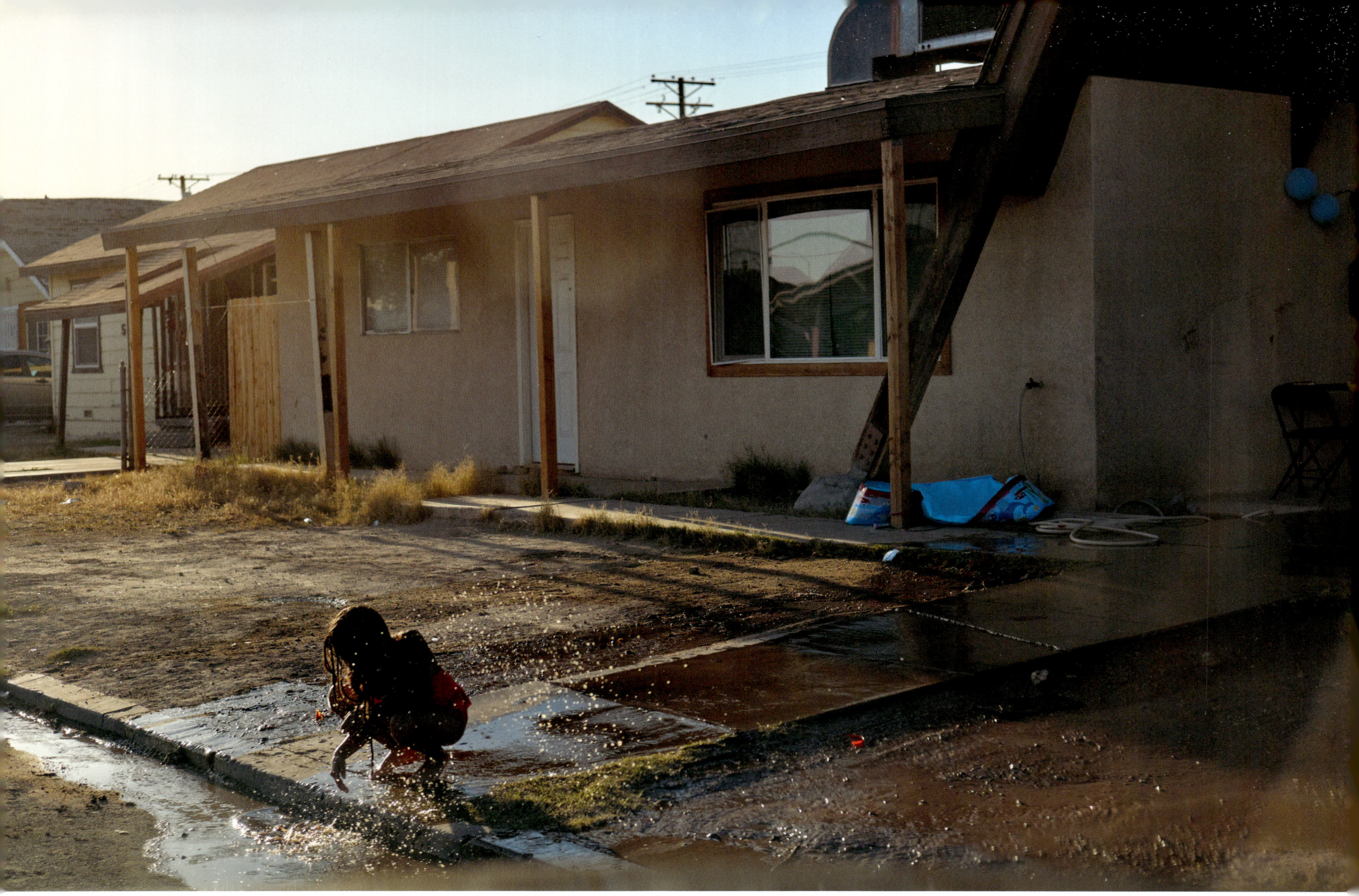

Abril playing at a water leakage, El Centro

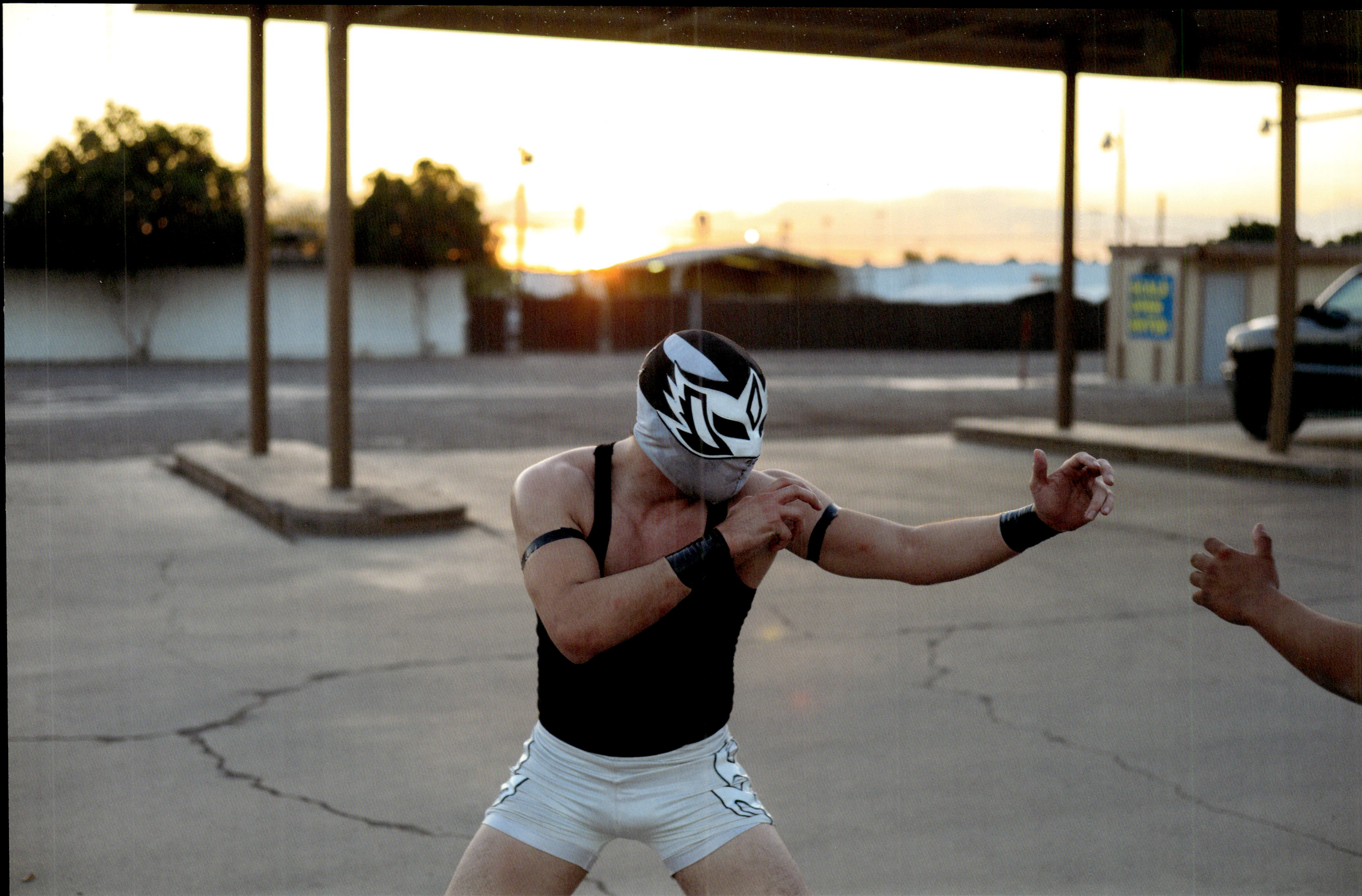

Lucha Libre fight, Holtville

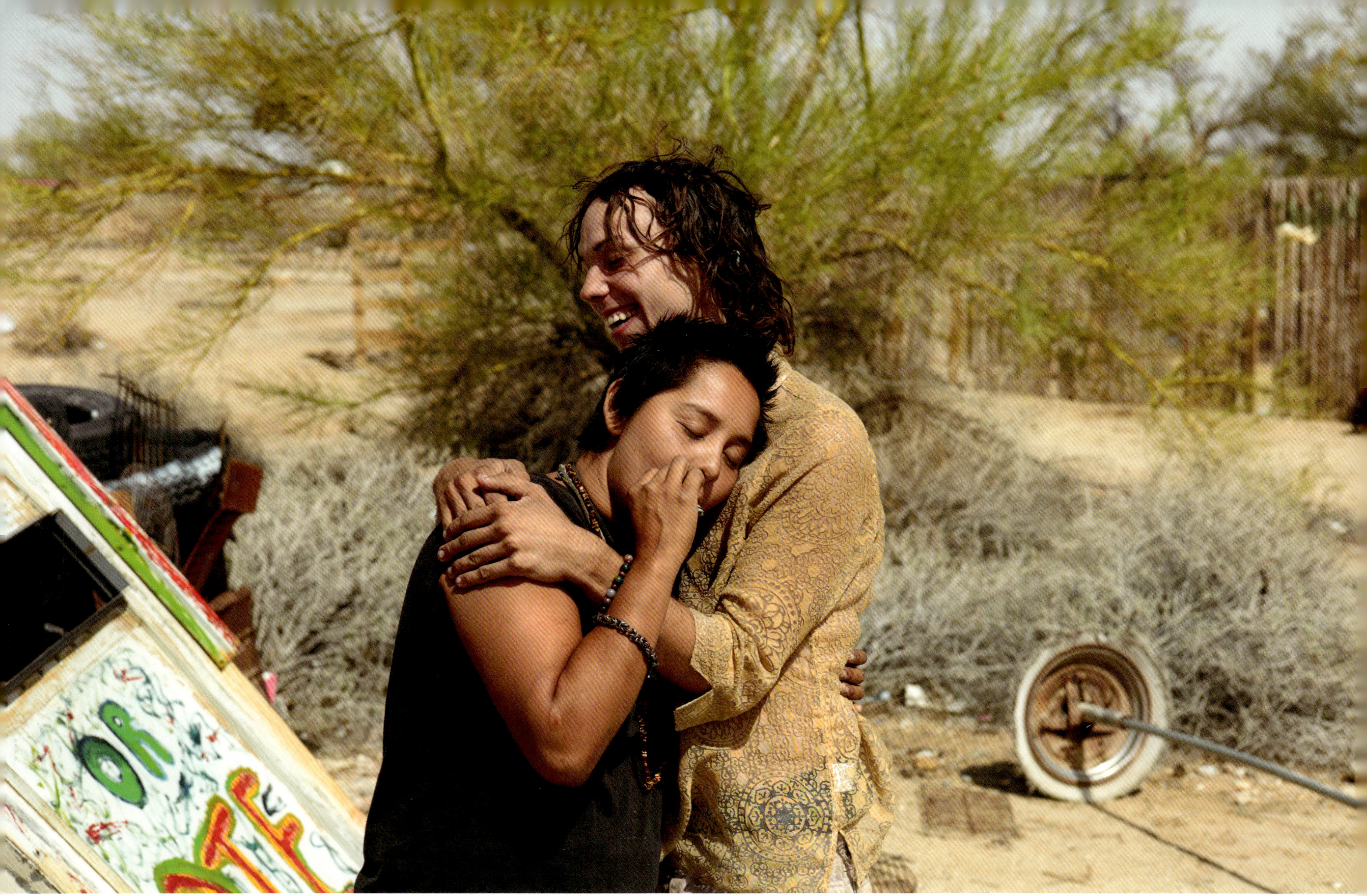

Christa and Conor by the skate pool, Slab City

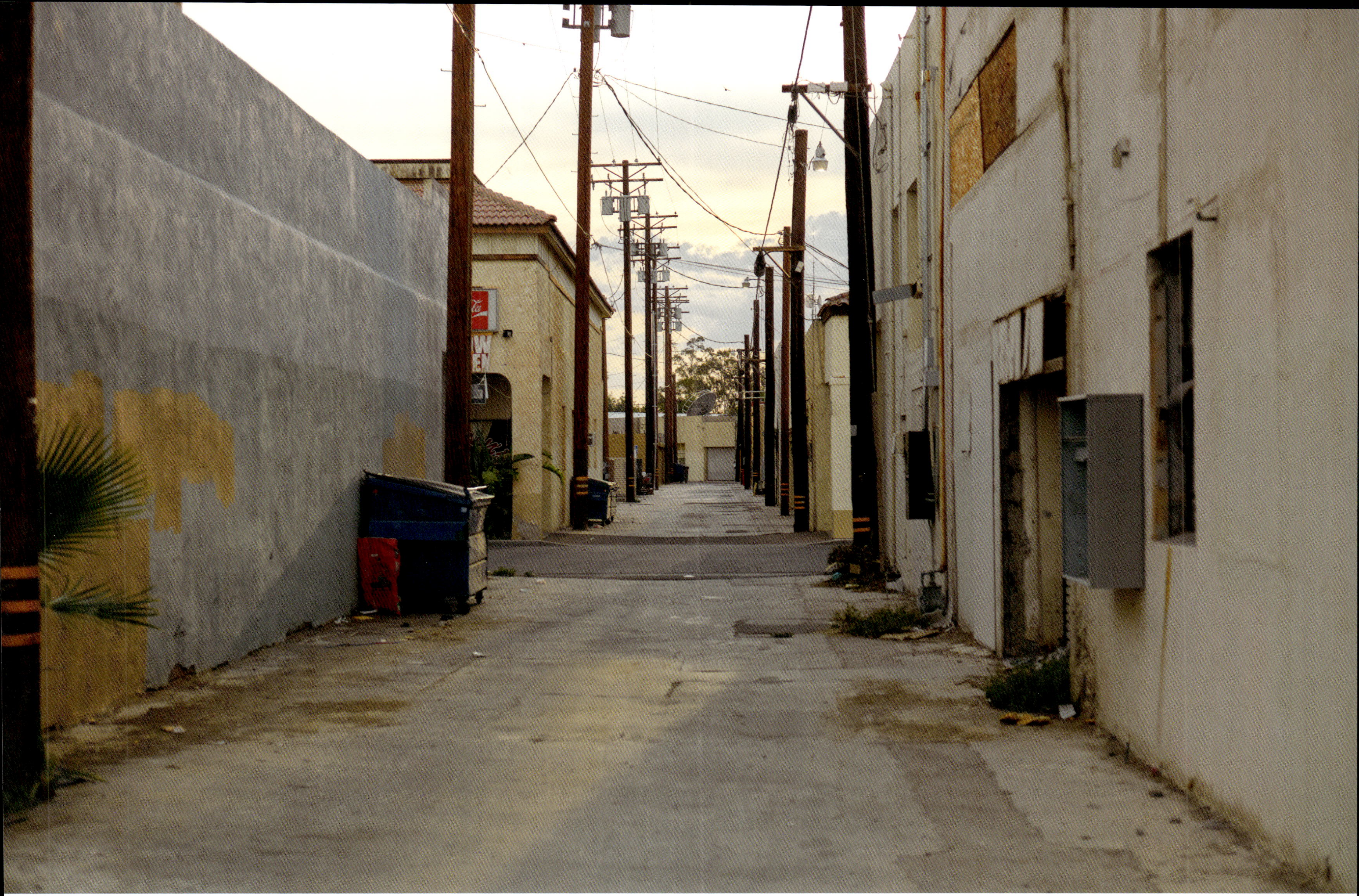

Alley, El Centro

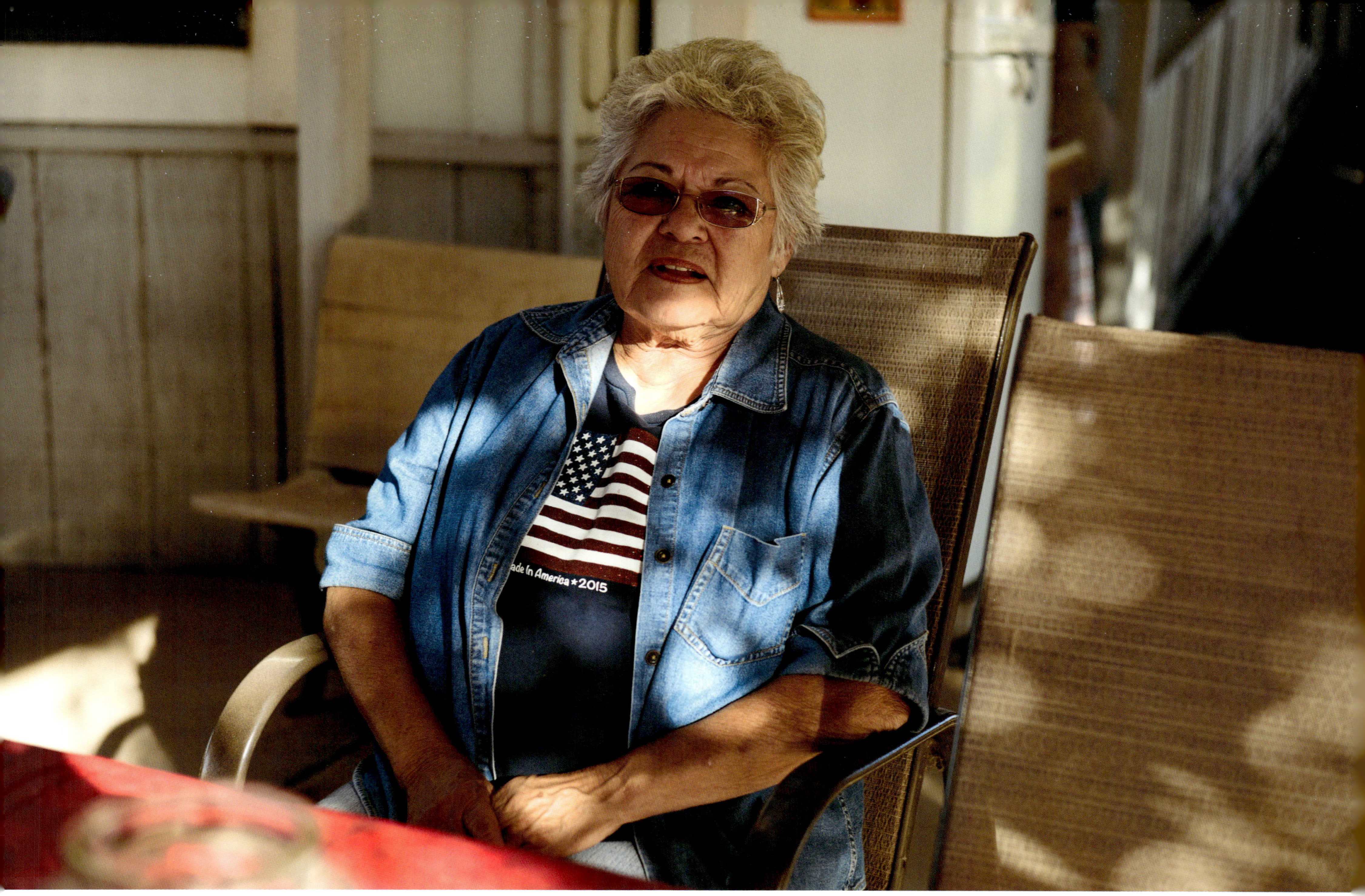

Ms. Castro on her farm, Holtville

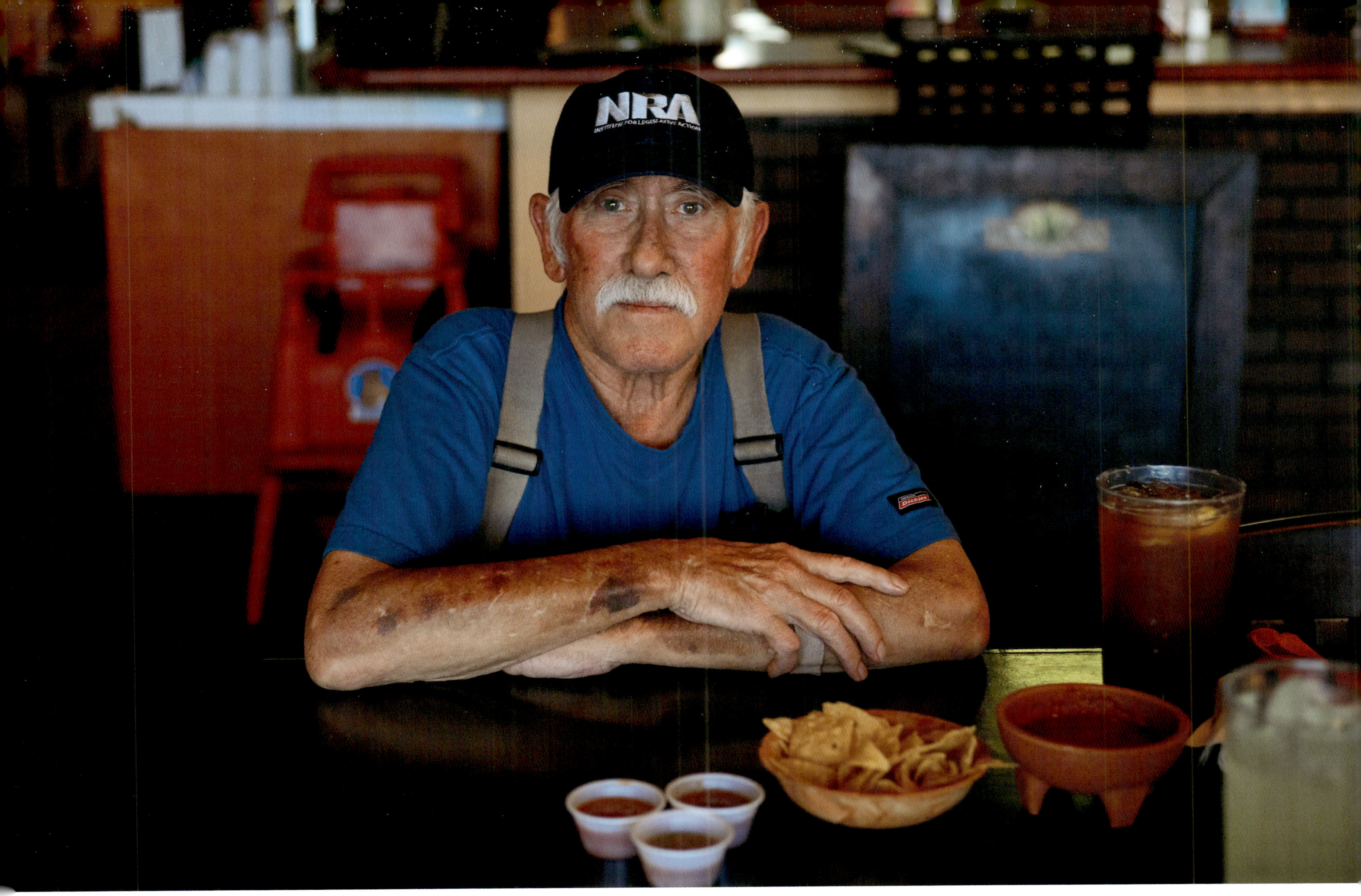

Mike at Jalisco's, El Centro

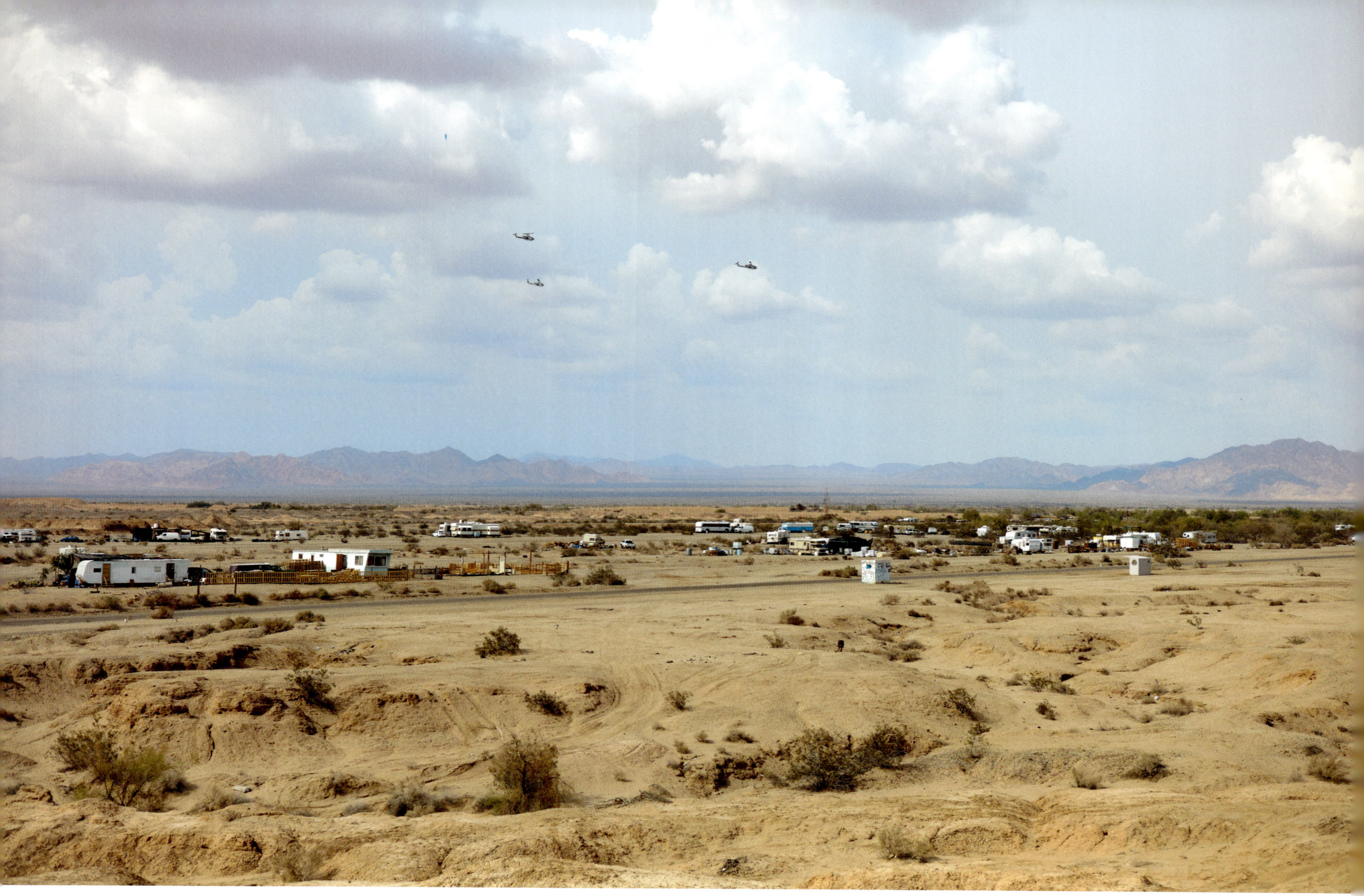

Helicopters flying towards bombing range, Slab City

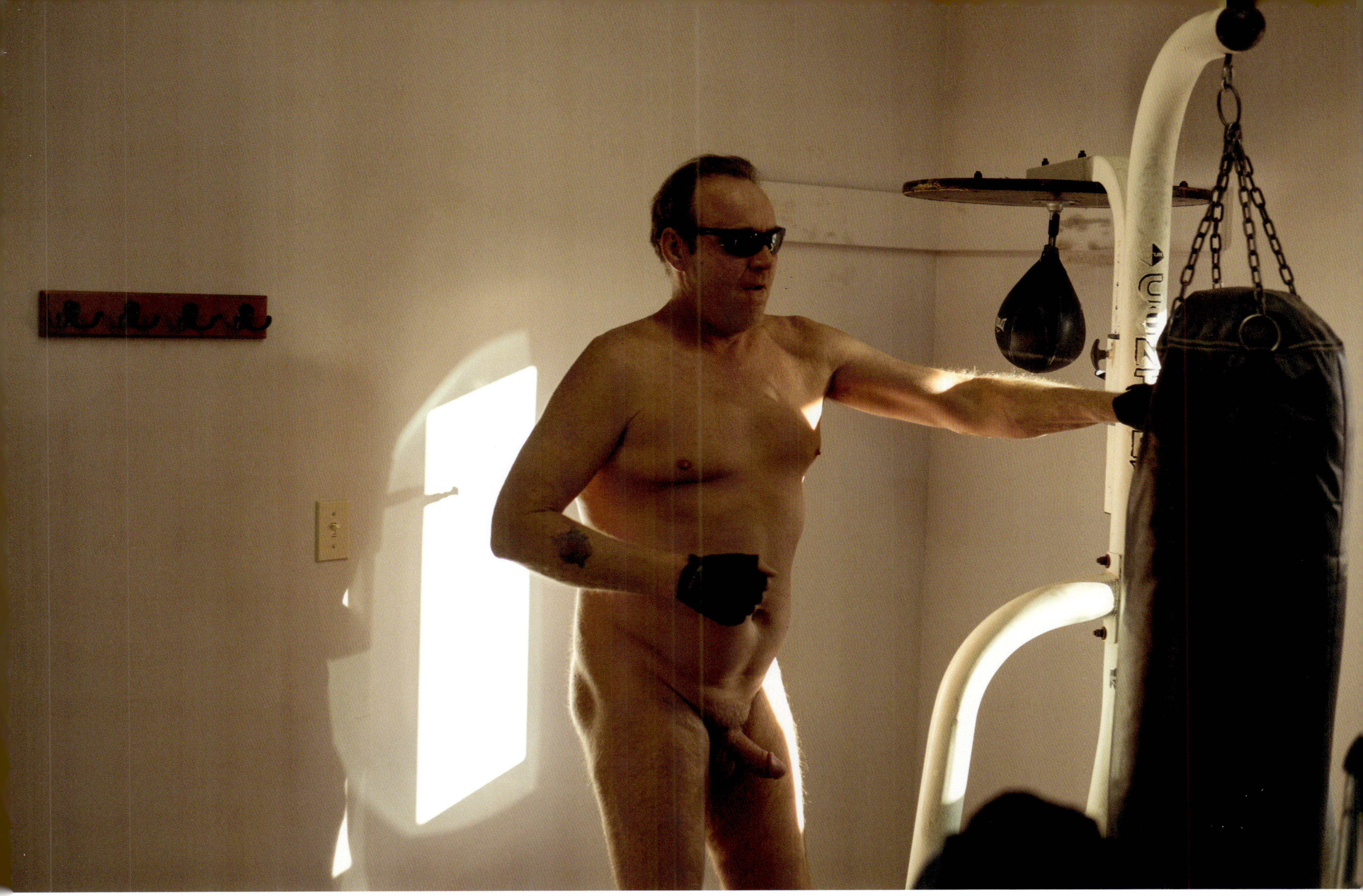

David, Ocotillo Mountains

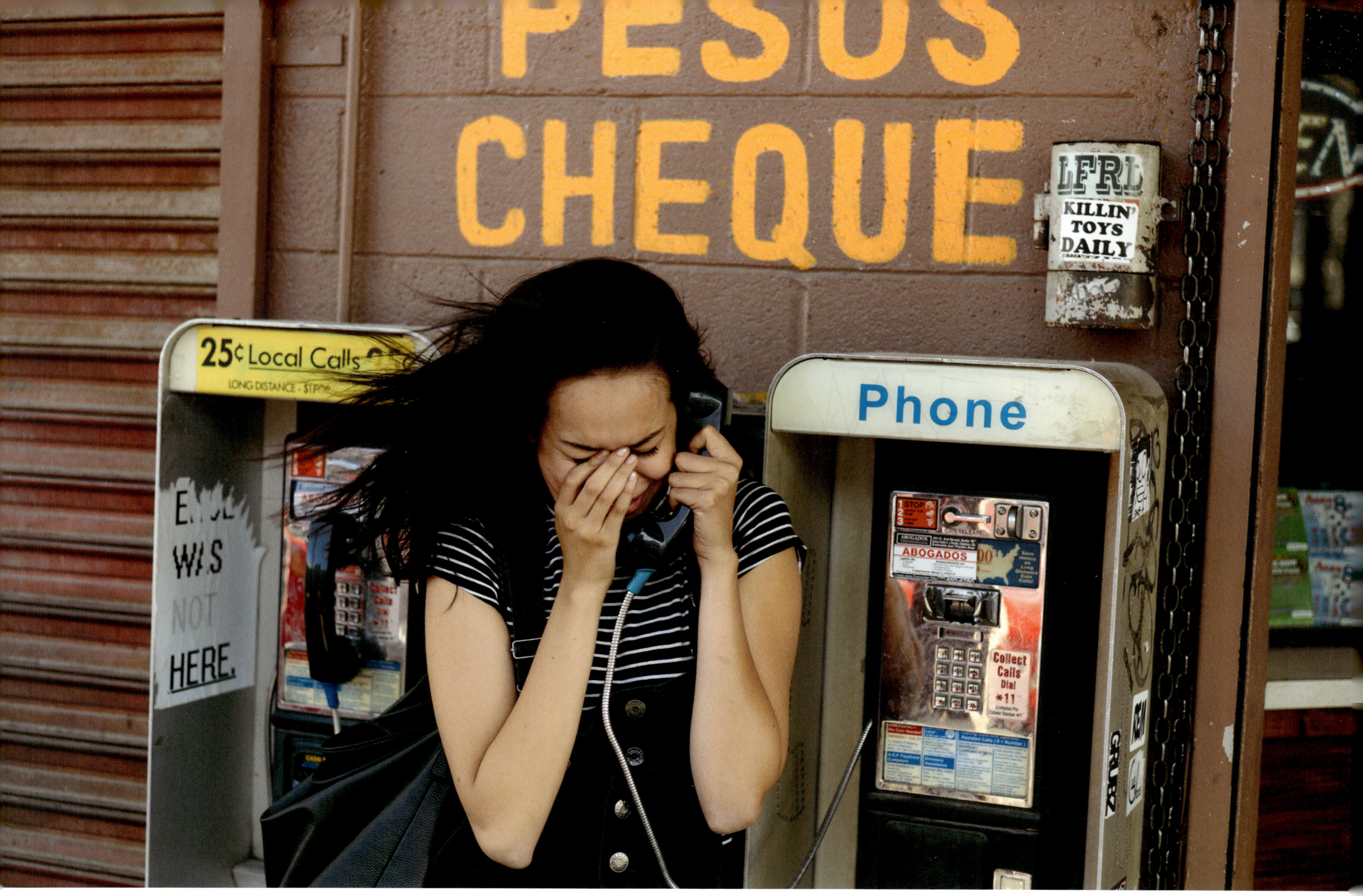

Sarah calling home, Calexico

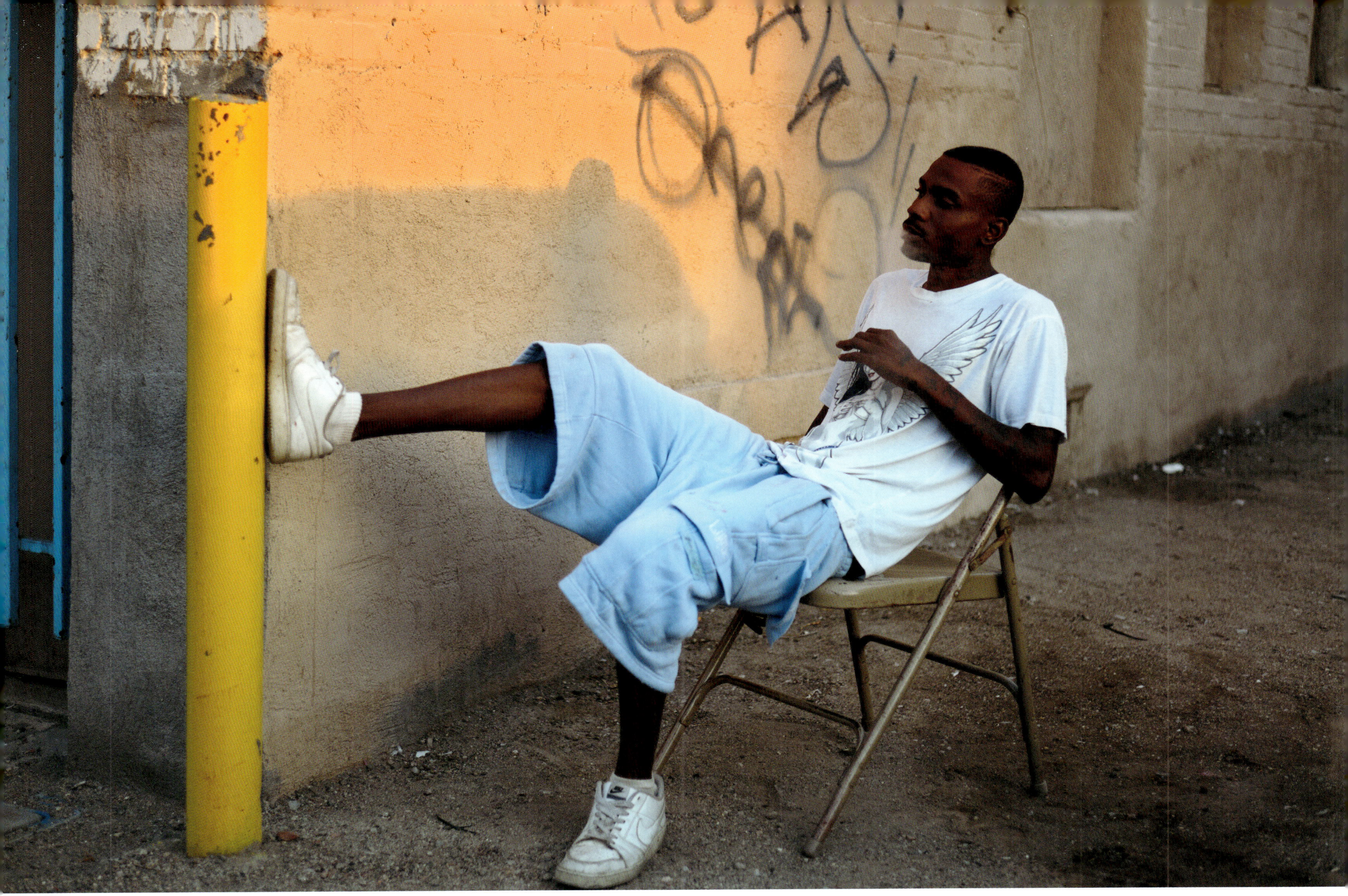

Chris having a break from work, El Centro

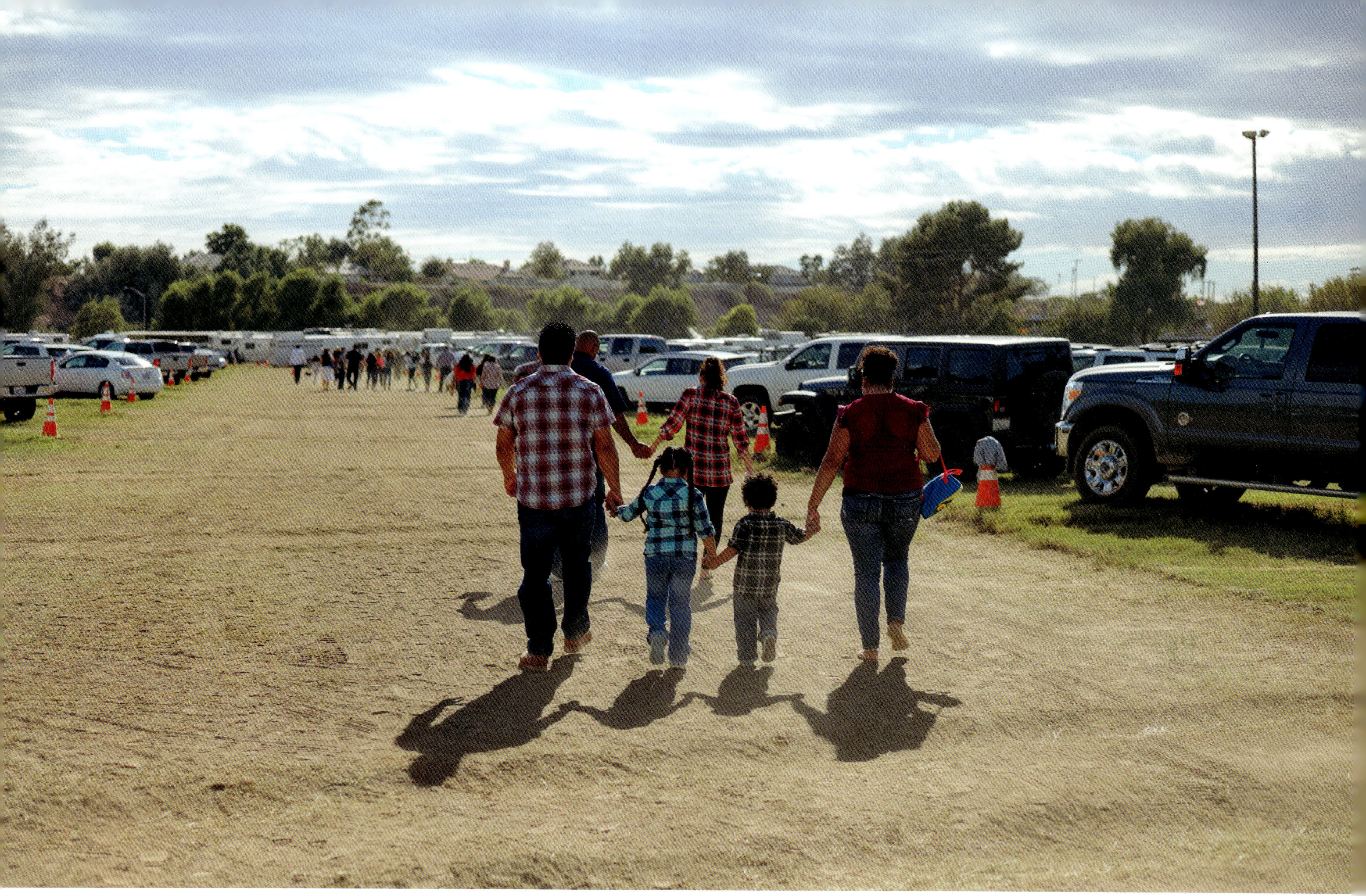

Cattle Call Arena, Brawley

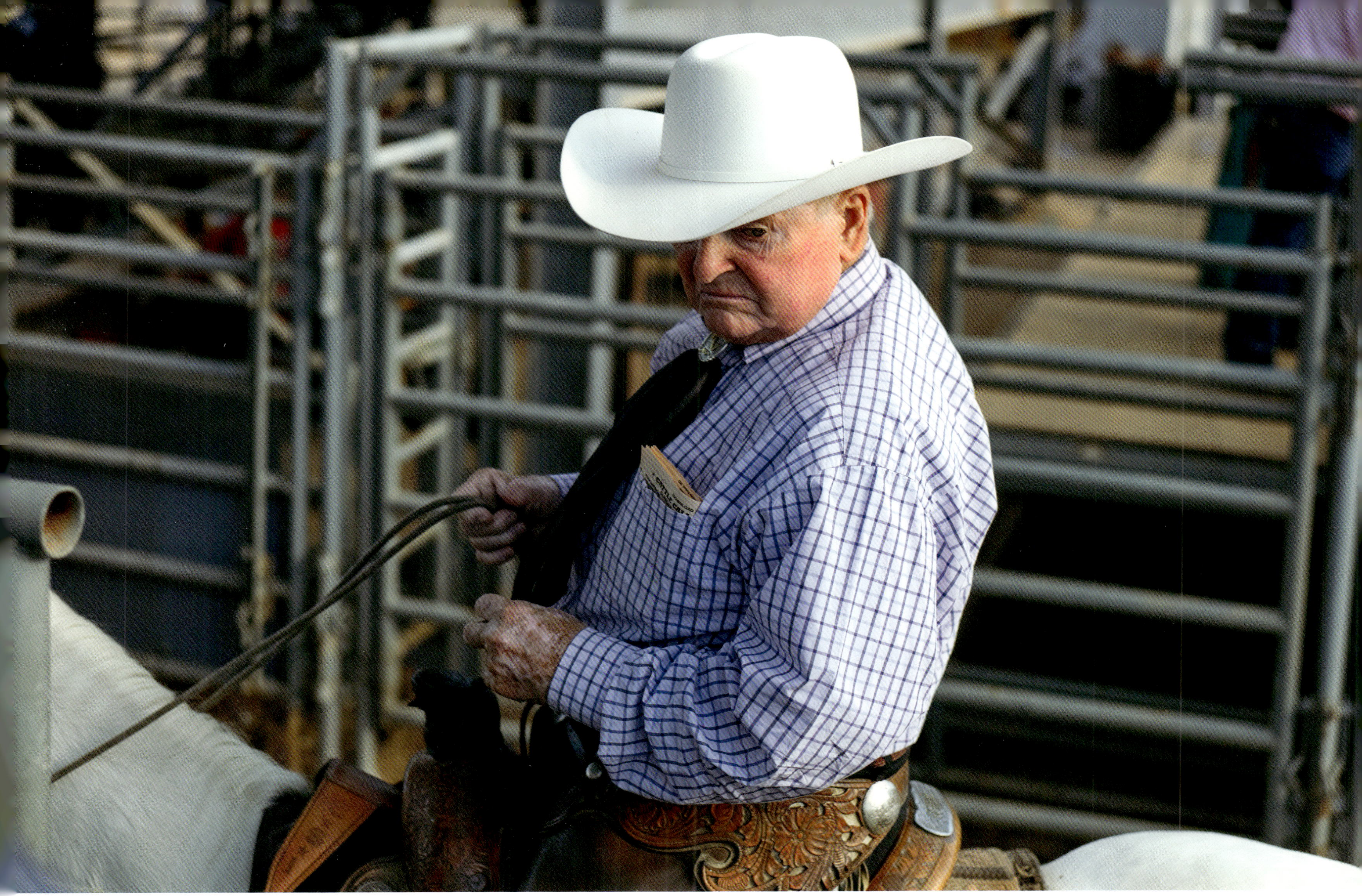

Supervisor at the rodeo, Brawley

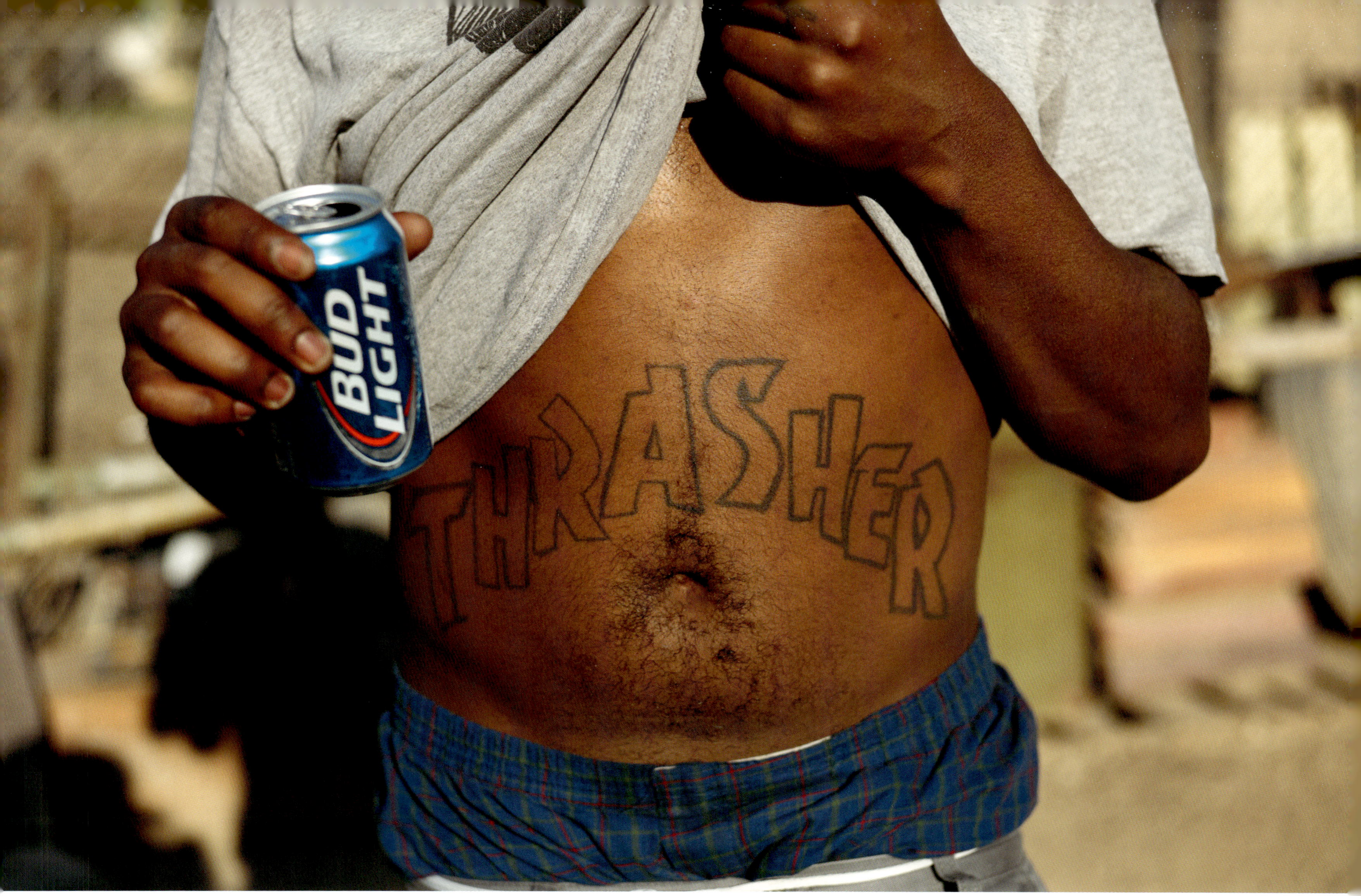

Shedon, El Centro

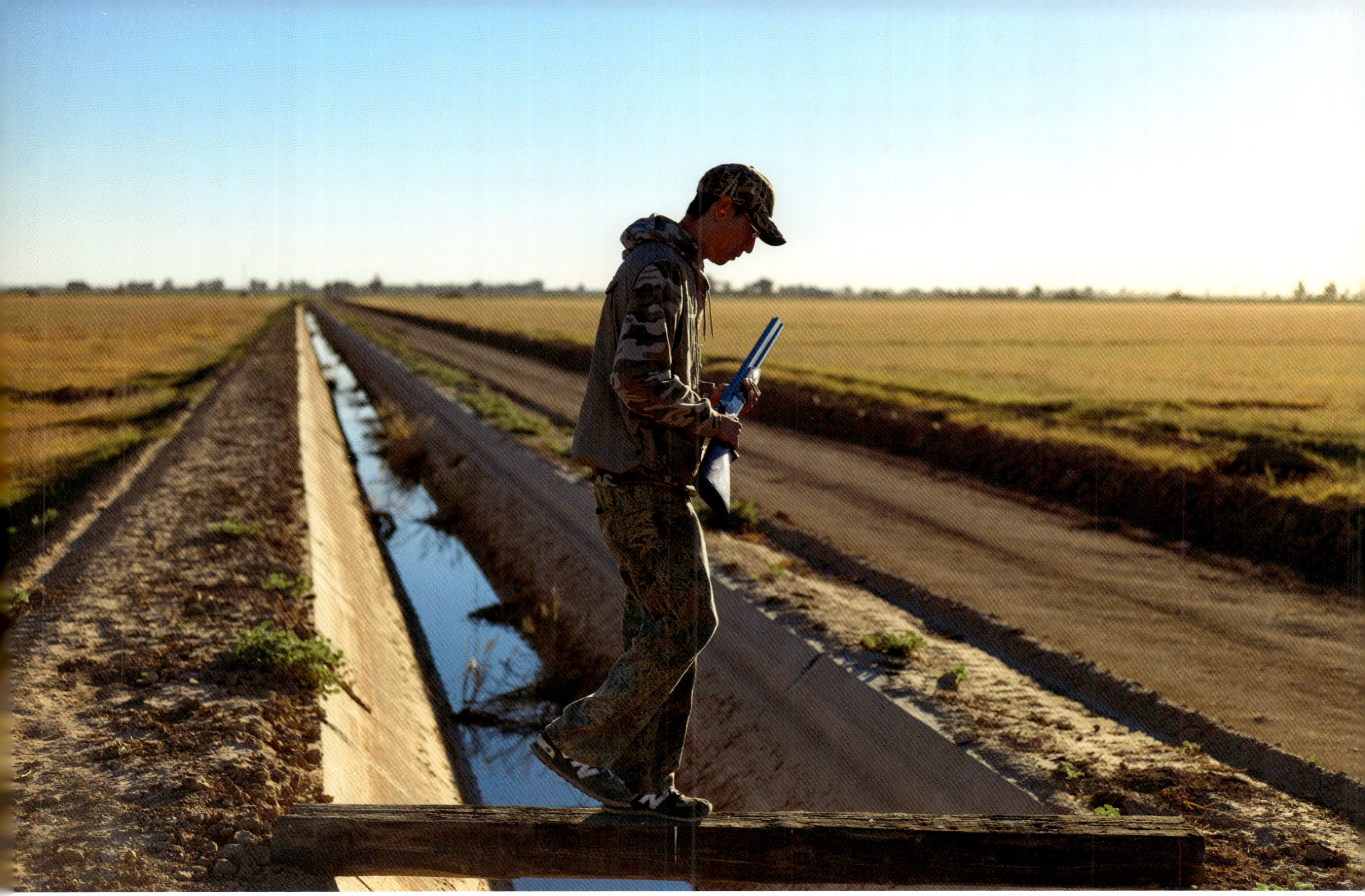

Andy bird hunting, near Heber

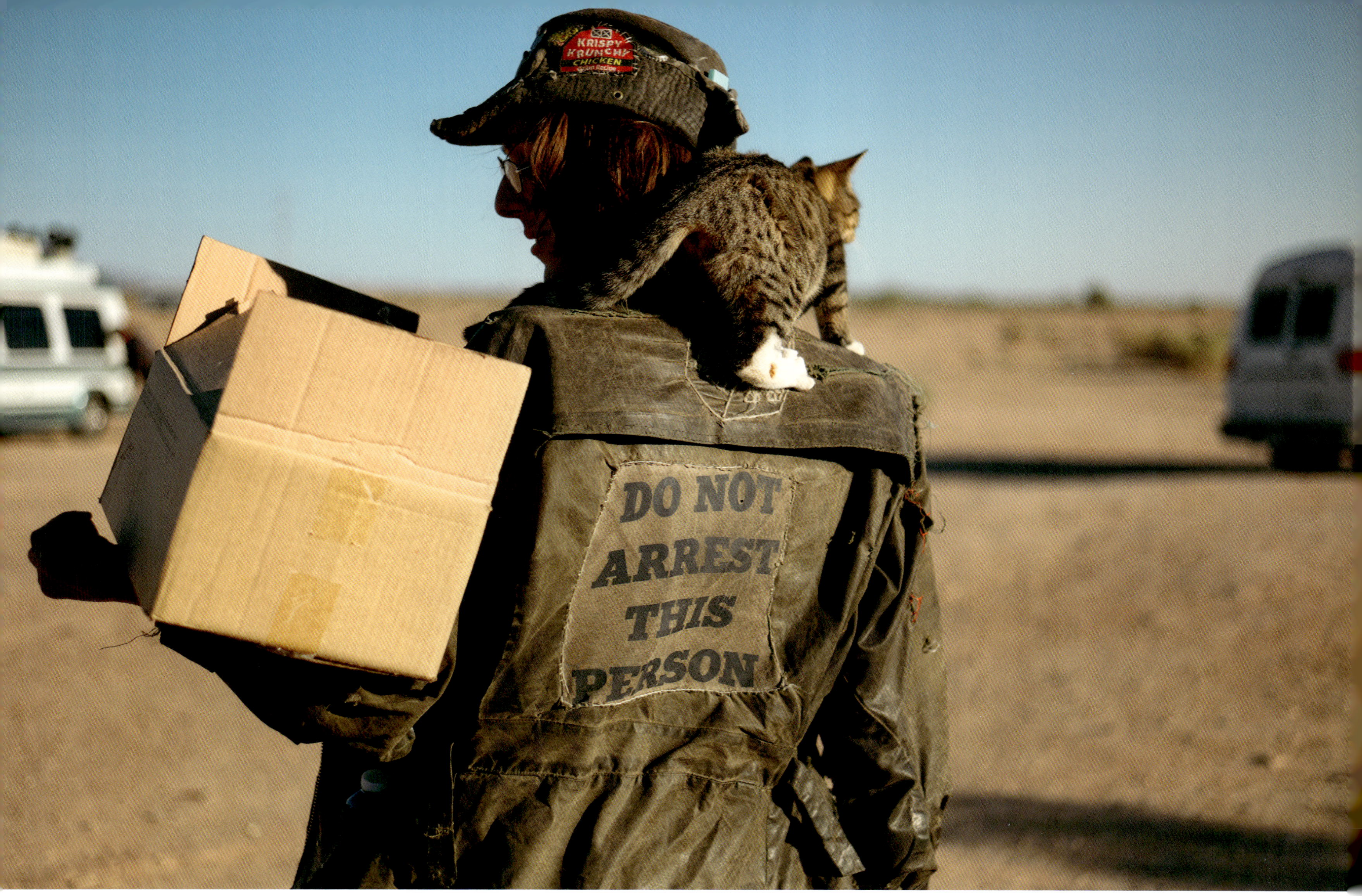

Therese, Poverty Flats

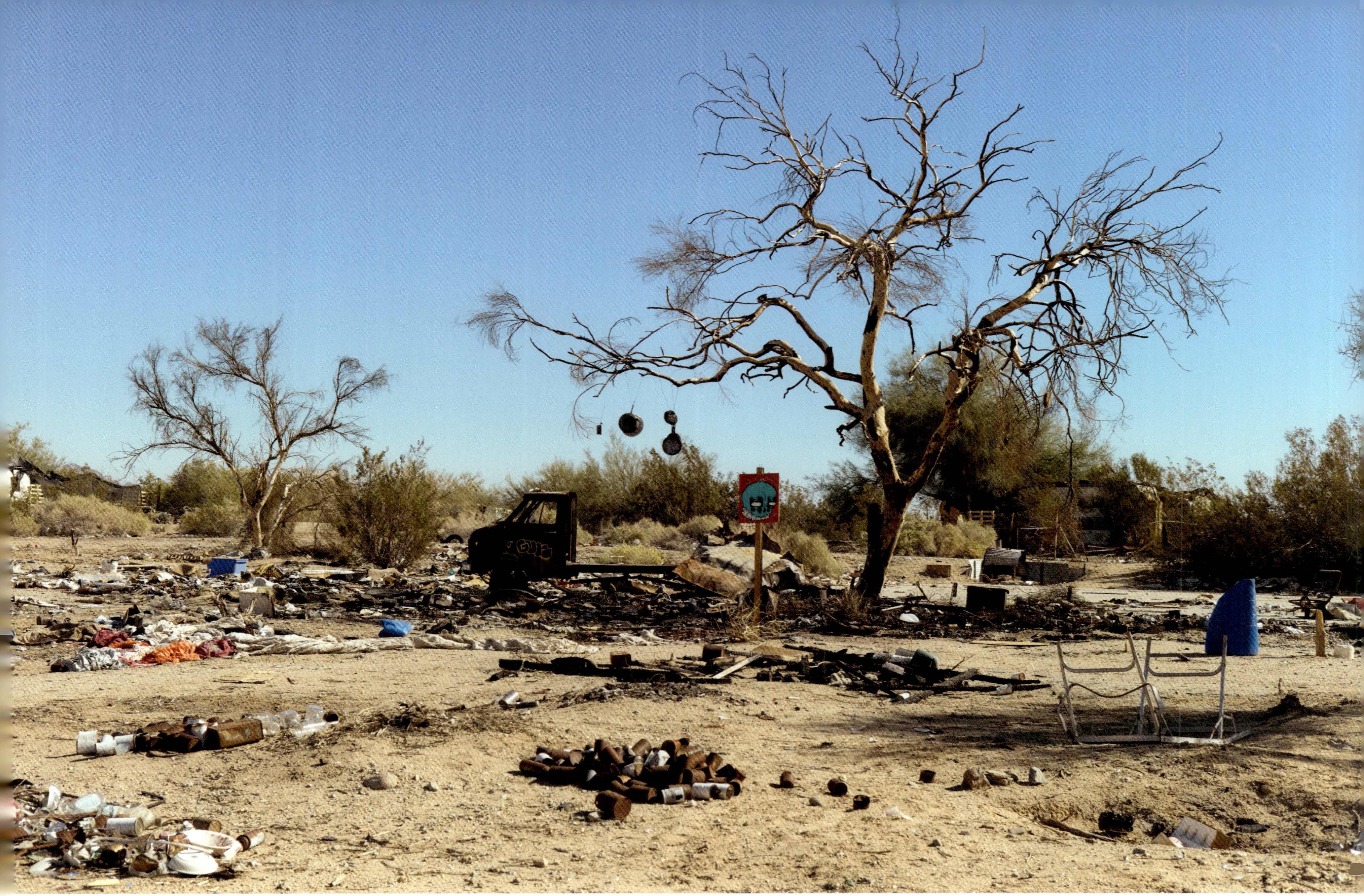

Burned down Camp in Area 5, Slab City

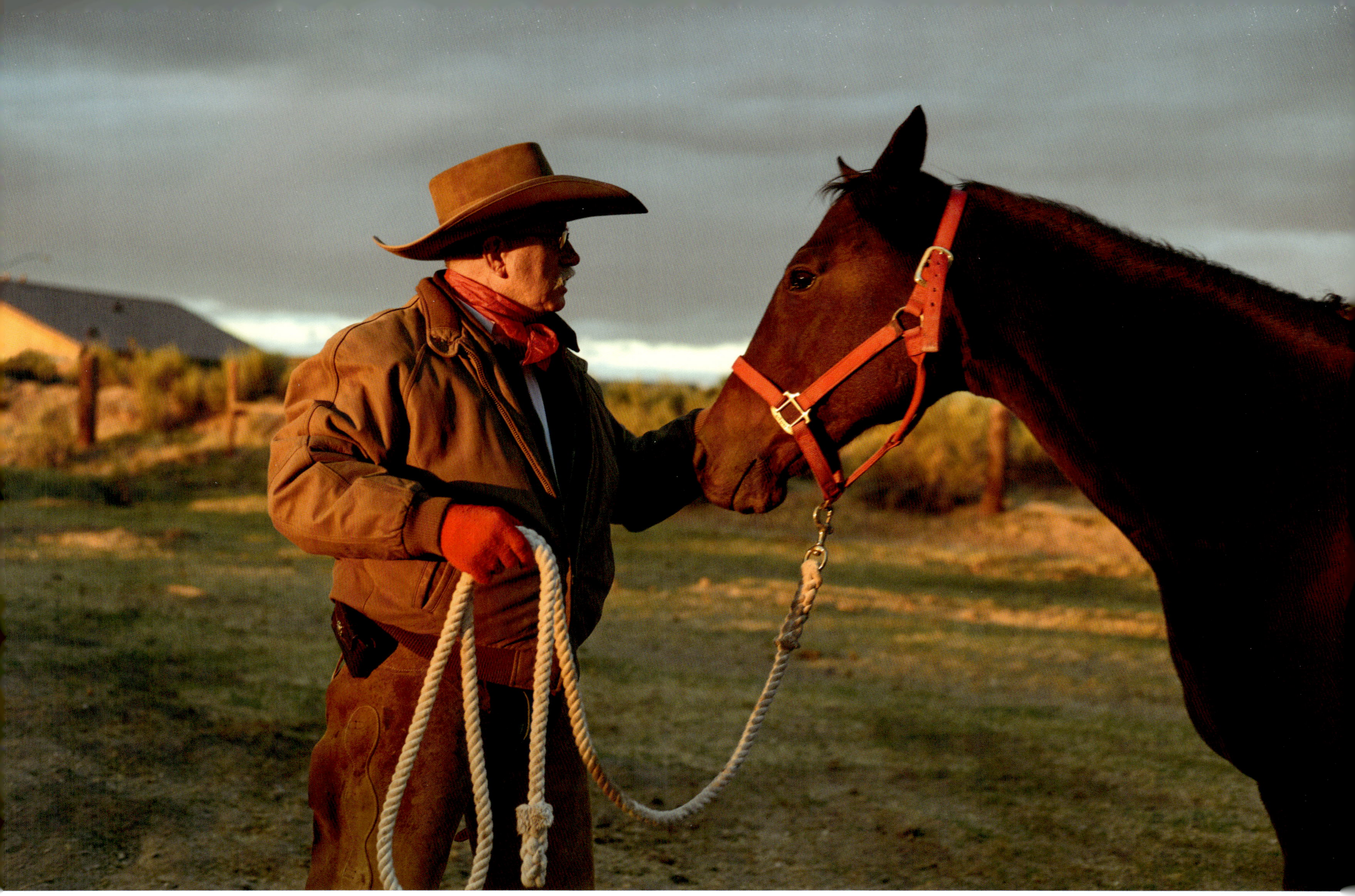

Mayor Mark Gran, Imperial

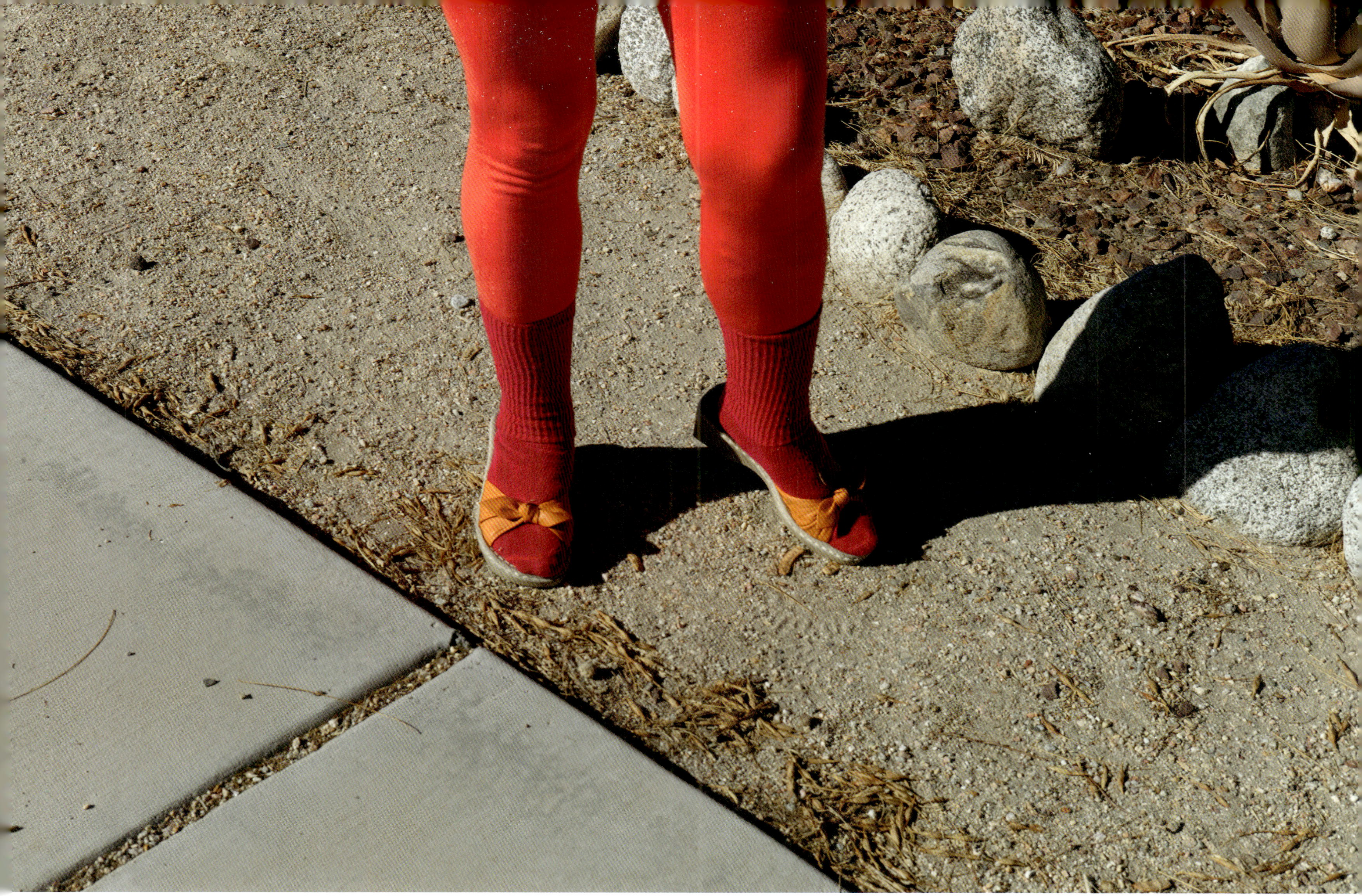

Cindy in her garden, Salton City

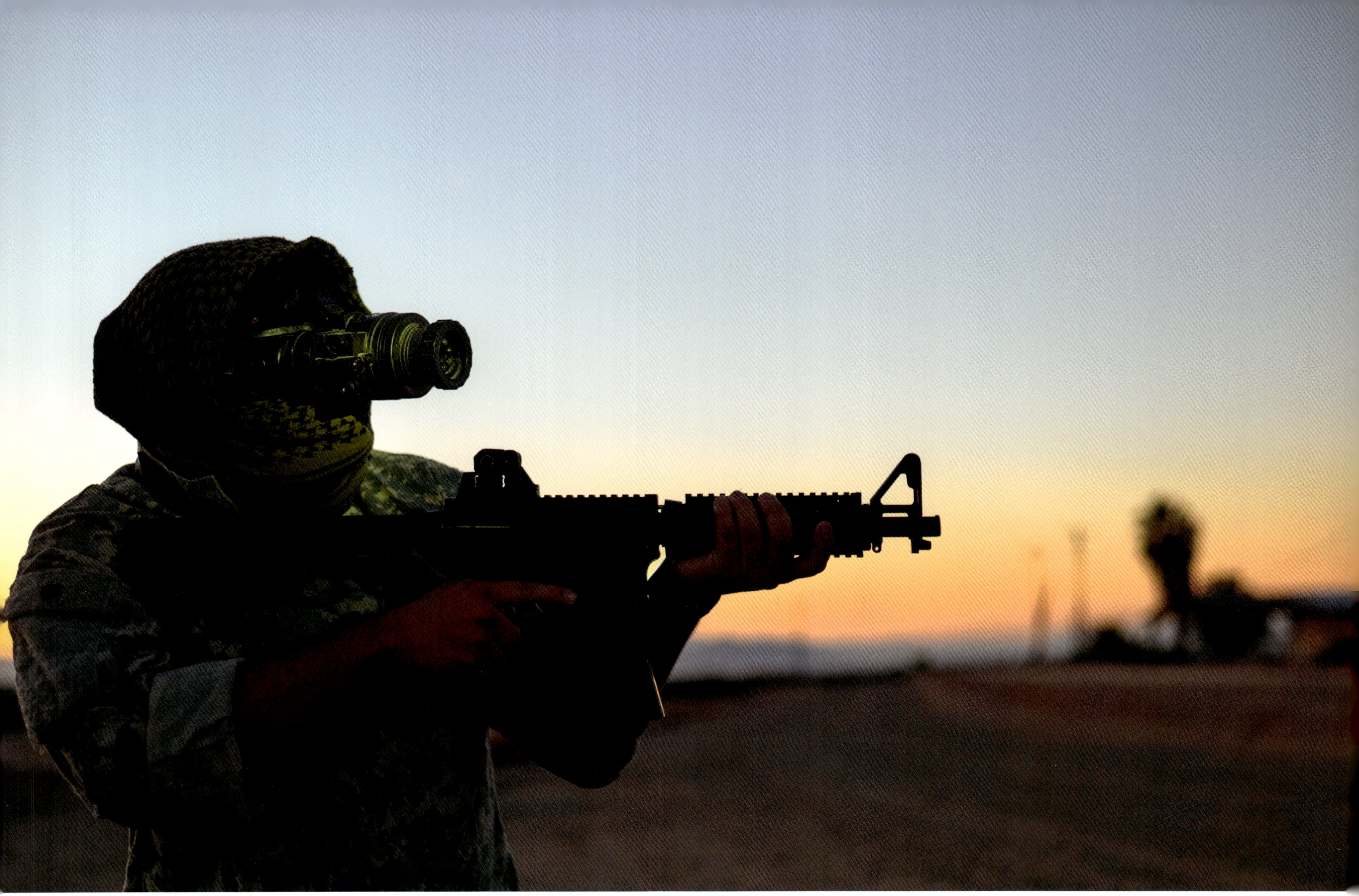

Hector at the mansion, Wilsie

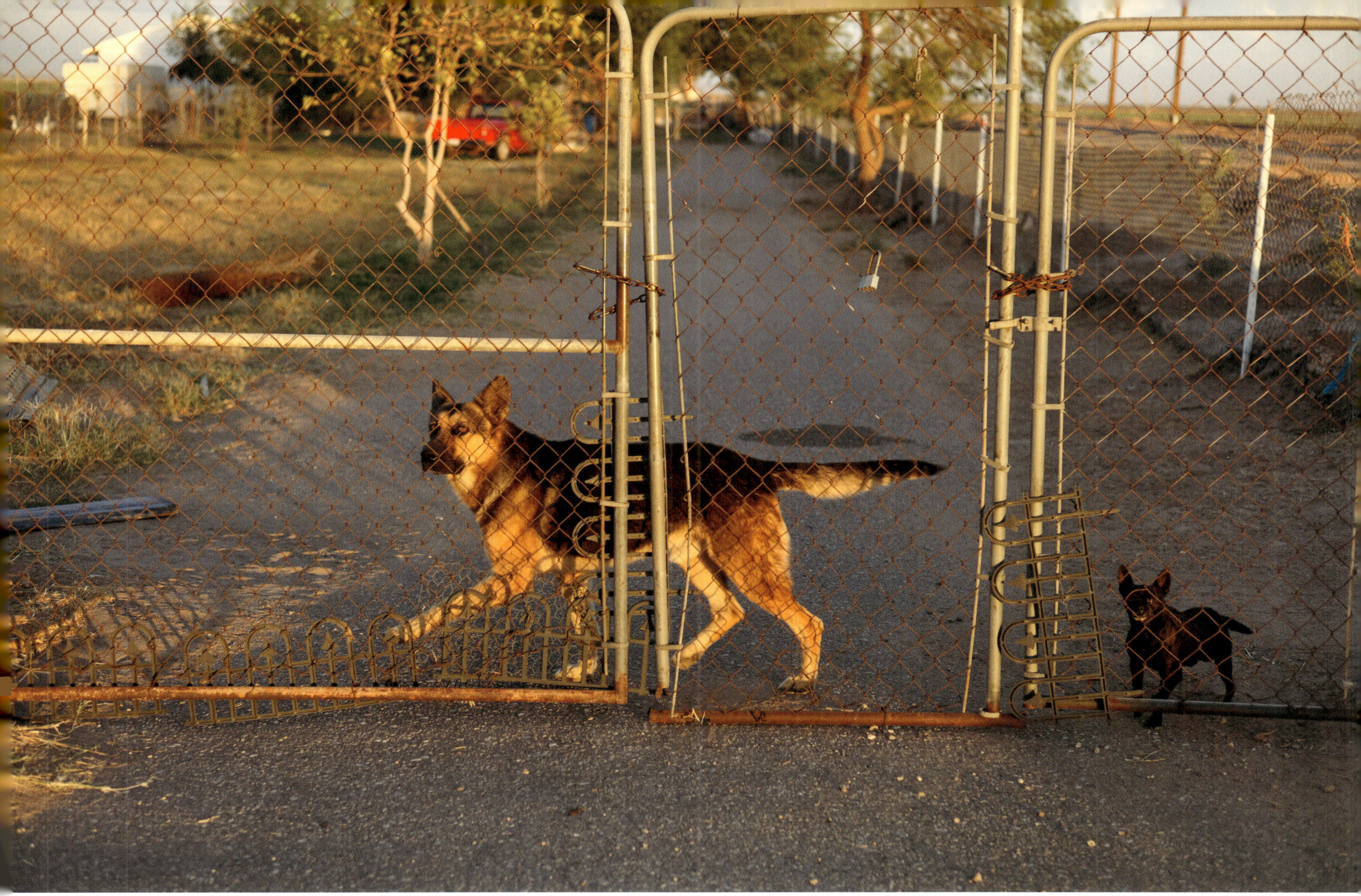

Farm at Highway 115, Fuller

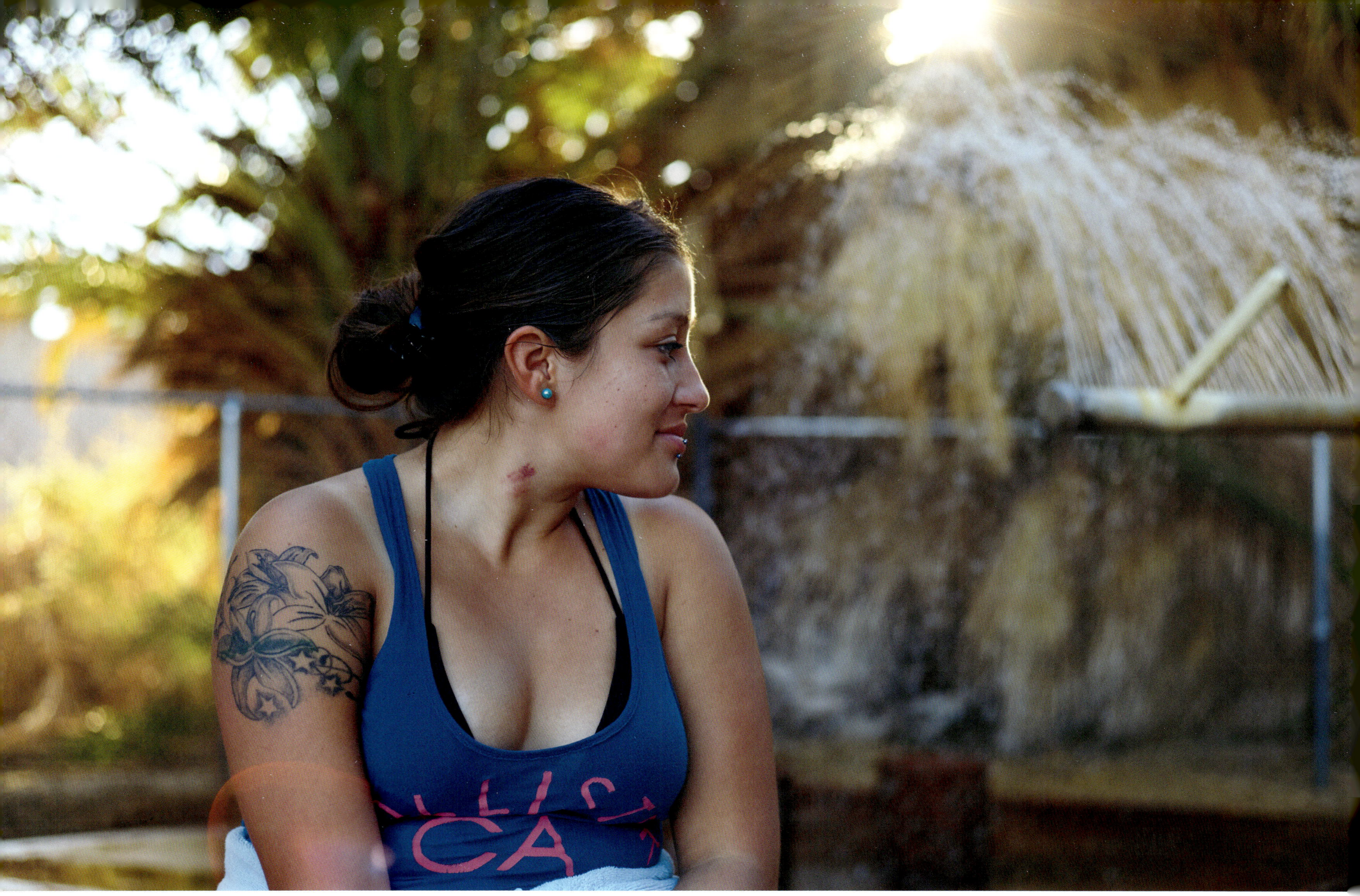

Lupe, Hot Springs

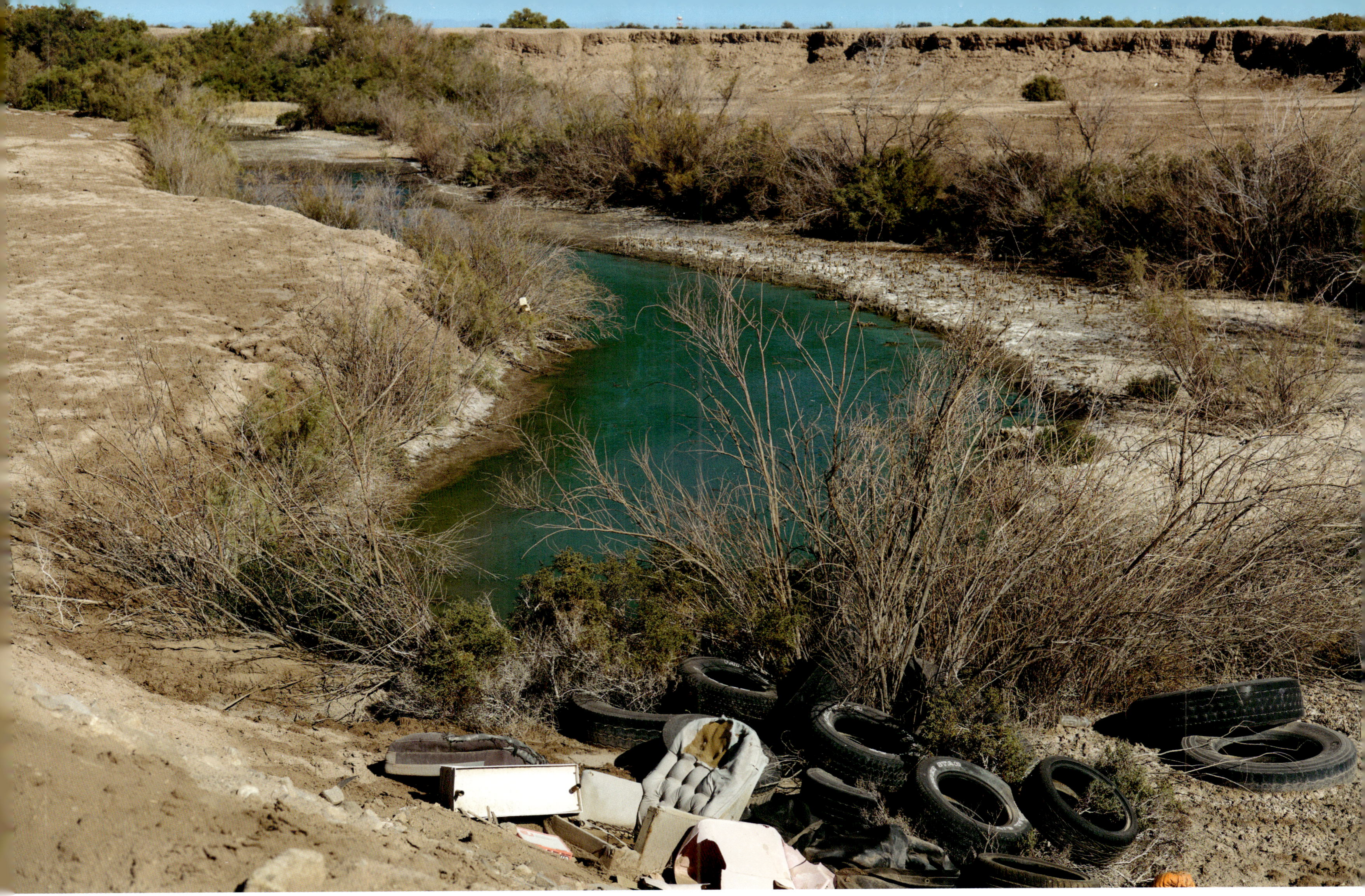

The New River, Greeson Wash

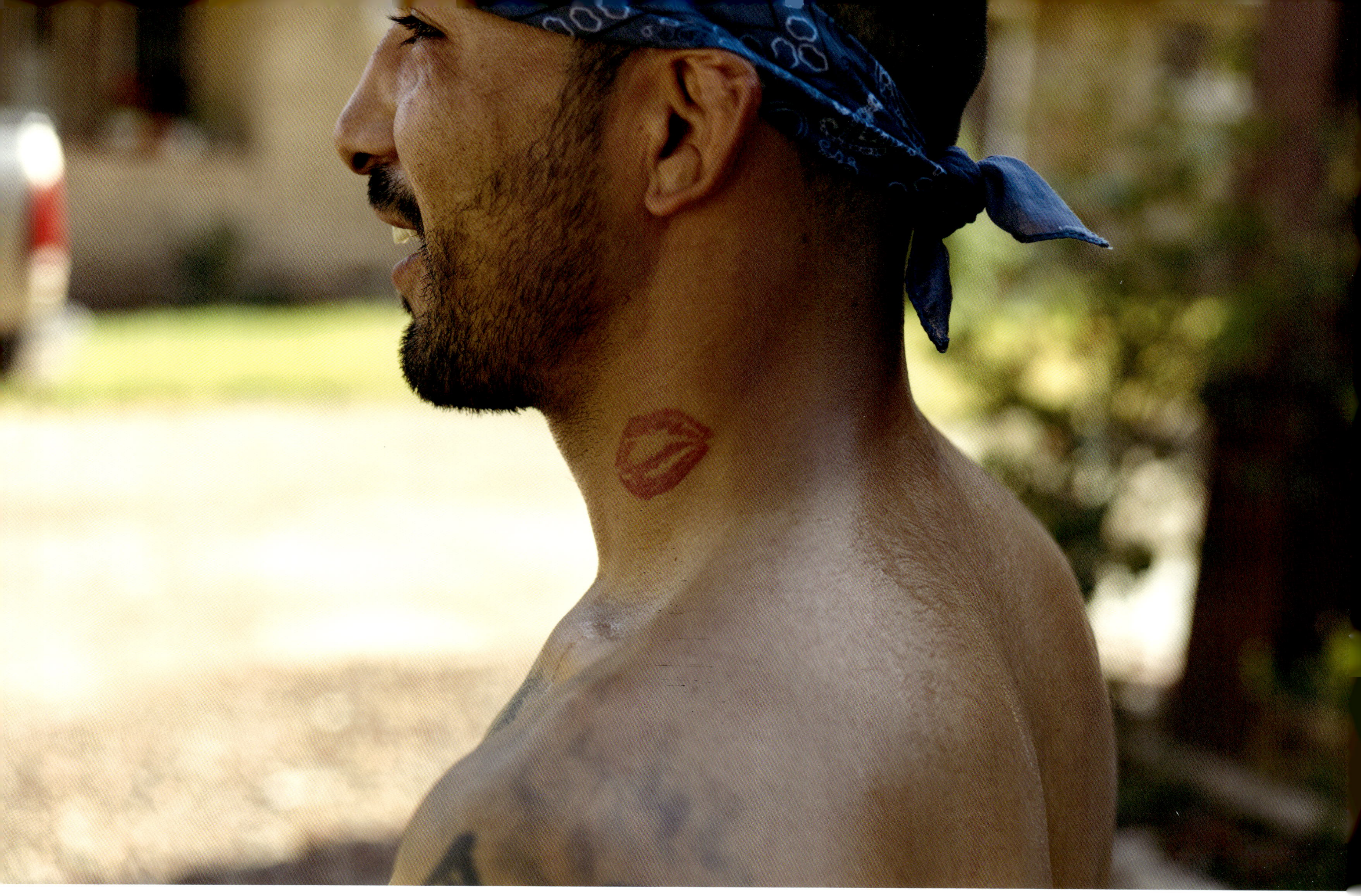

Jorge, Holtville

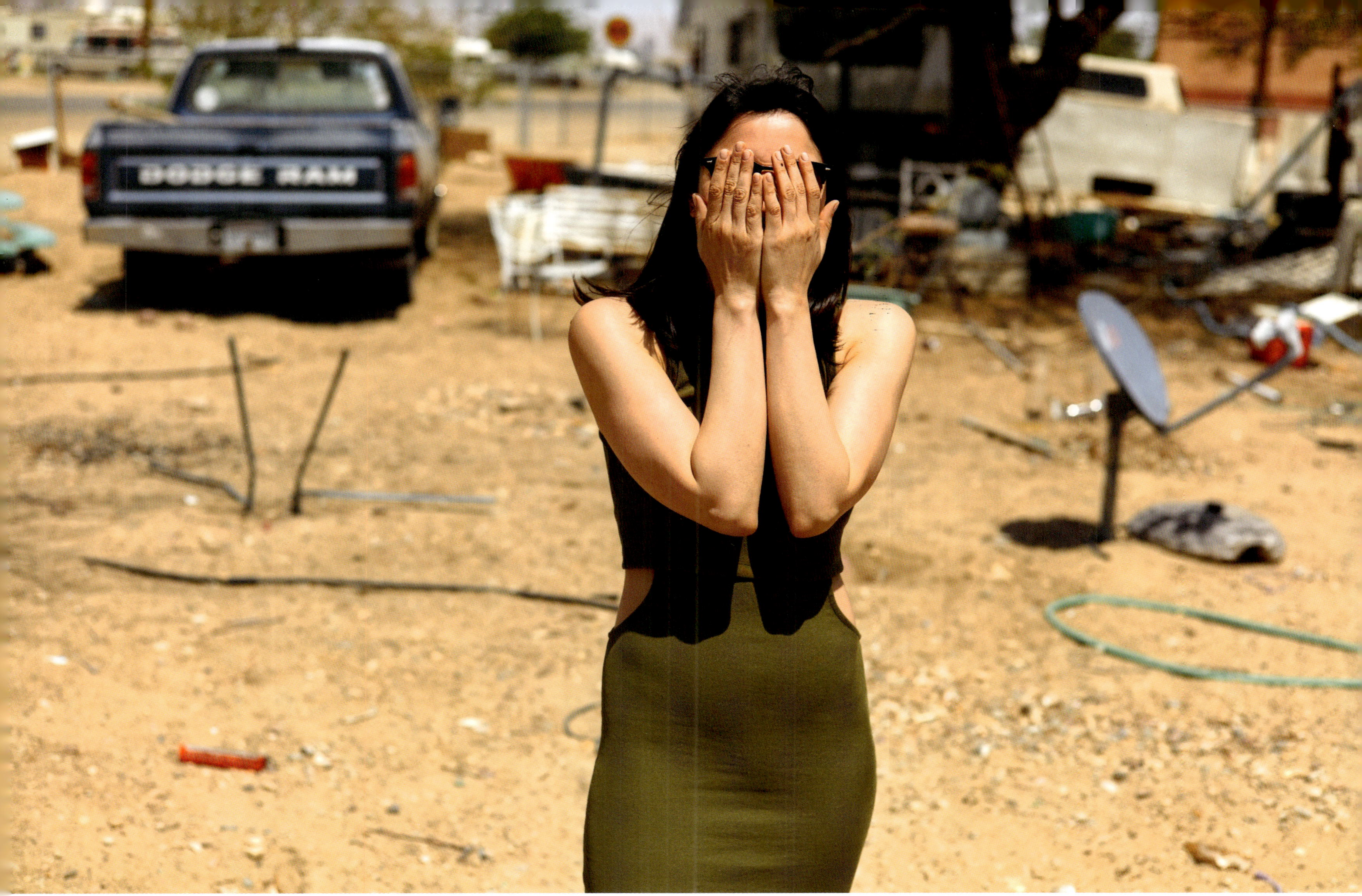

Steff, near Niland

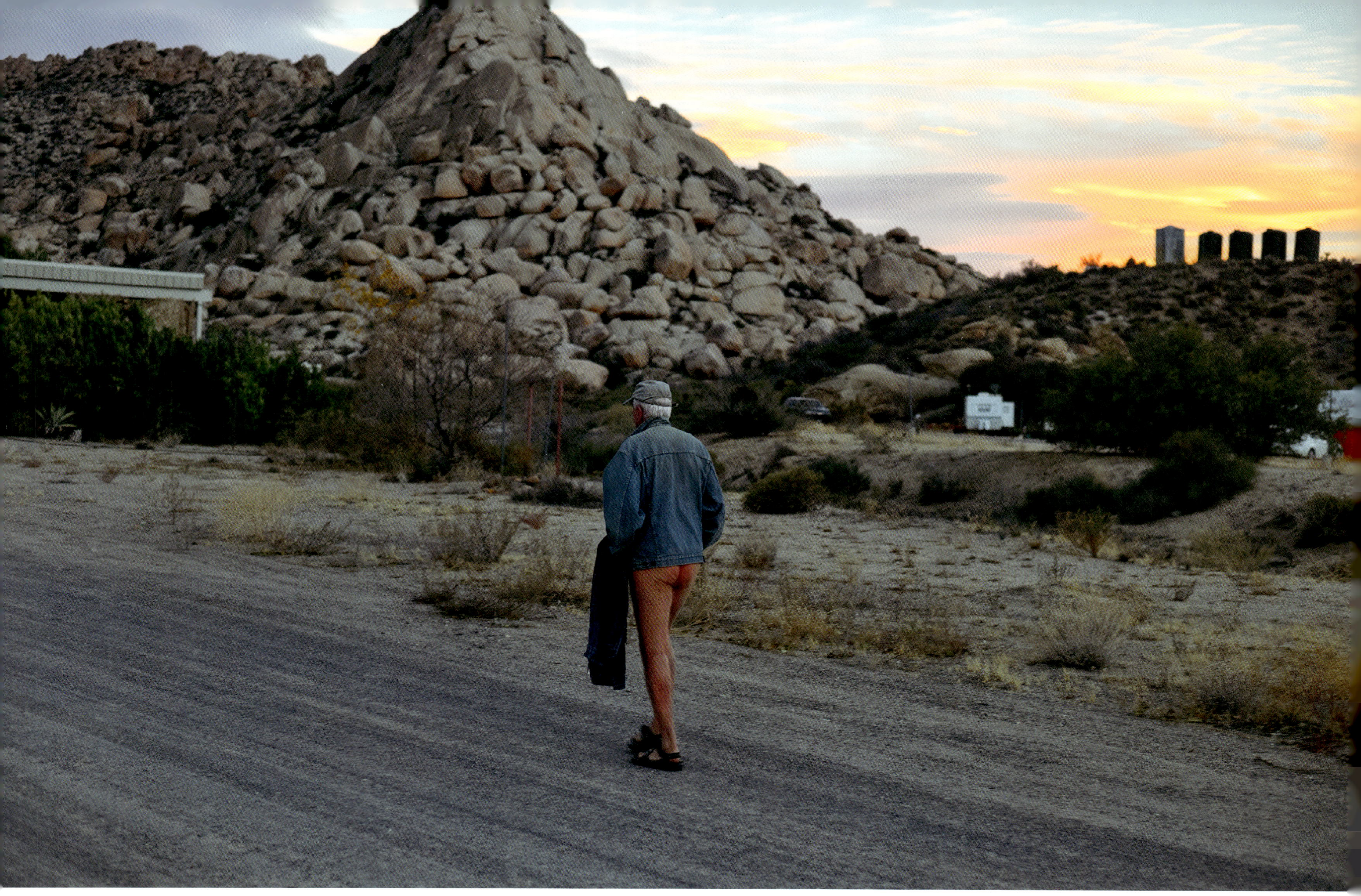

Don, Ocotillo Mountains

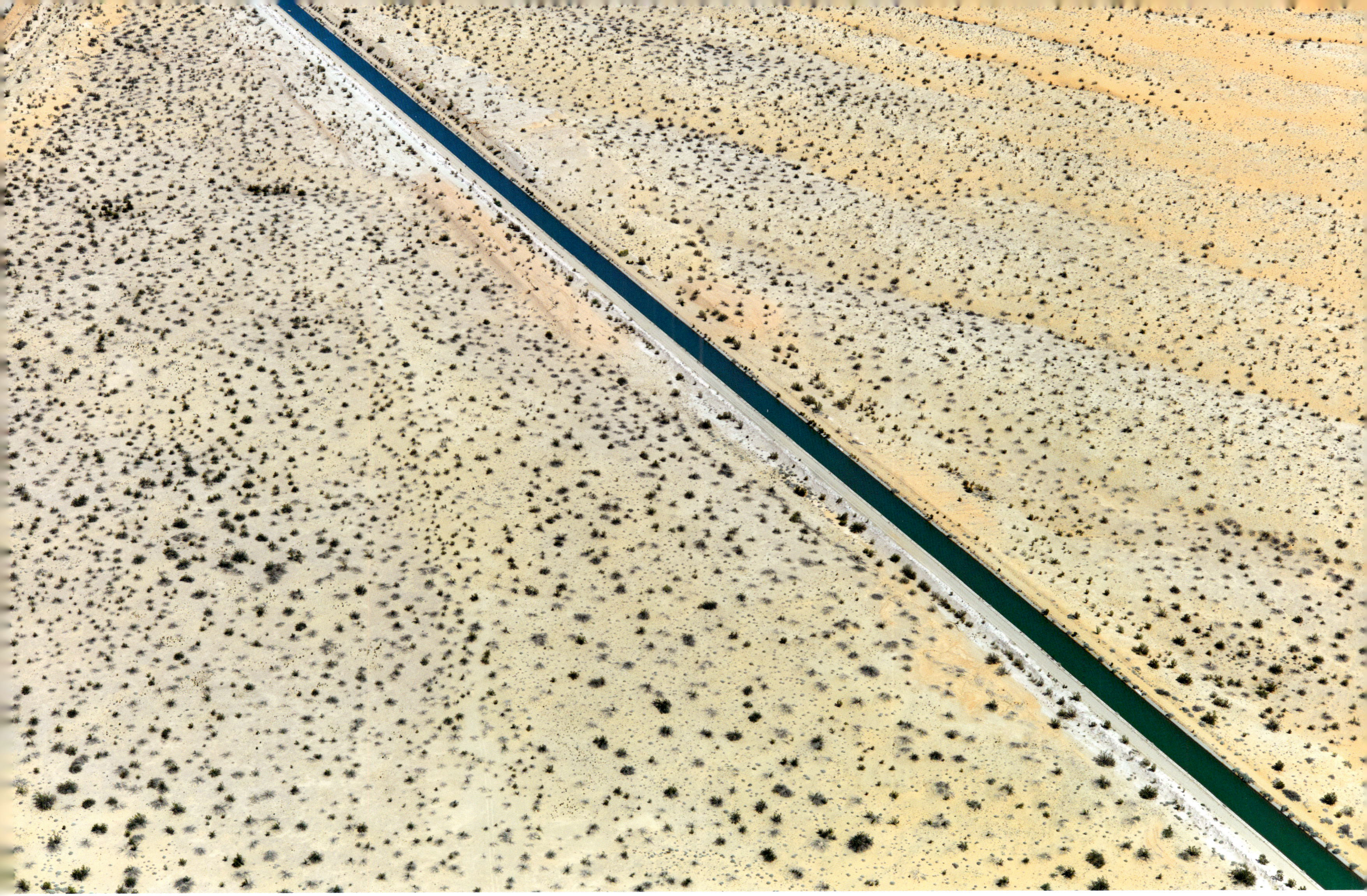

The All-American Canal, near Felicity

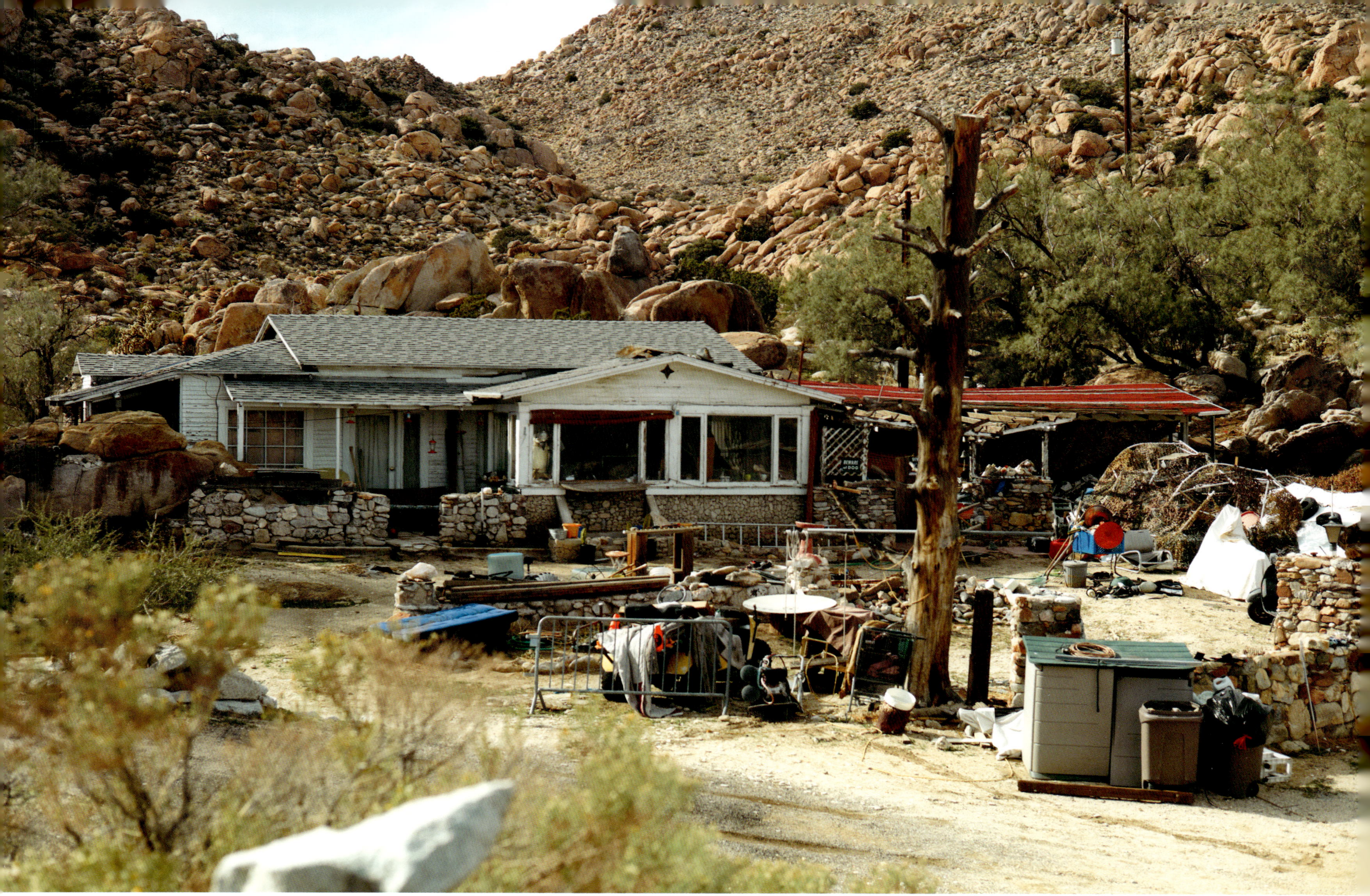

Mountain home, Boulder Oaks

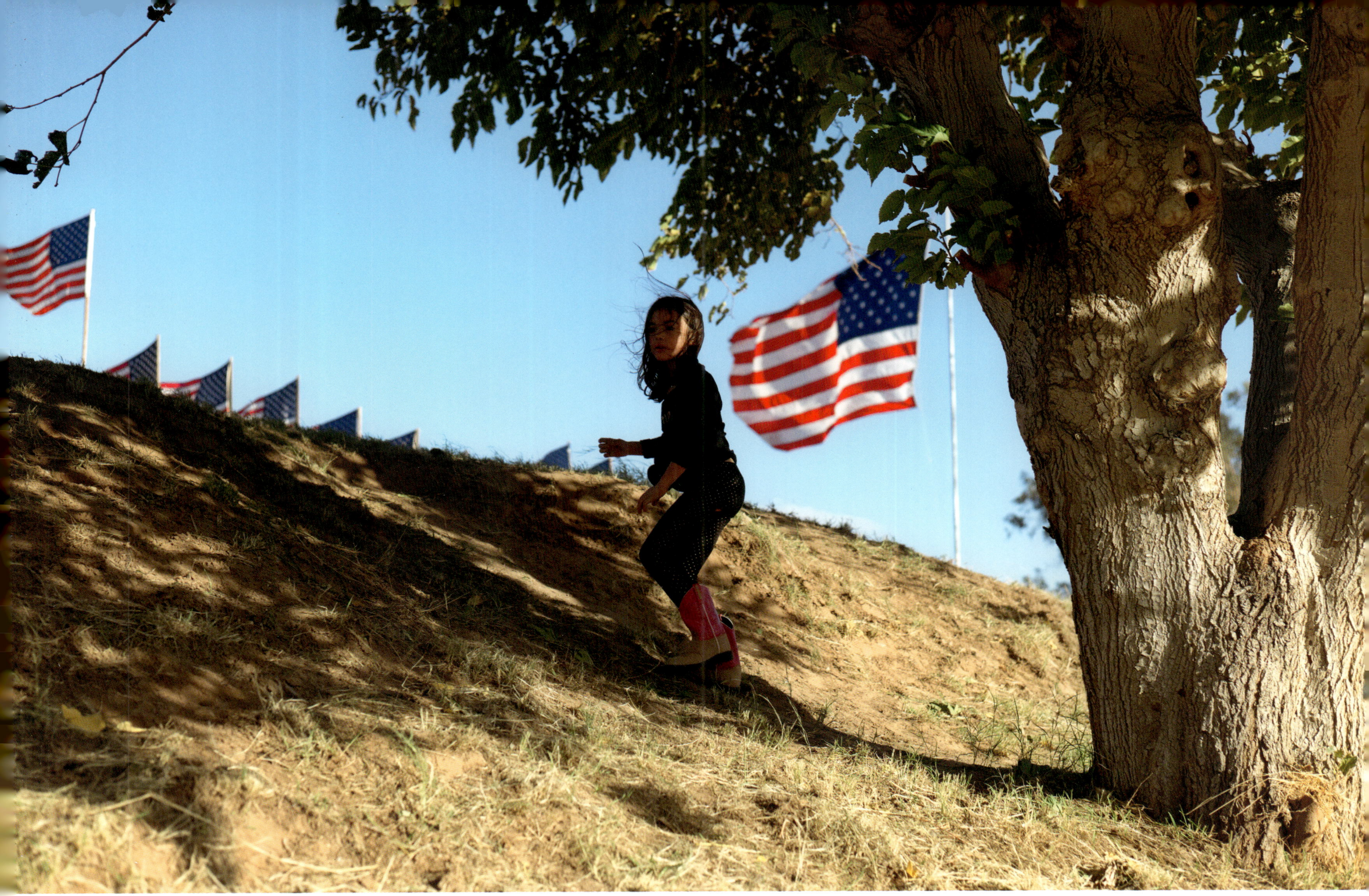

Eleadora on the 4th of July, Brawley

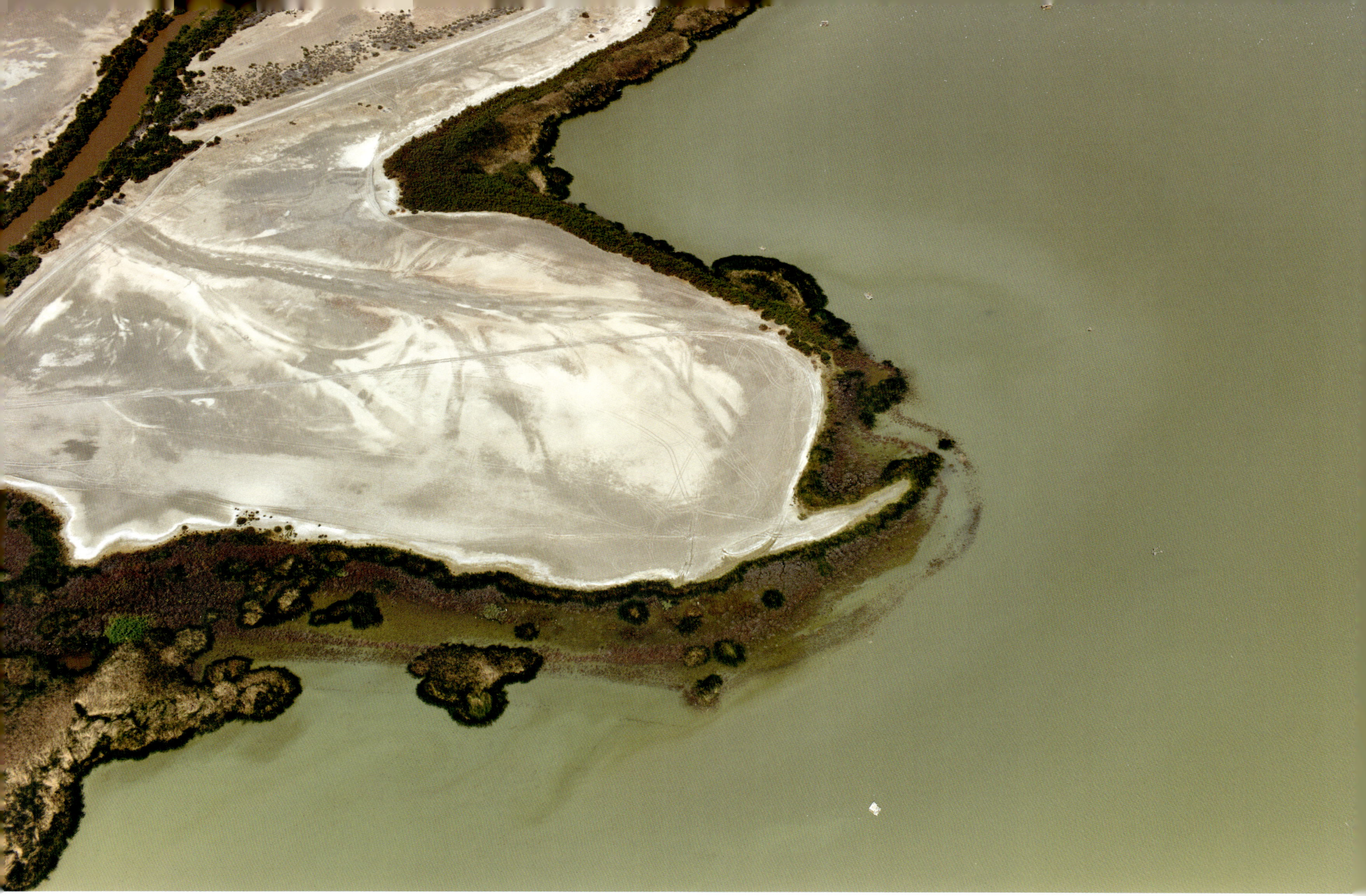

New River Delta, Salton Sea

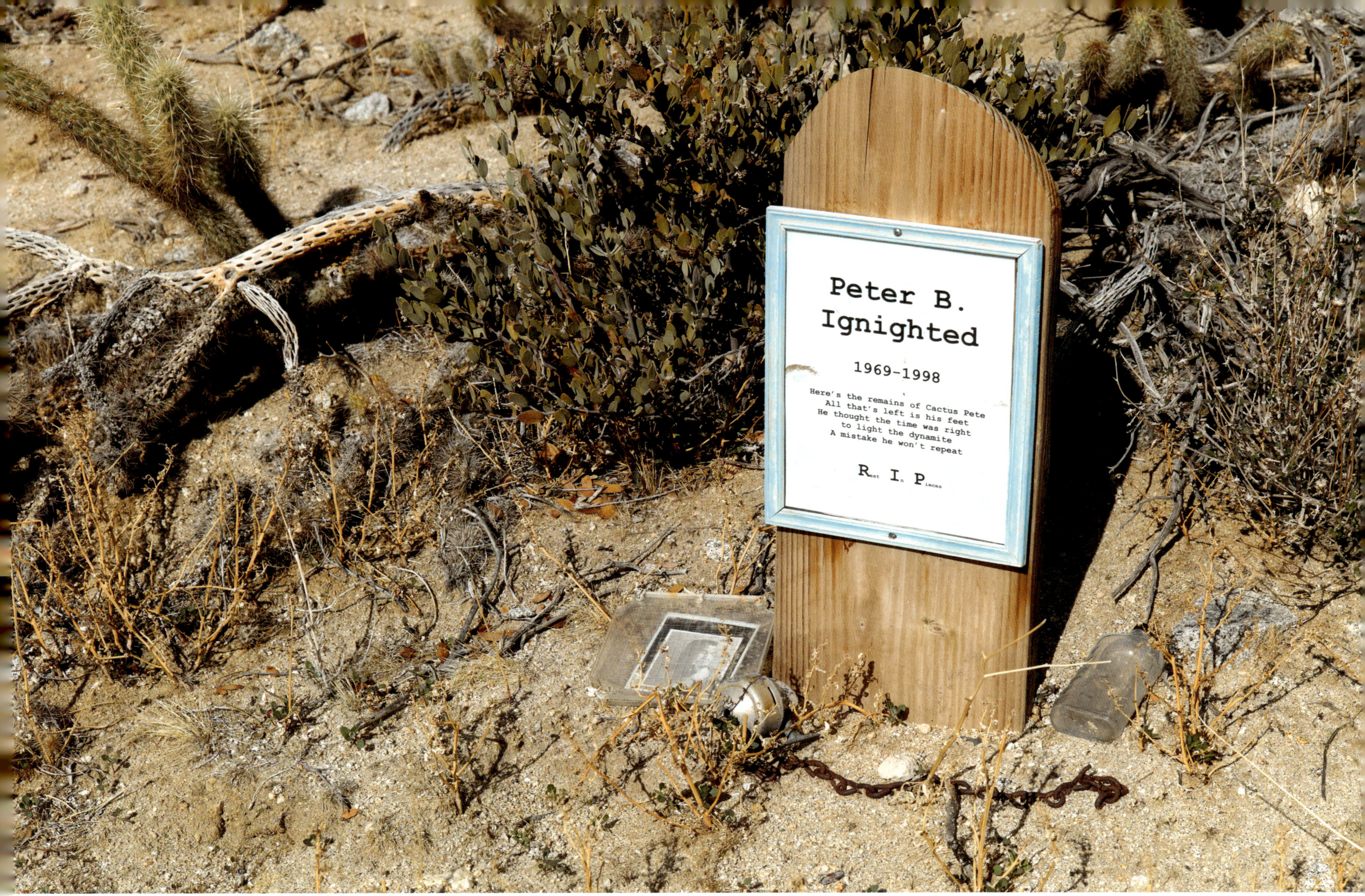
Peter B.
Ignighted
1969-1998
Here's the remains of Cactus Pete
All that's left is his feet
He thought the time was right
to light the dynamite
A mistake he won't repeat
Rest In Pieces

Peter's grave, Desert View Tower

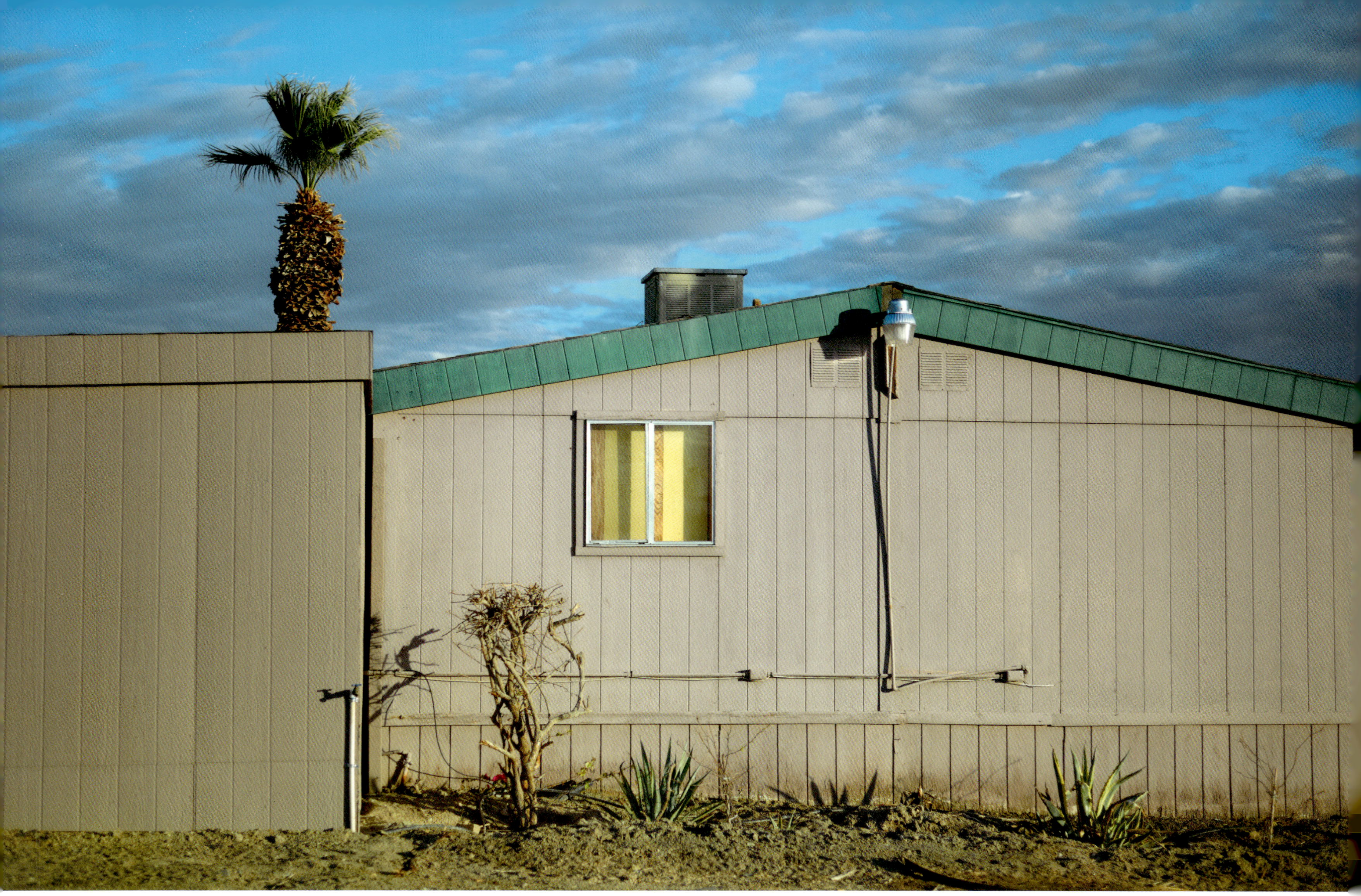

Cabin, Chocolate Mountains

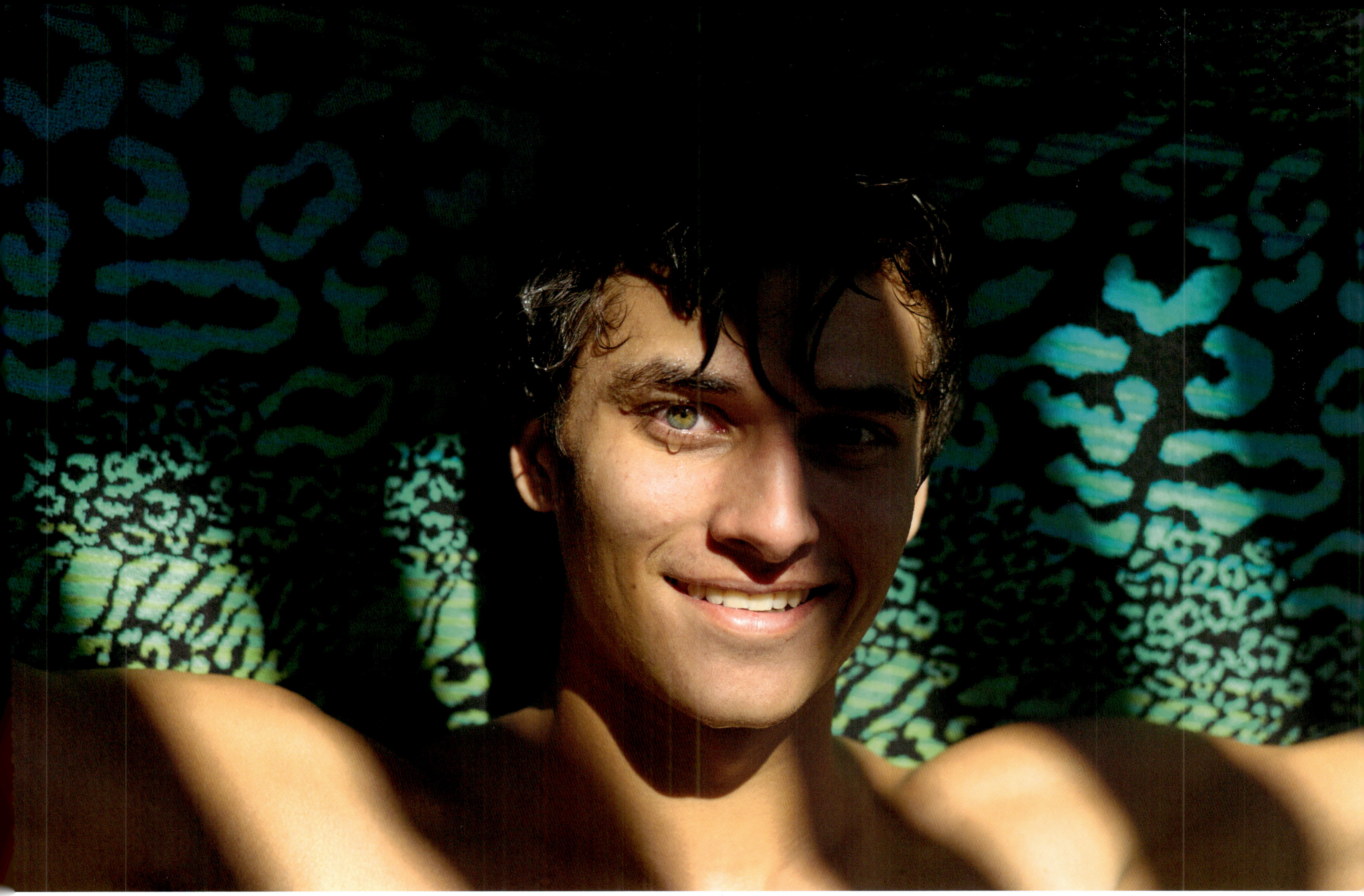

Trey by his family pool, Heber

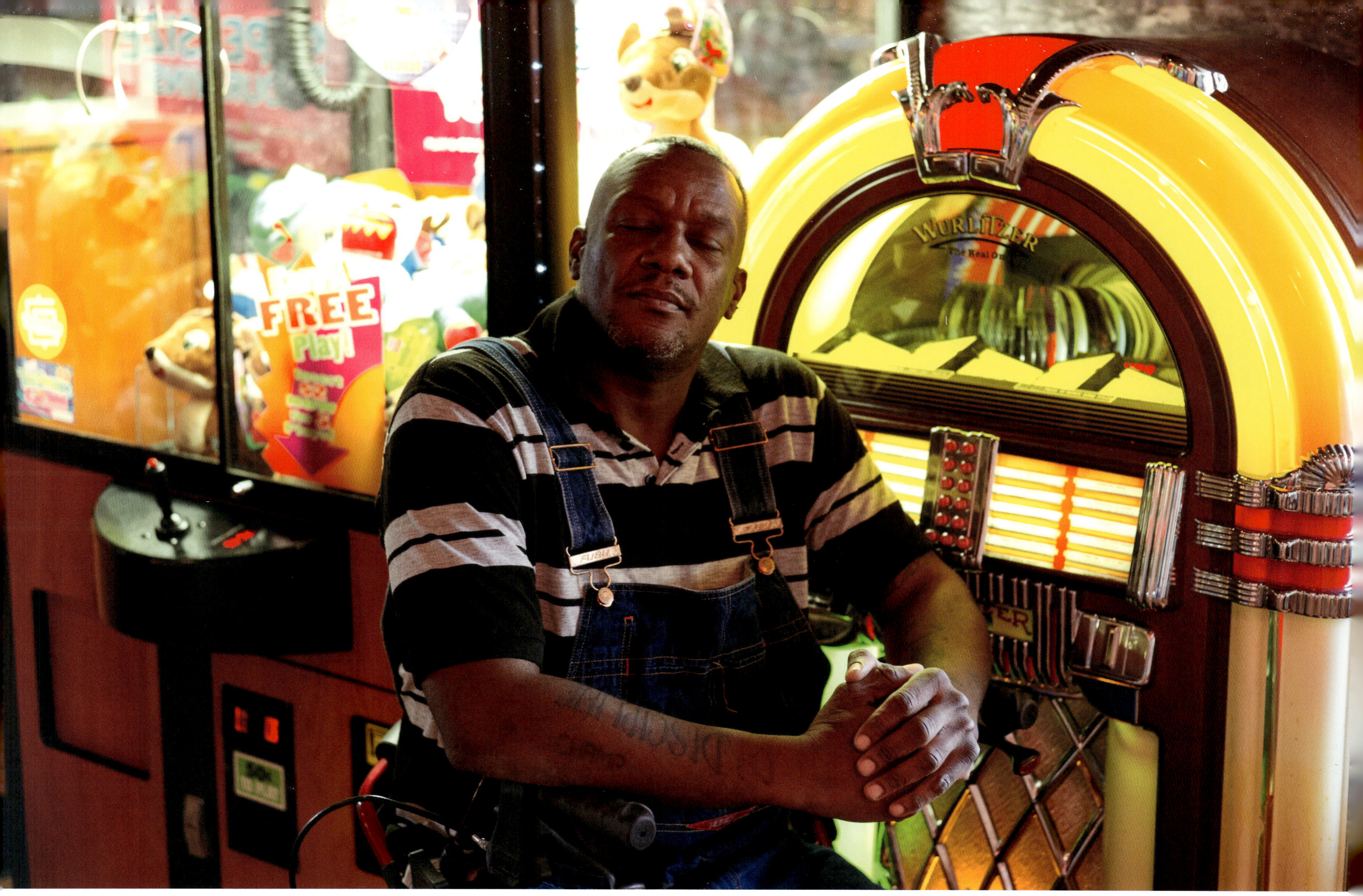

Champ in the sports bar, El Centro

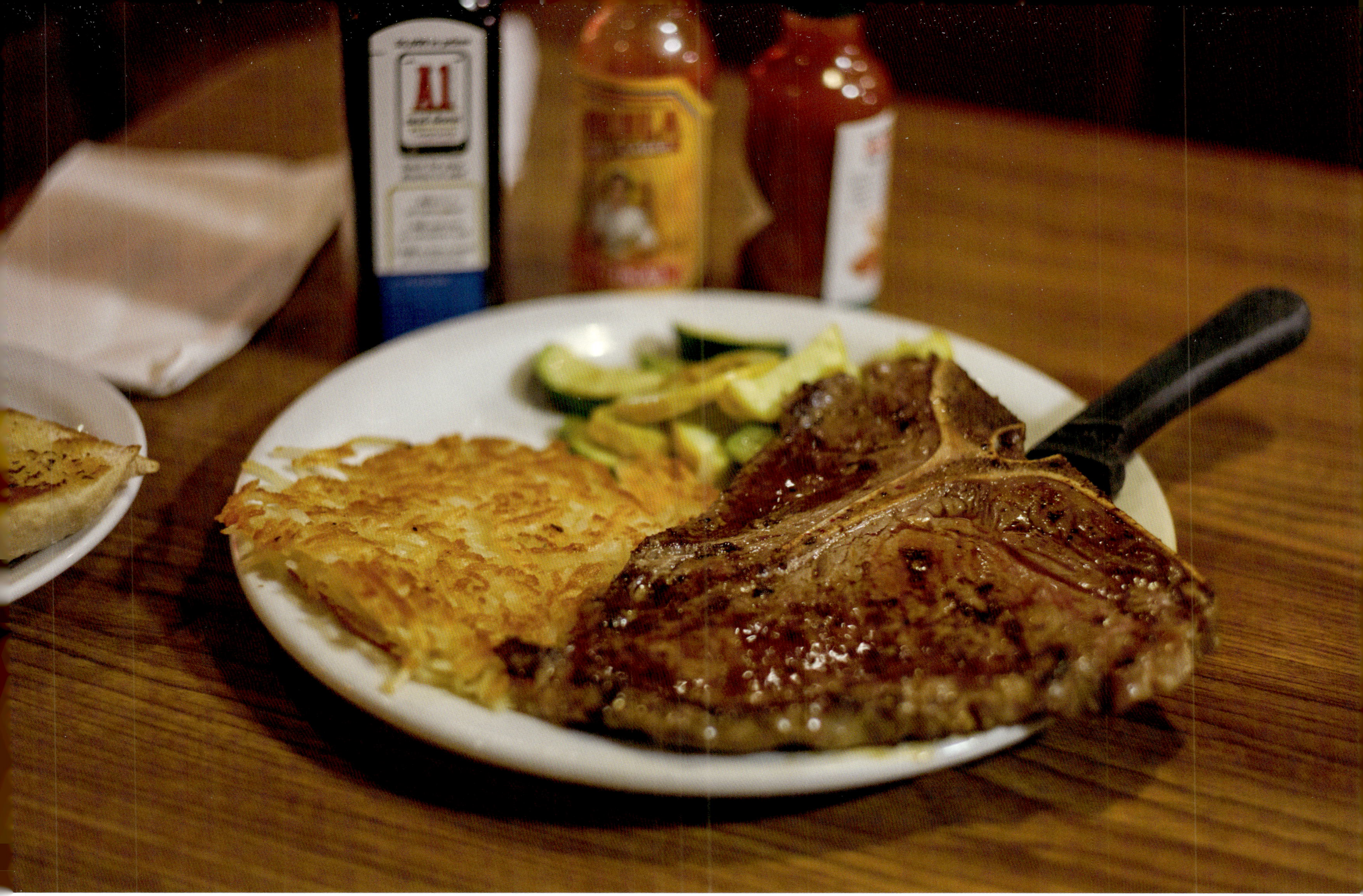

T-Bone Steak Special, El Centro

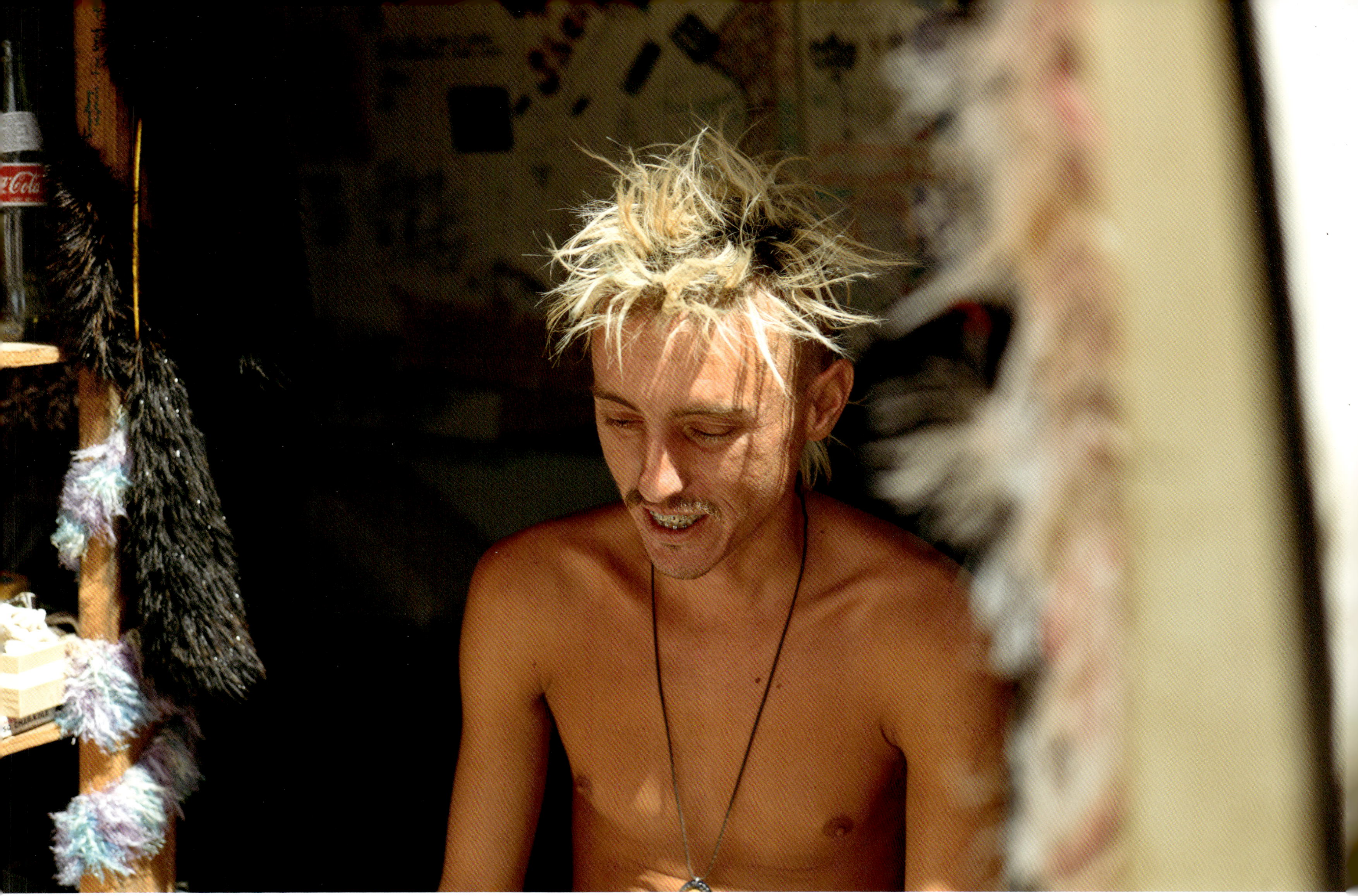

Jordan in his camper van, Slab City

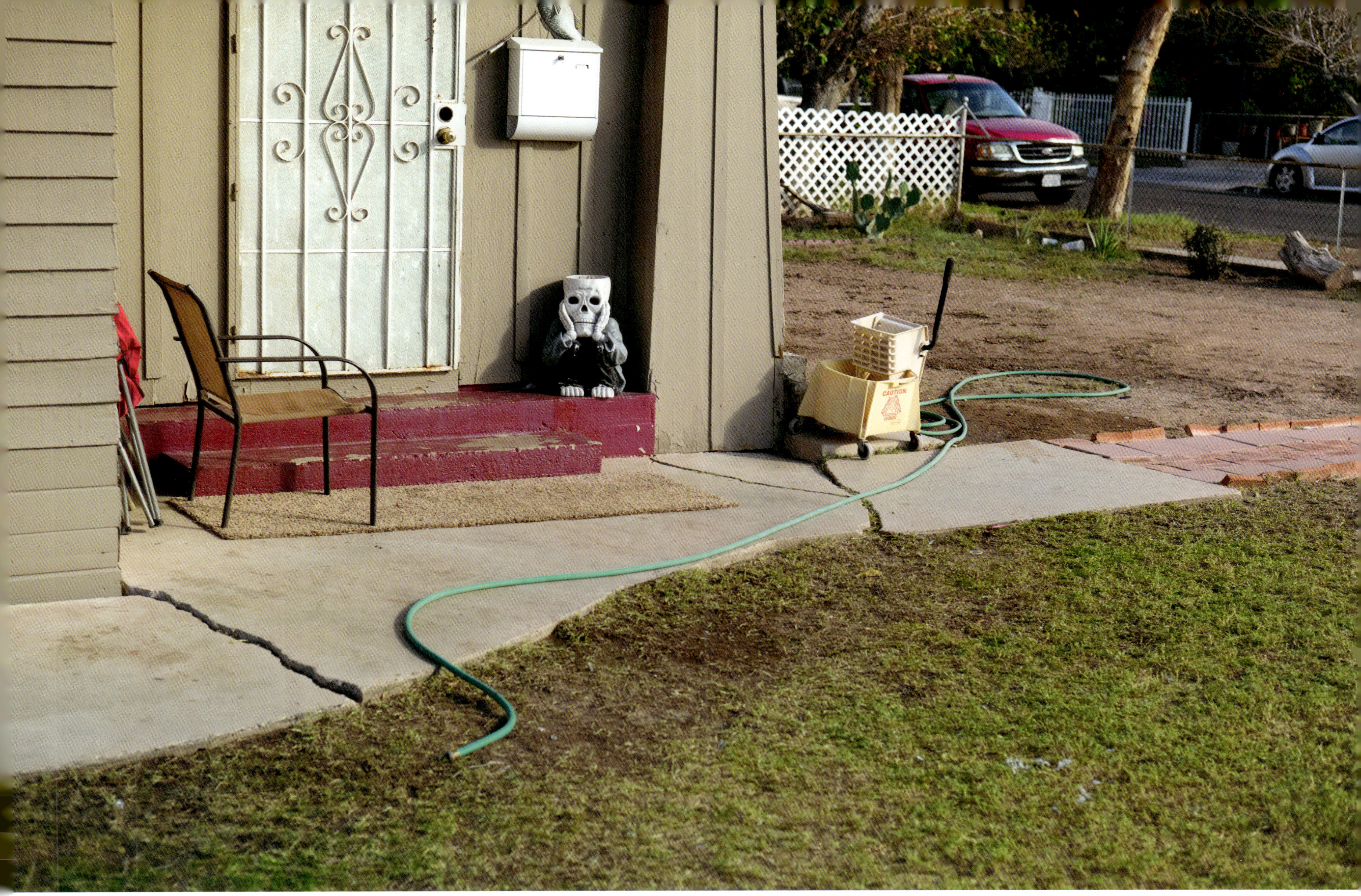

8th Street, El Centro

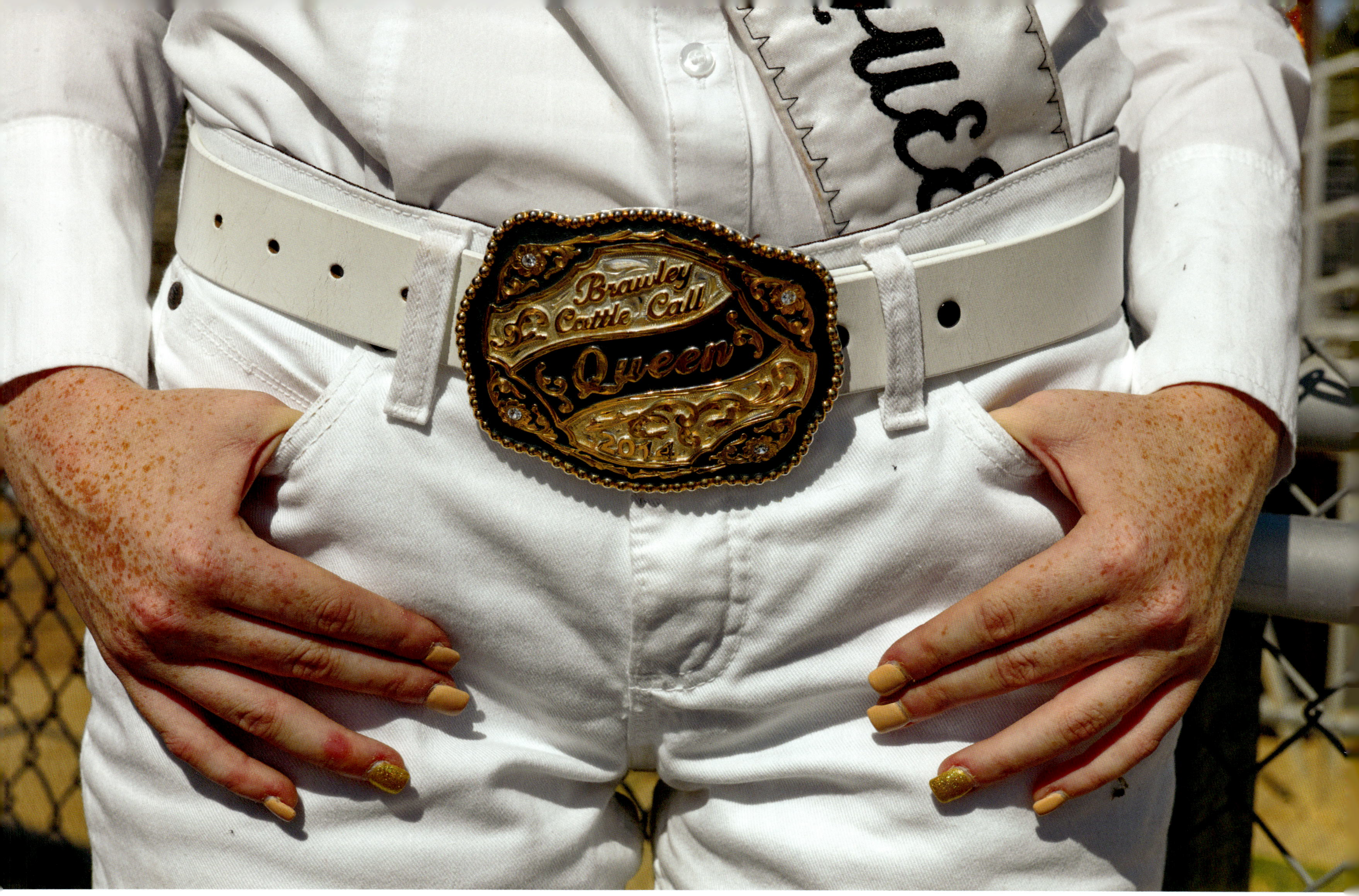

Alex, Brawley

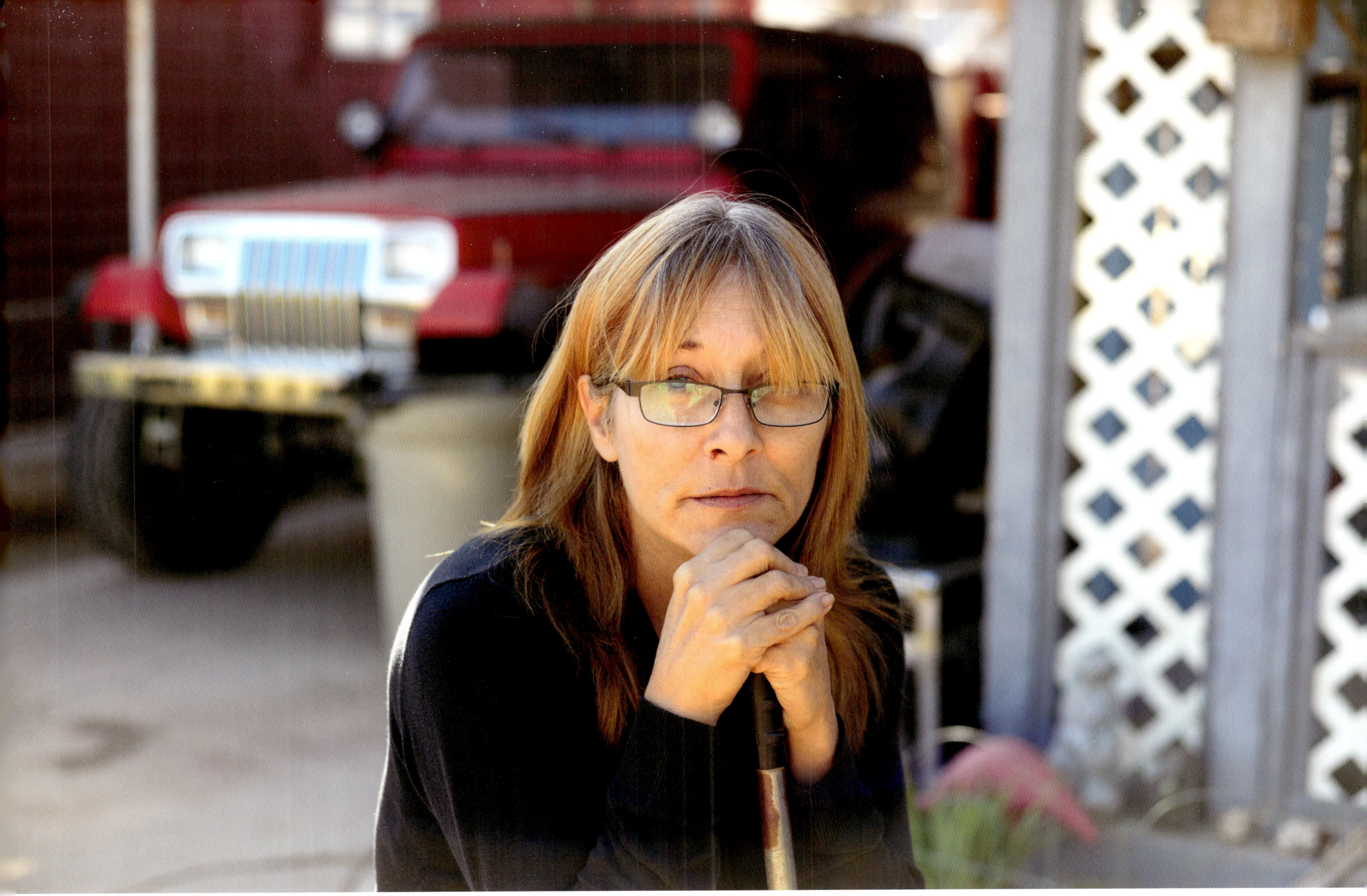

Sherri, El Centro

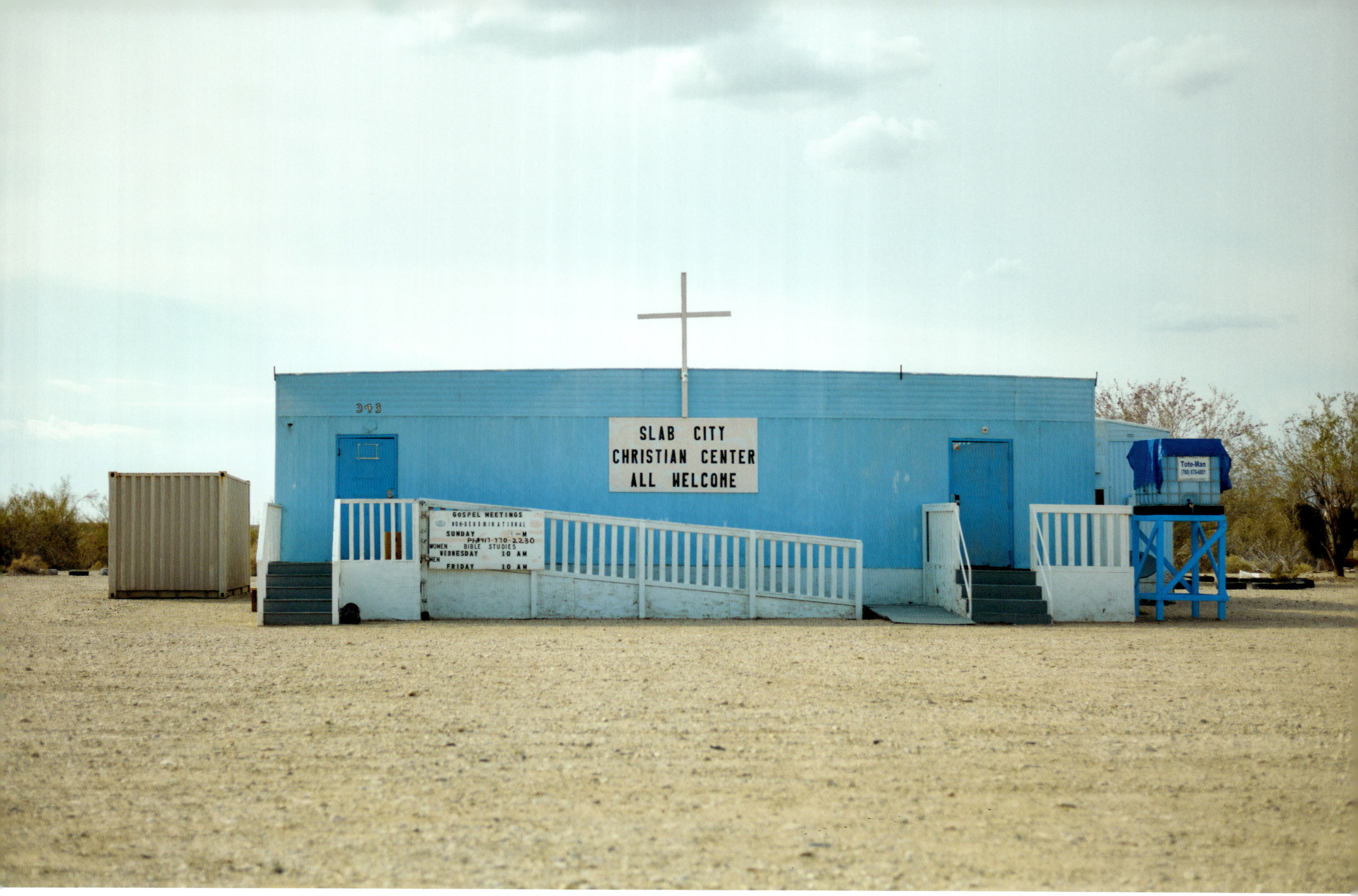

Church, Slab City

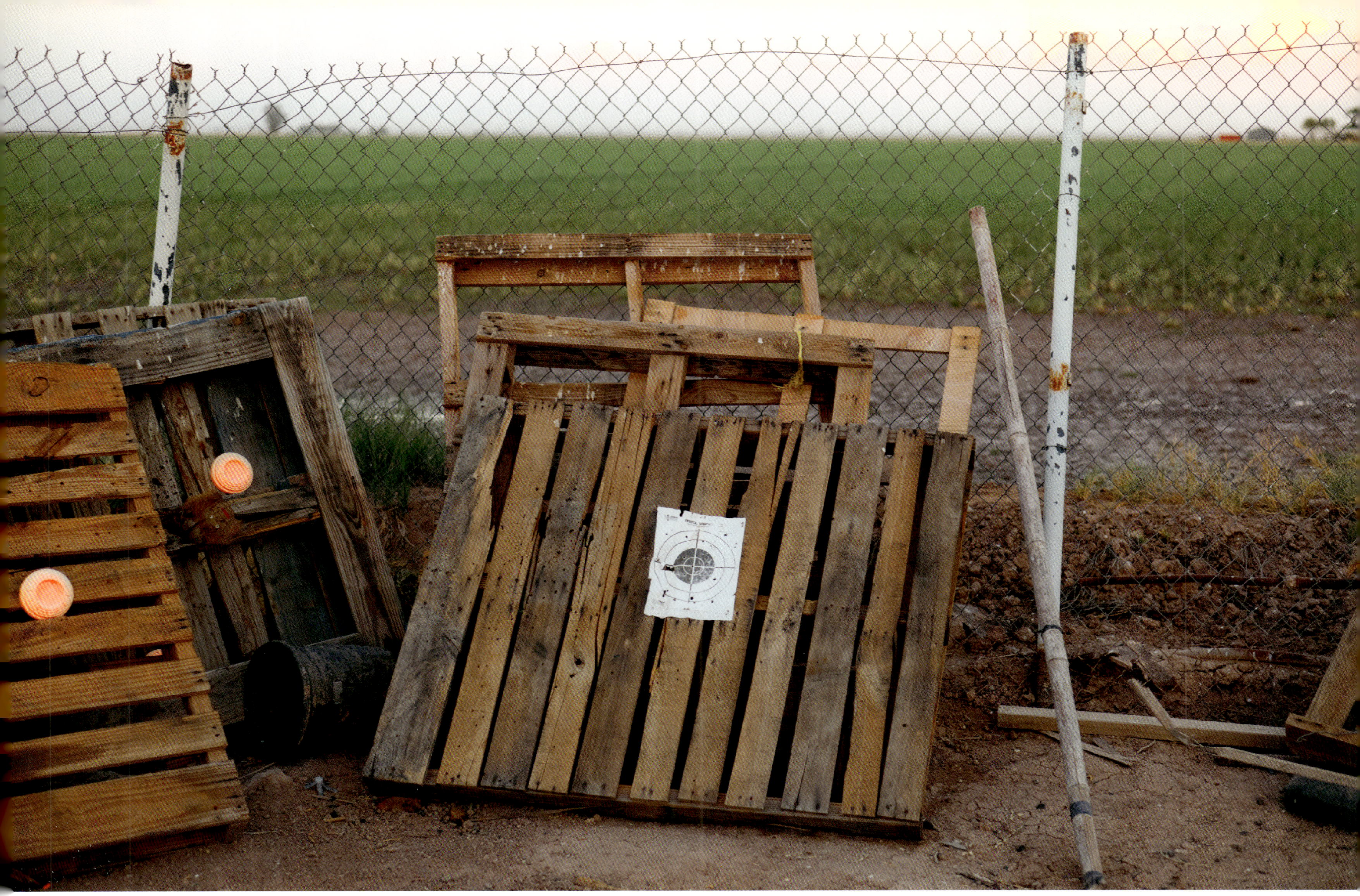

Yard, Sandia

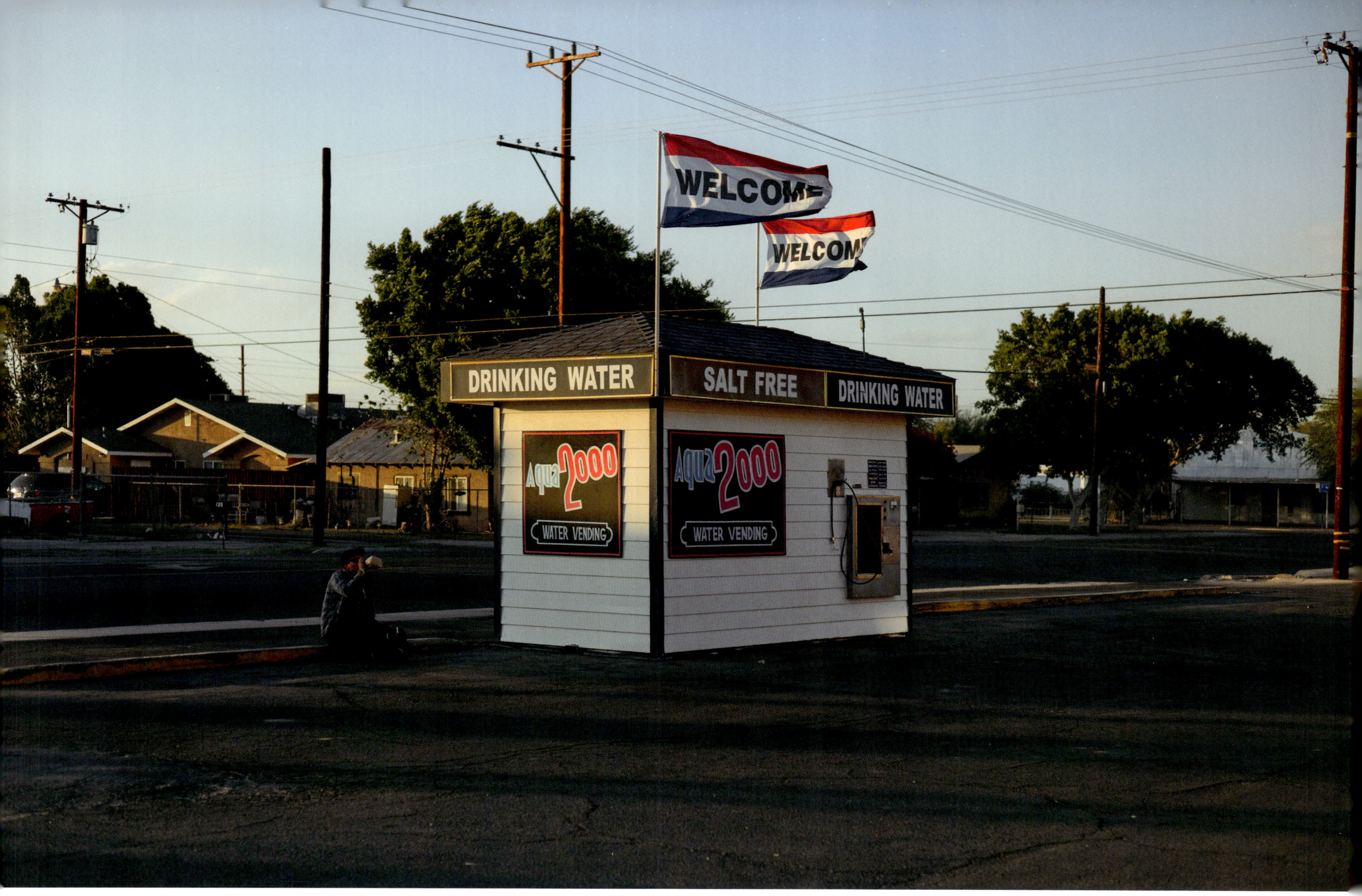

Albert at the liquor store car park, Brawley

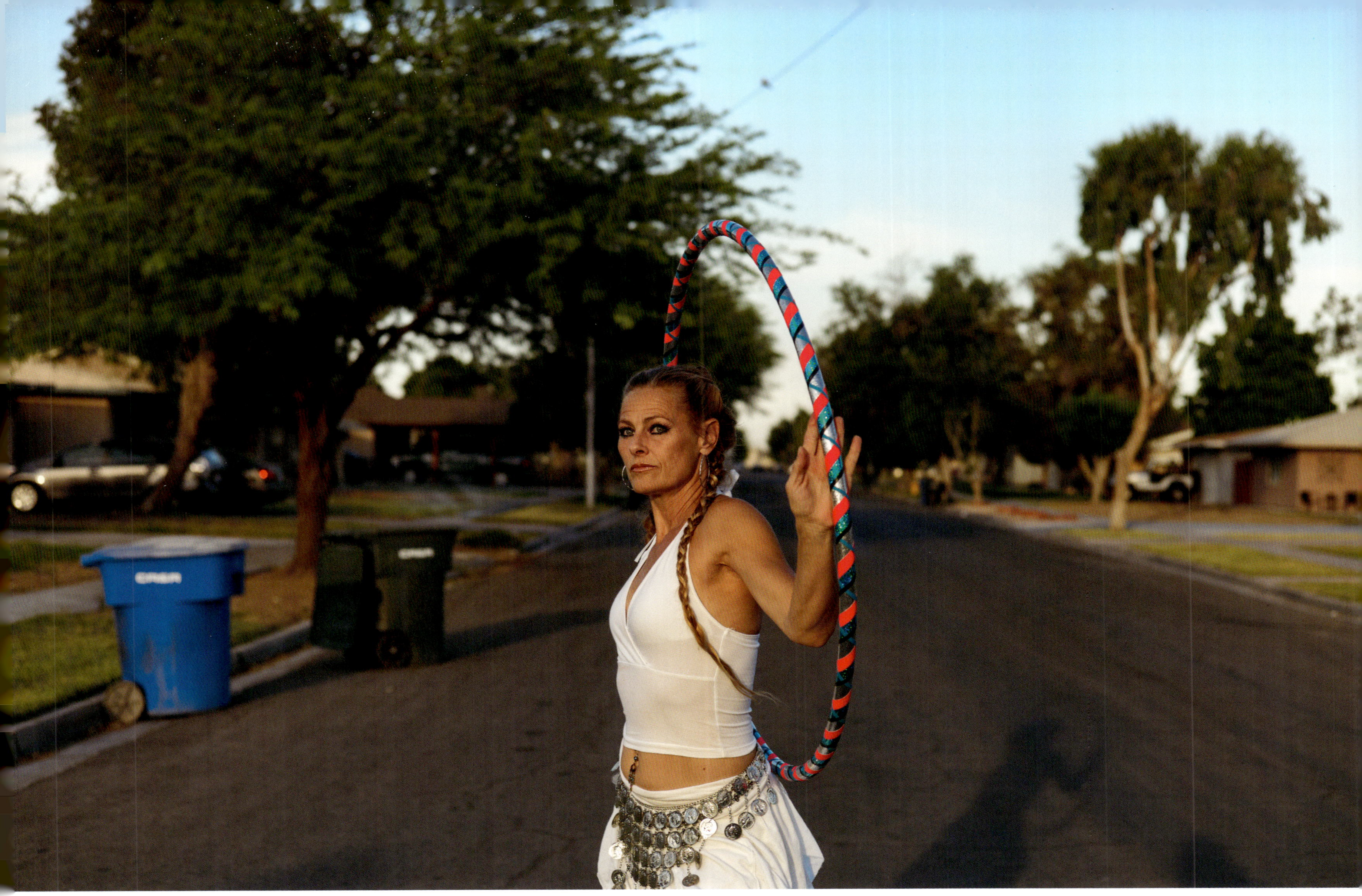

Sunshine on Desert Gardens Drive, El Centro

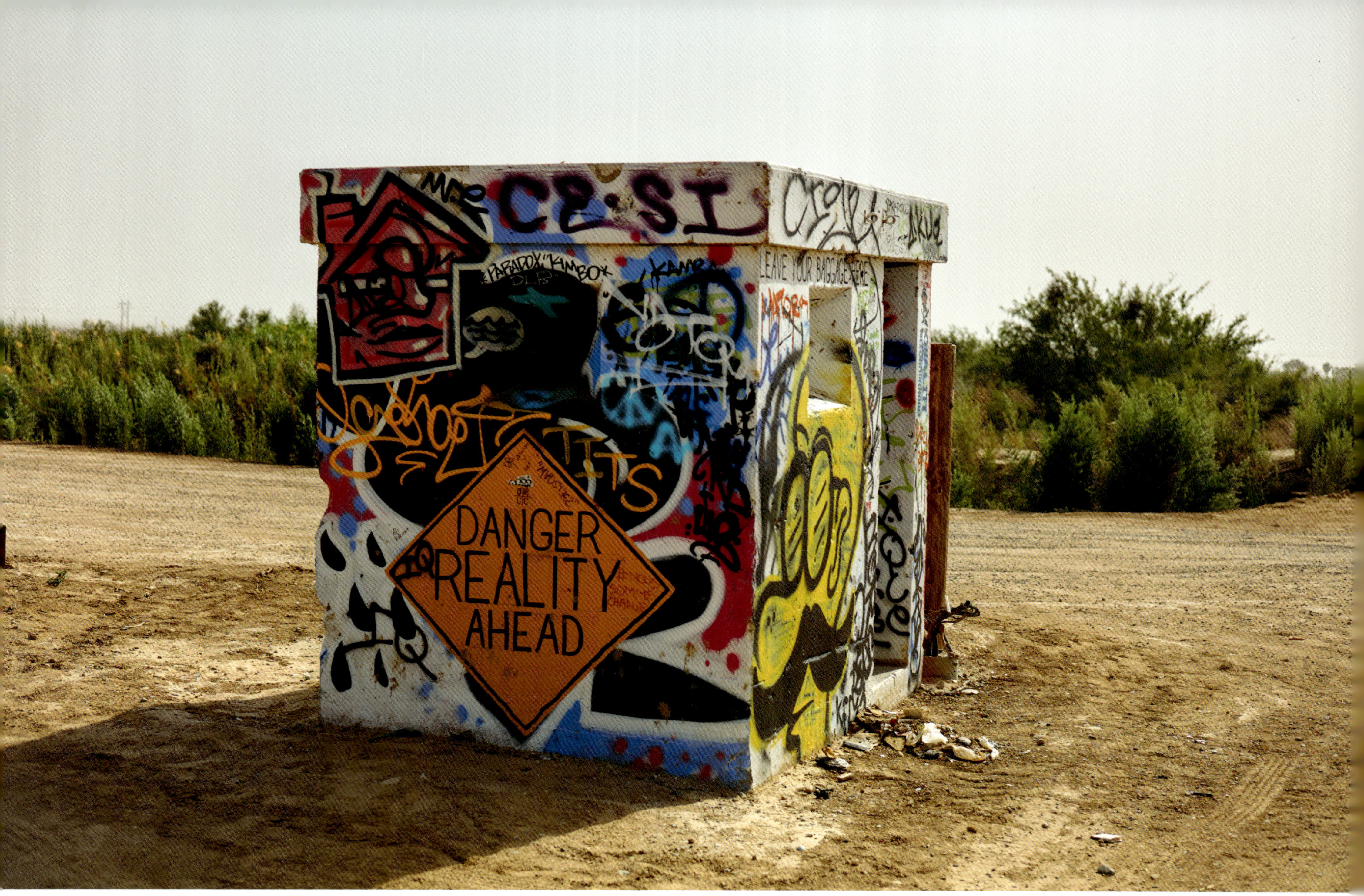

The Slabs guard house, near Salvation Mountain

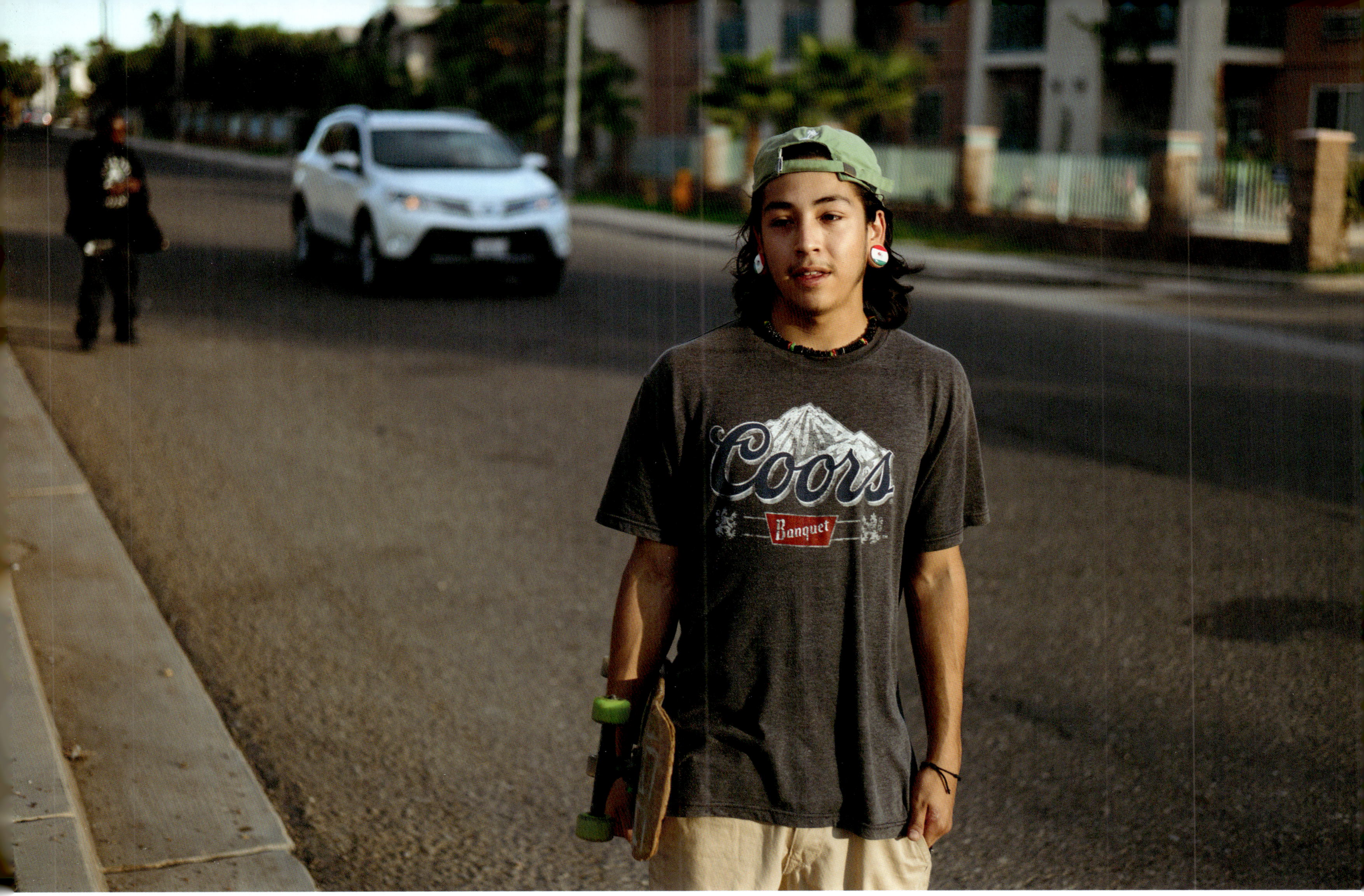

Carlos on his way to Sidewinder Skatepark, El Centro

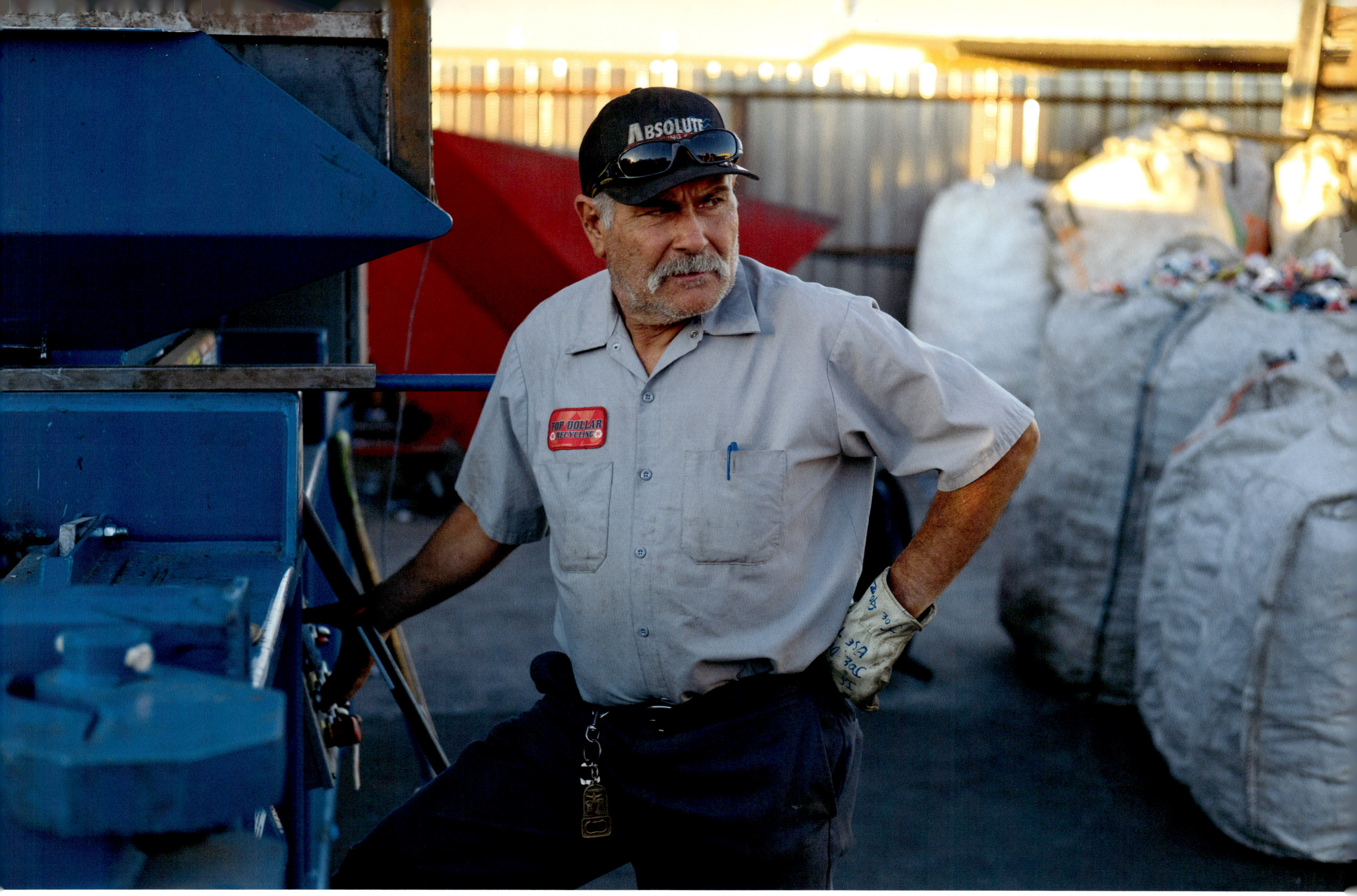

Joe at the Top Dollar Recycling Center, El Centro

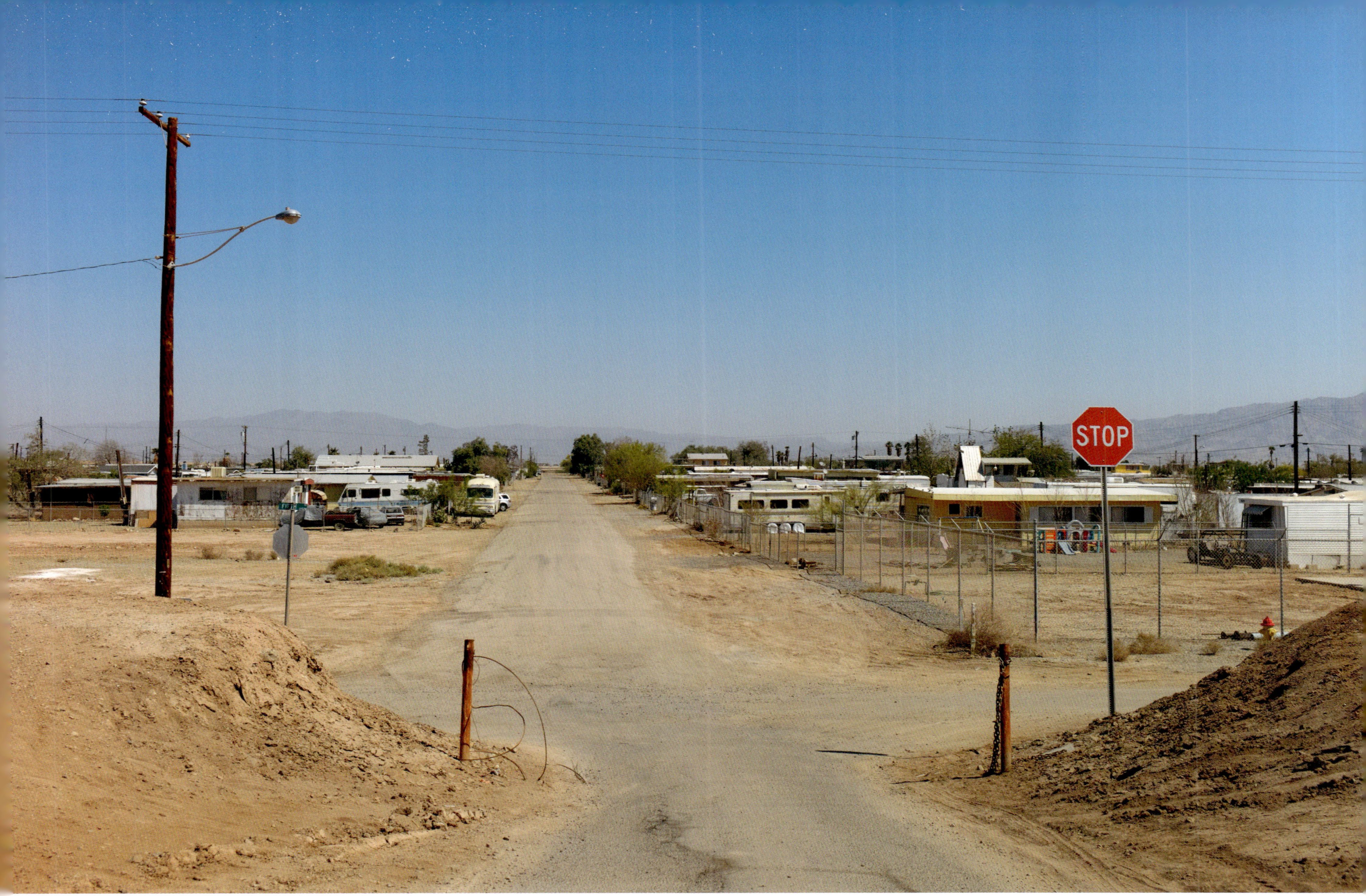

Main Street, Bombay Beach

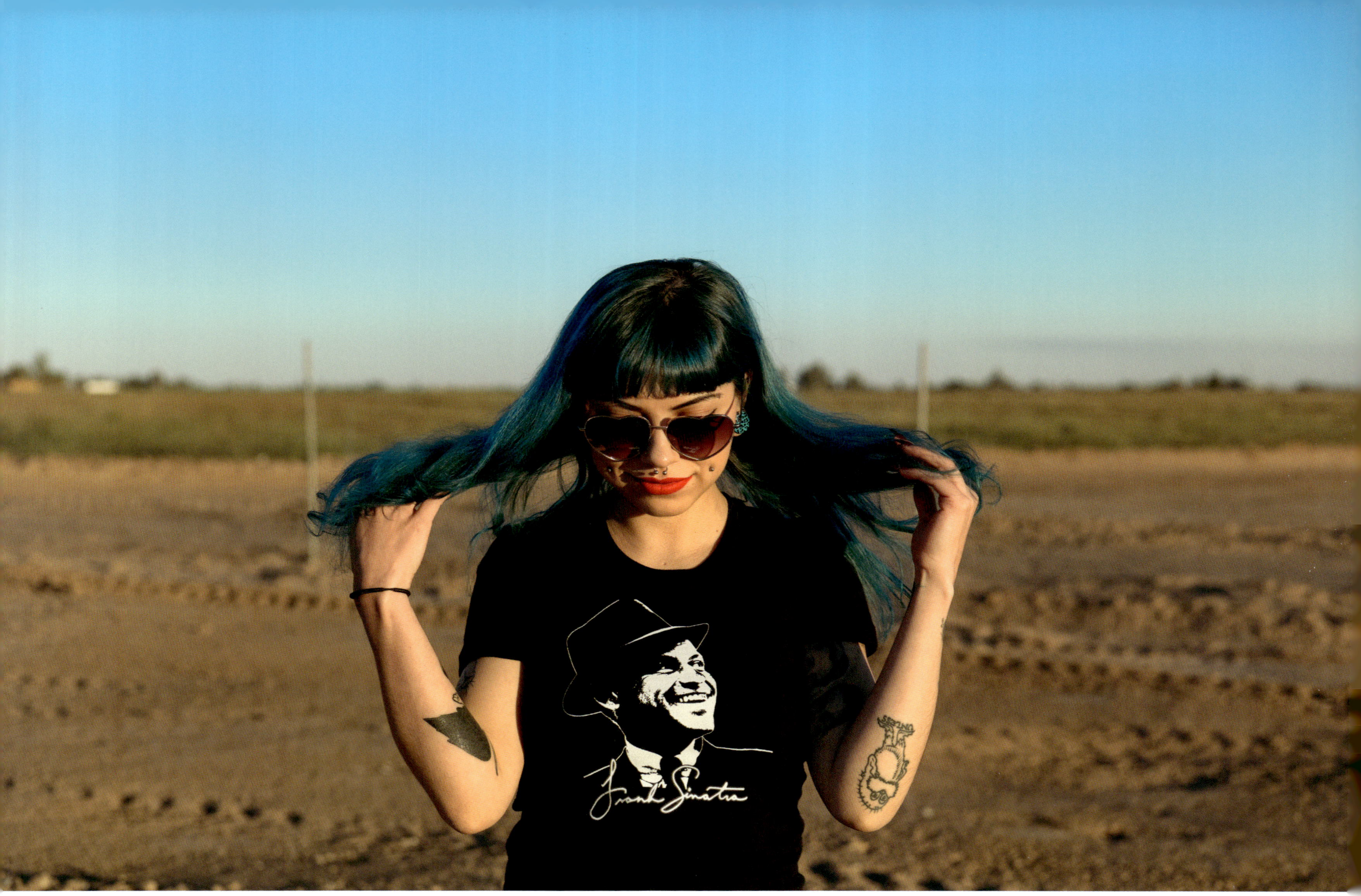

Araceli, Dixieland

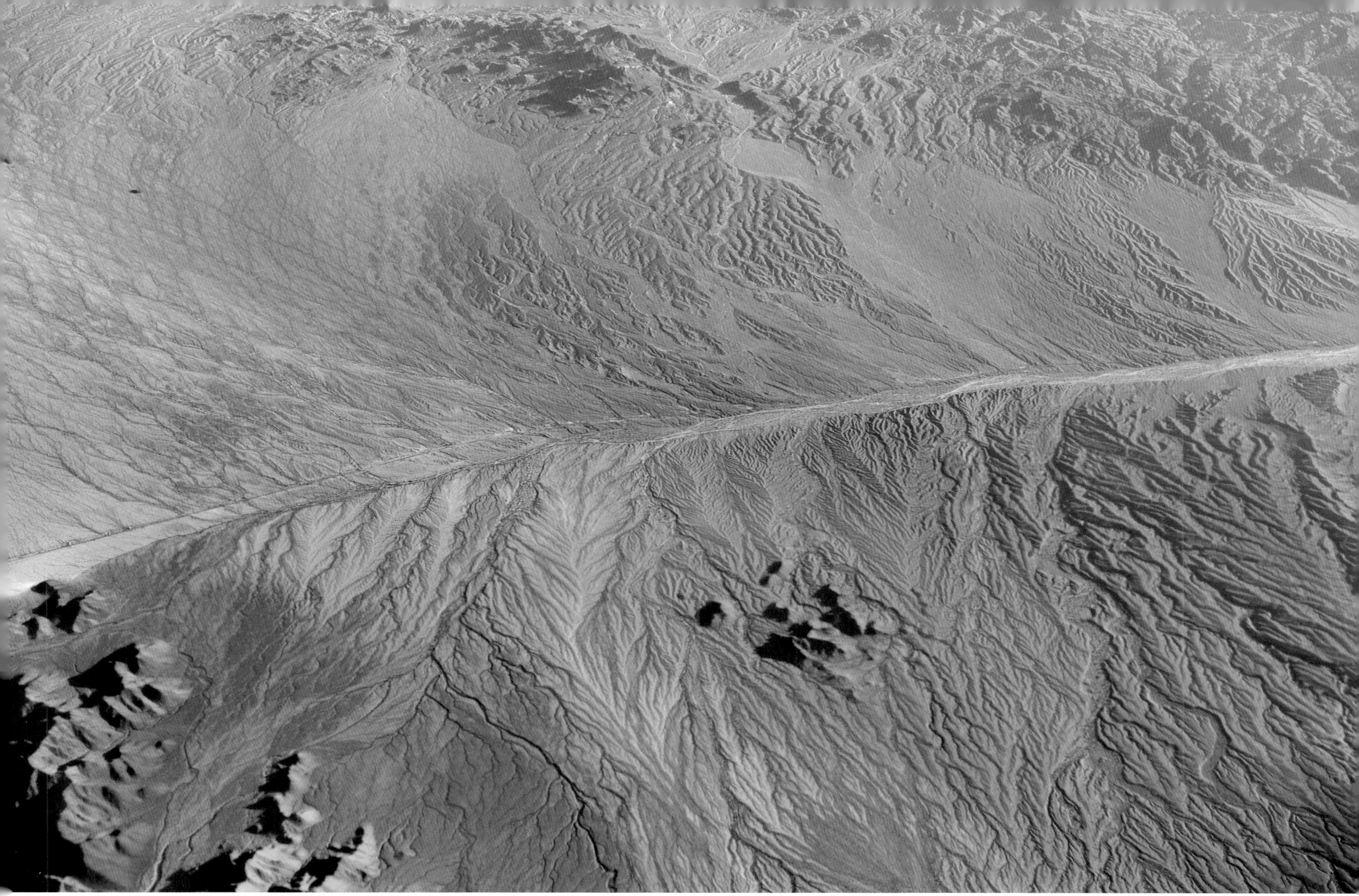

Wash outs, east of Tortuga

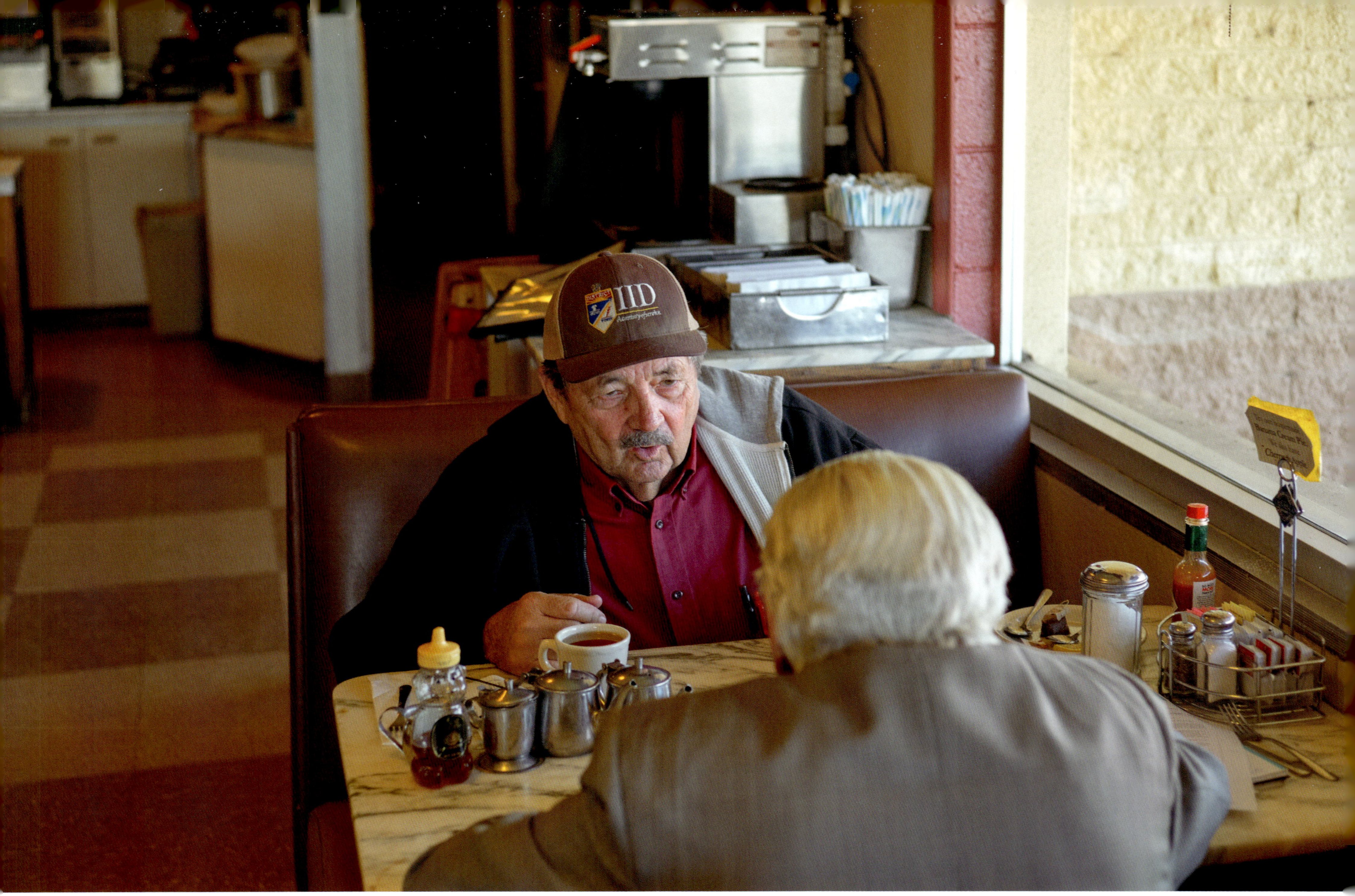

Mr. Hanks and Mr. Havens negotiating a water deal, Brawley

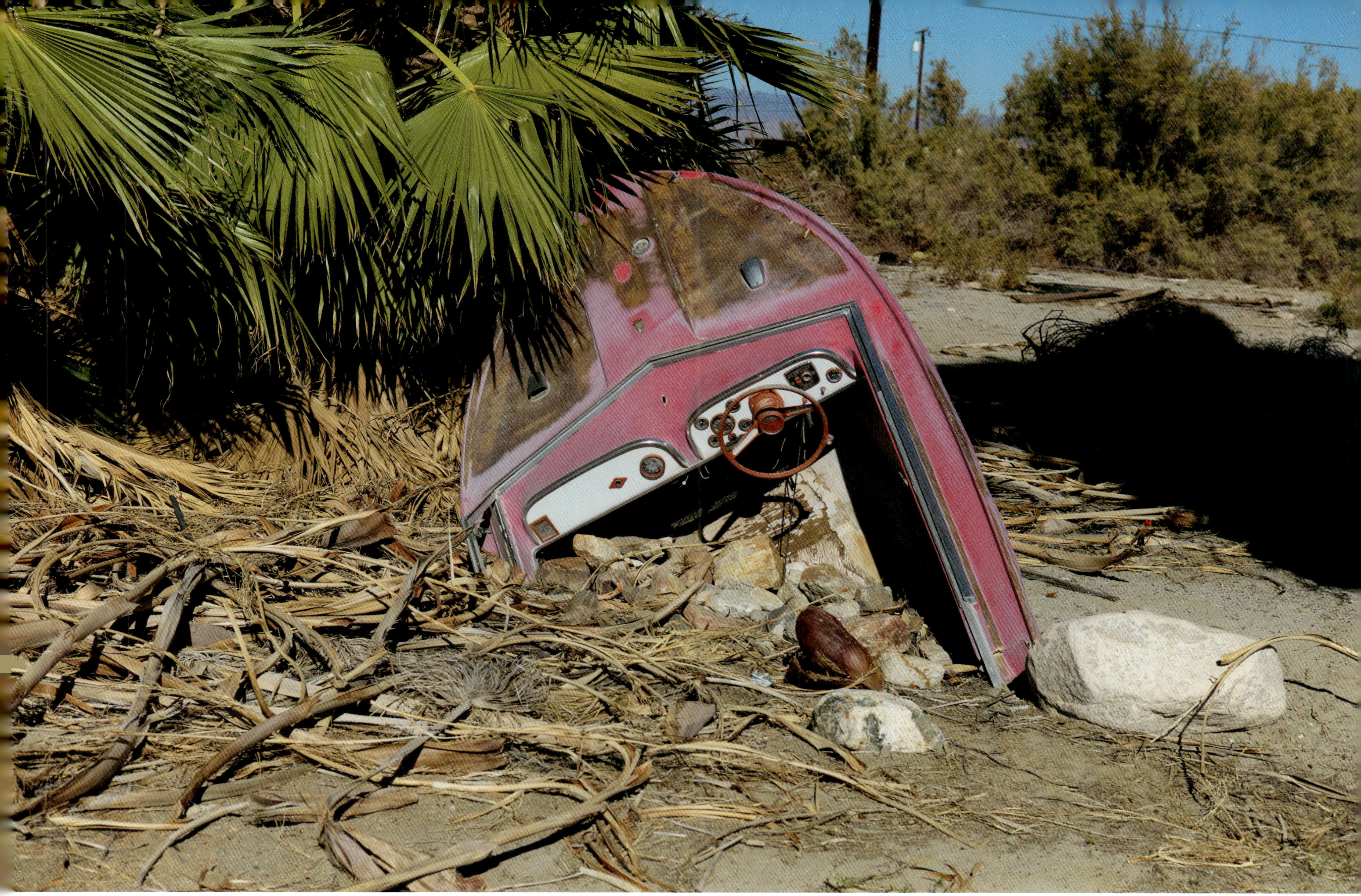

Marina Drive, Salton City

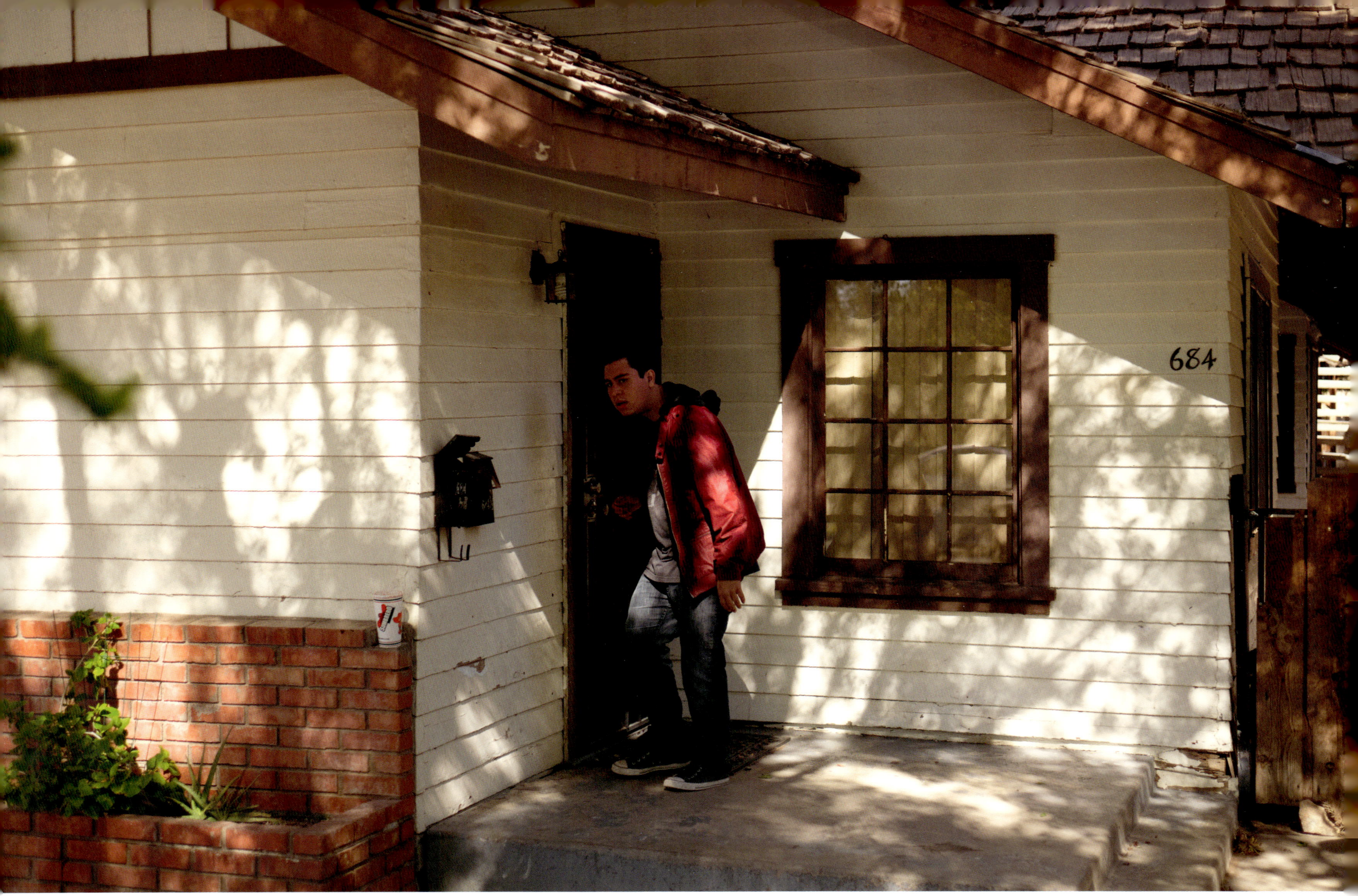

Adam at Moonies house, El Centro

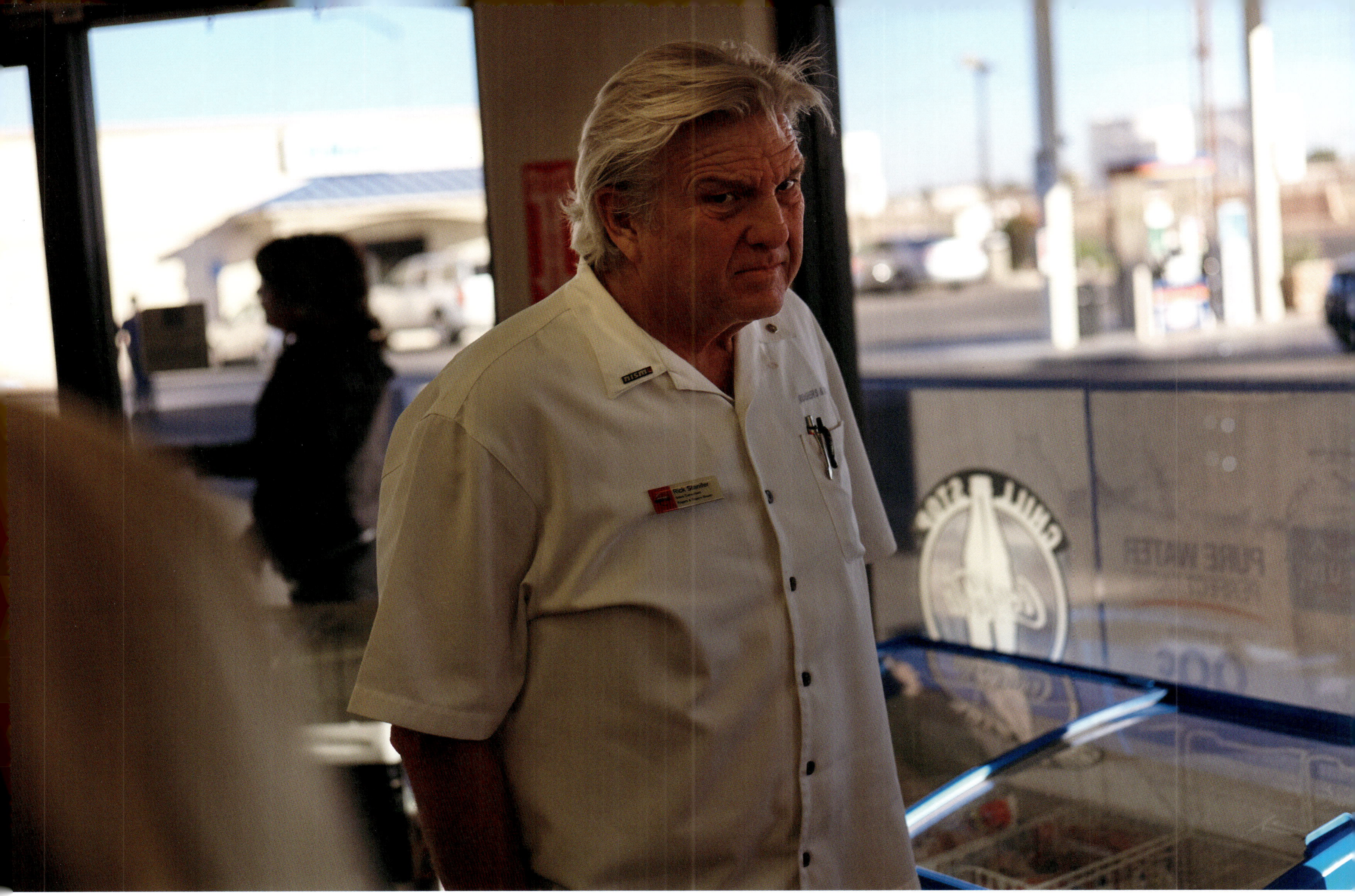

Rick at the gas station, Imperial

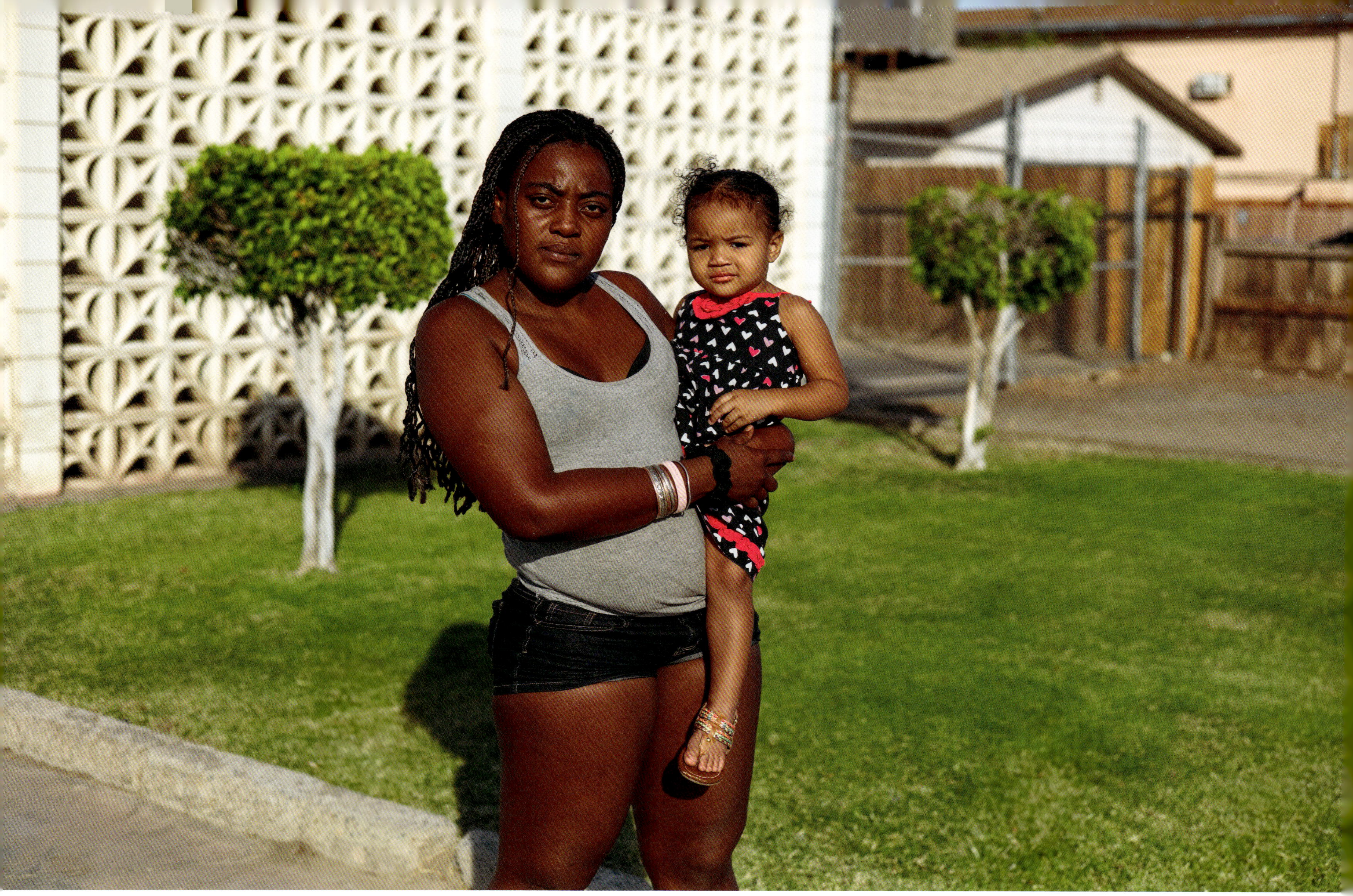

Kim and Genesis on Adams Avenue, El Centro

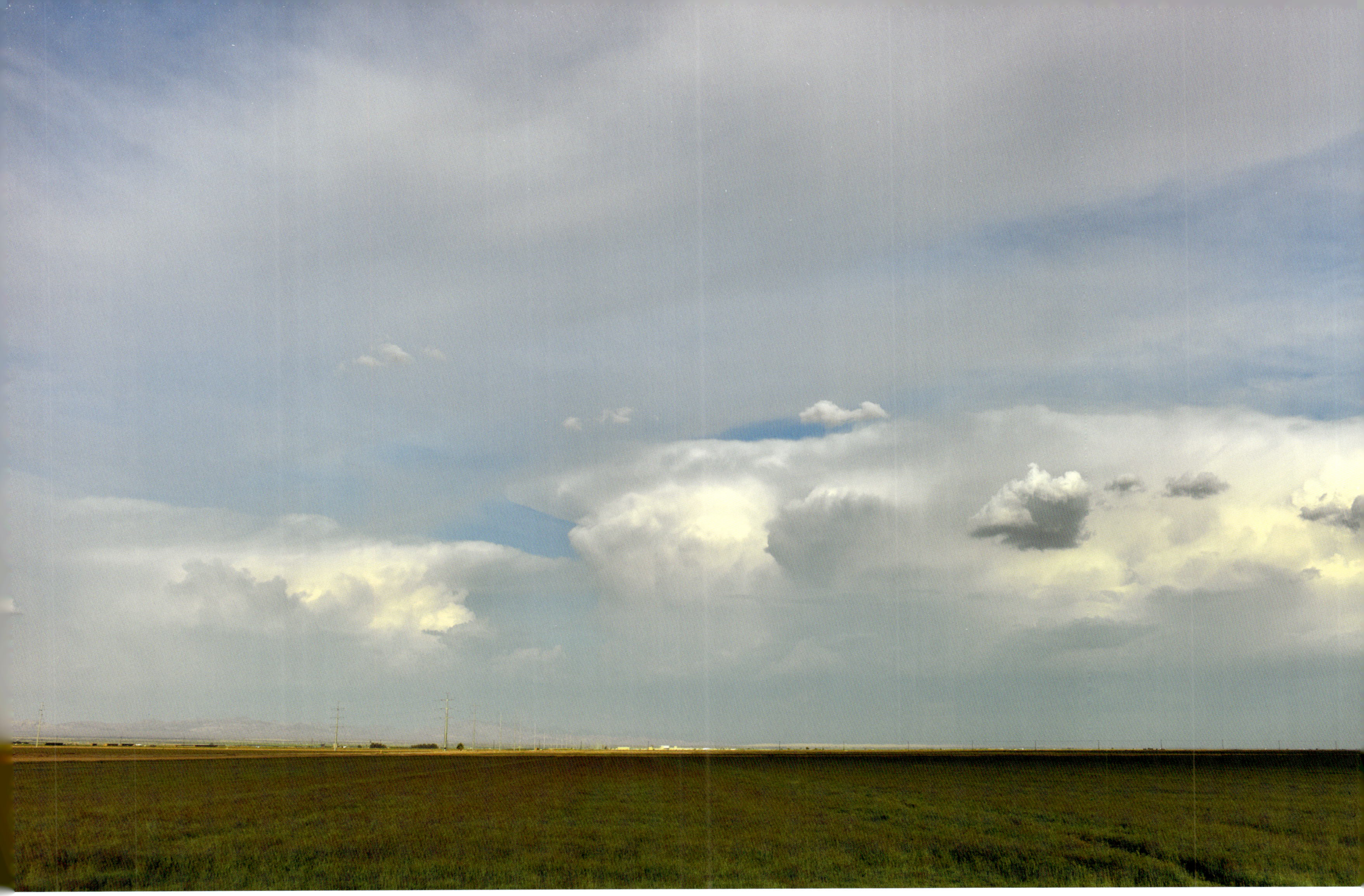

Alfalfa field, near Holtville

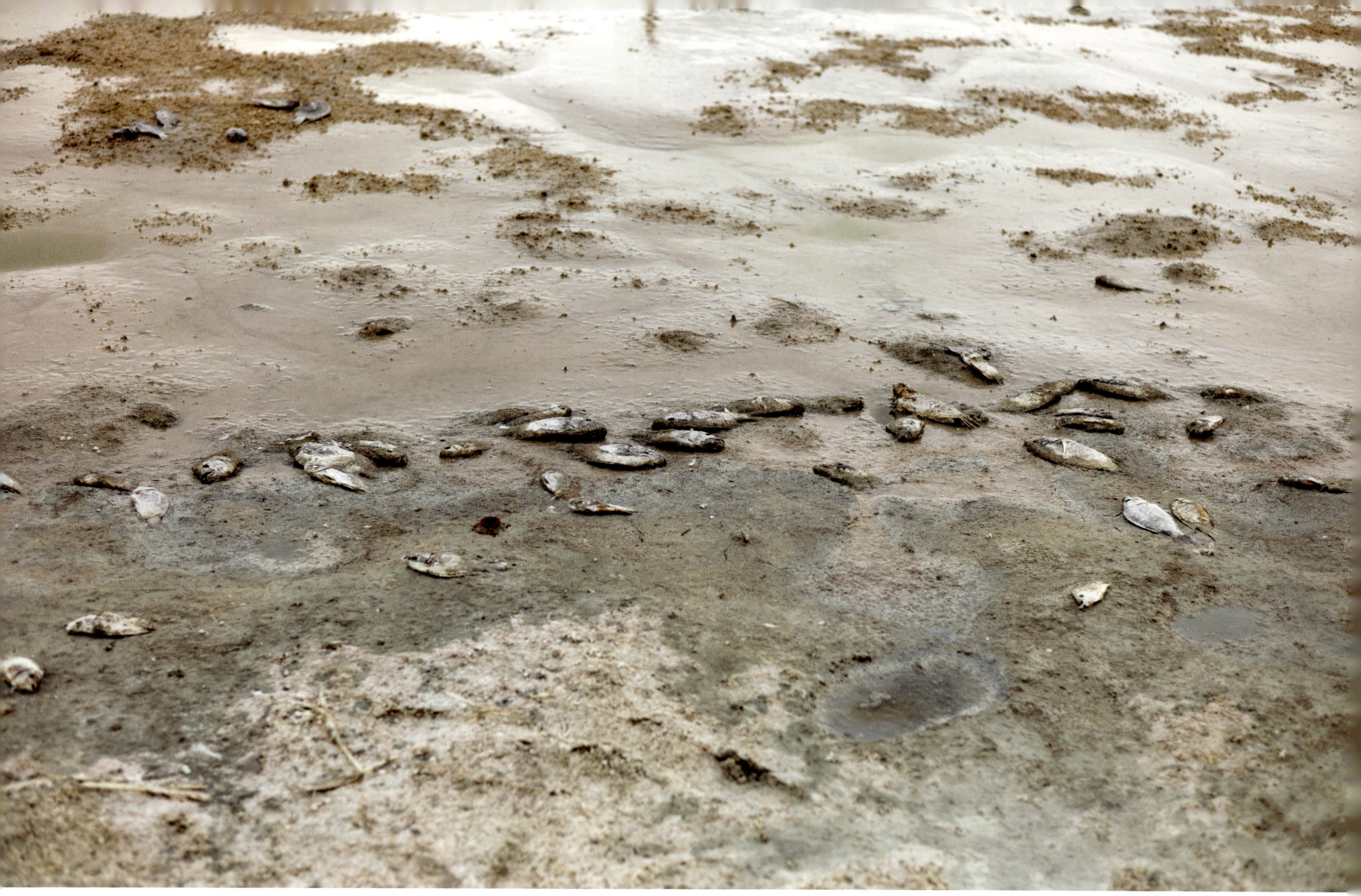

Dead Tilapia, Bombay Beach

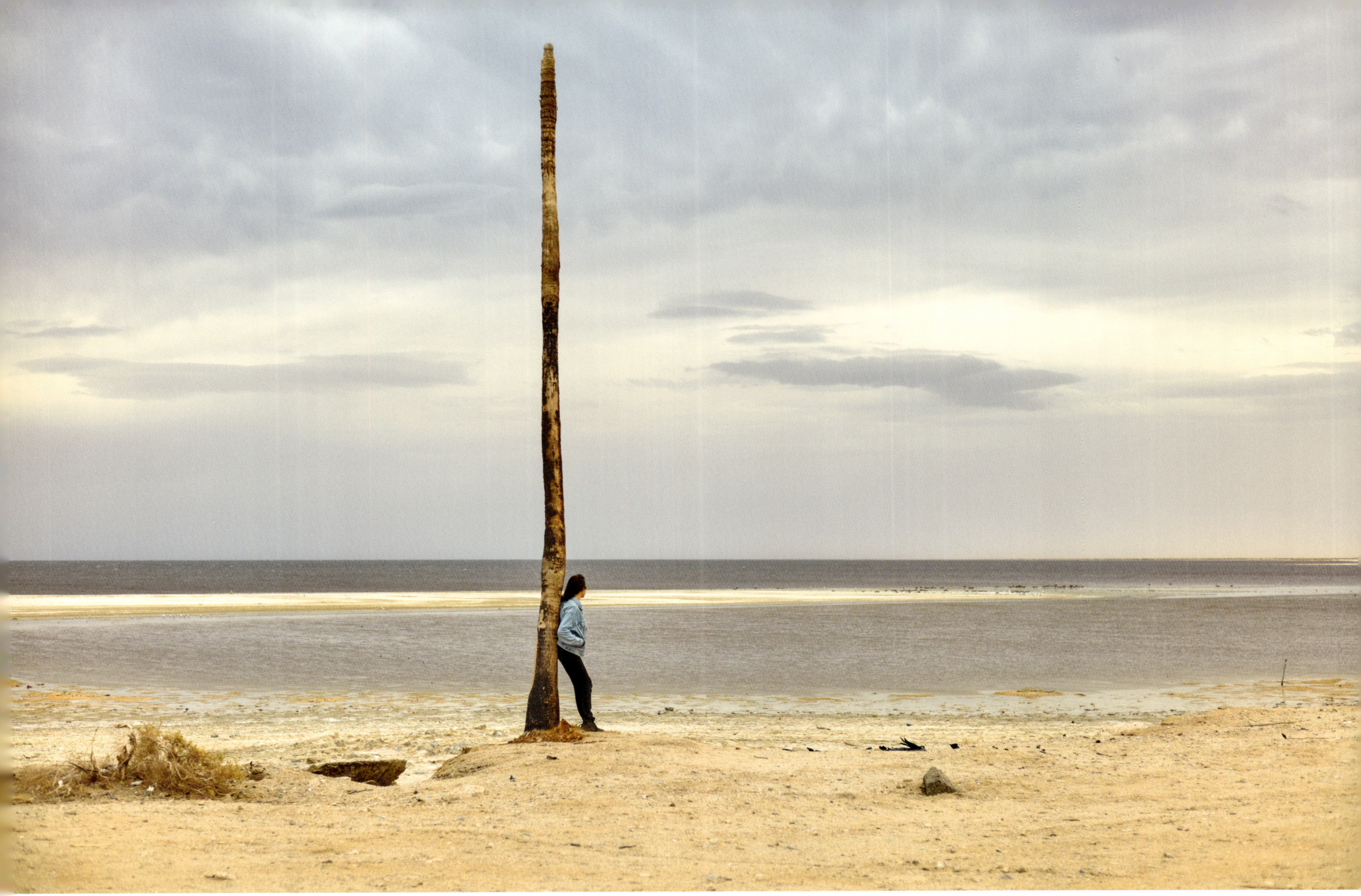

Sarah, Salton Sea Beach

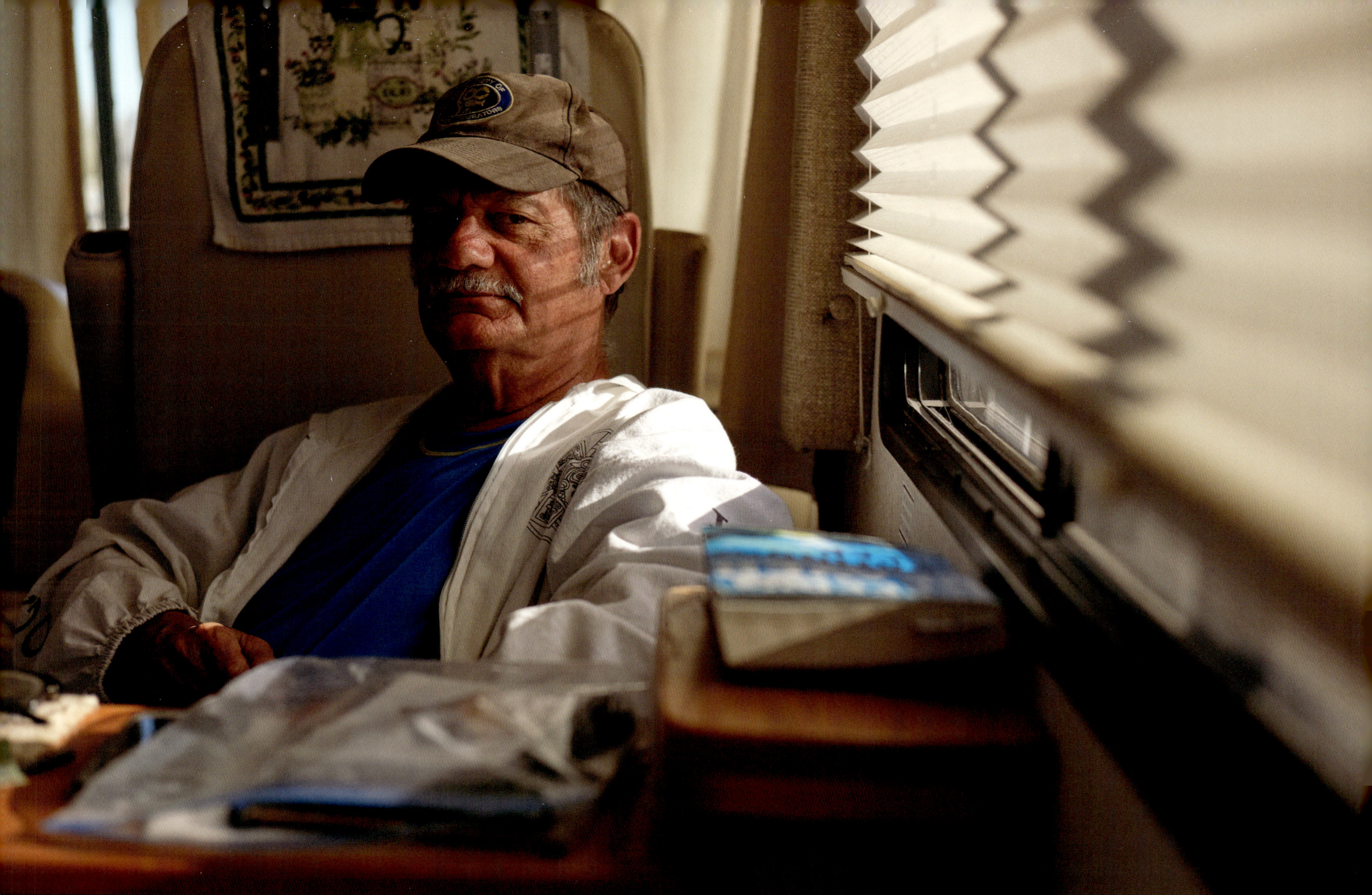

Bob in his RV, Slab City Suburbs

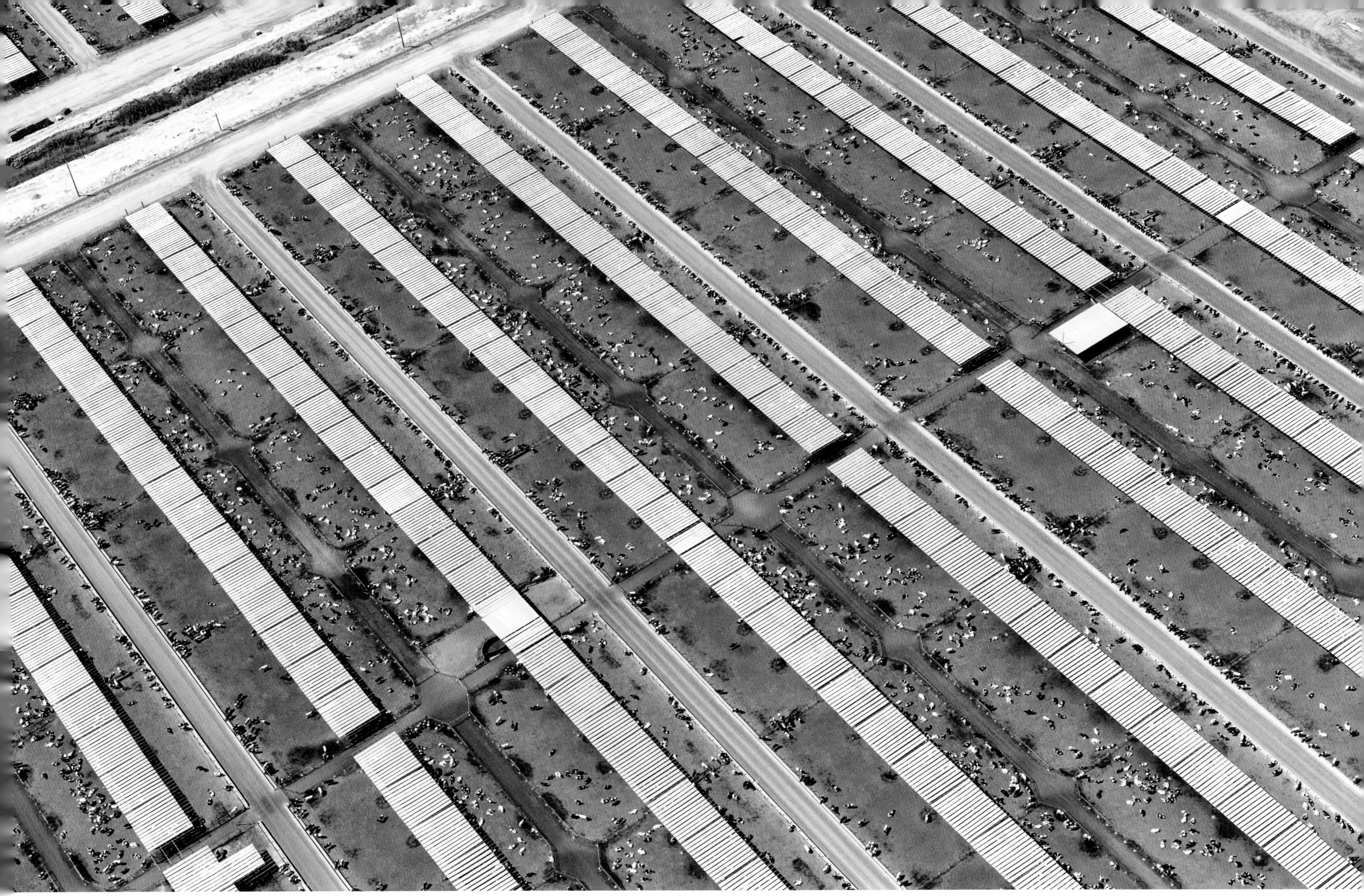

Brandt Cattle Co, Calipatria

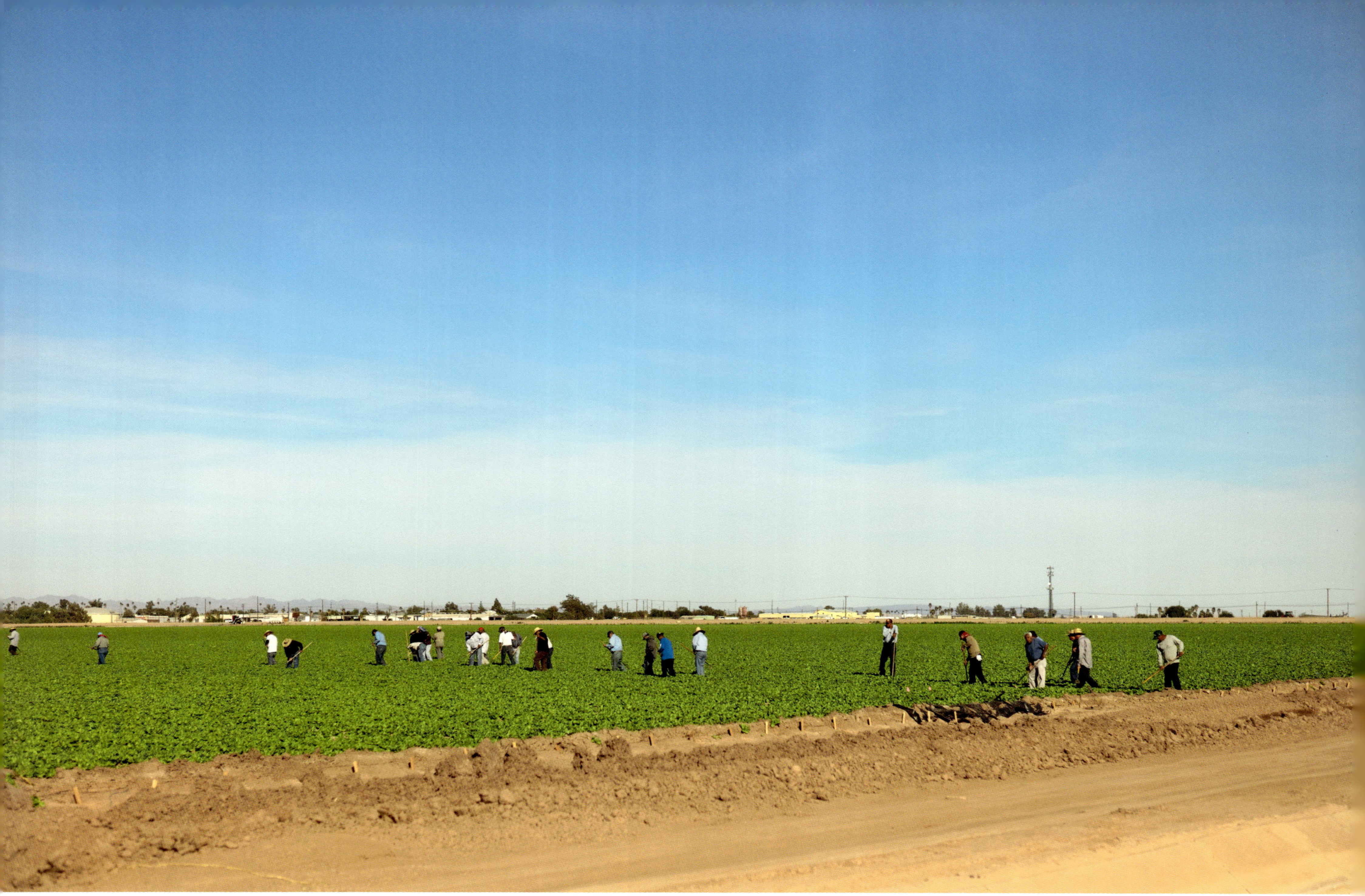

Salad field, Orita

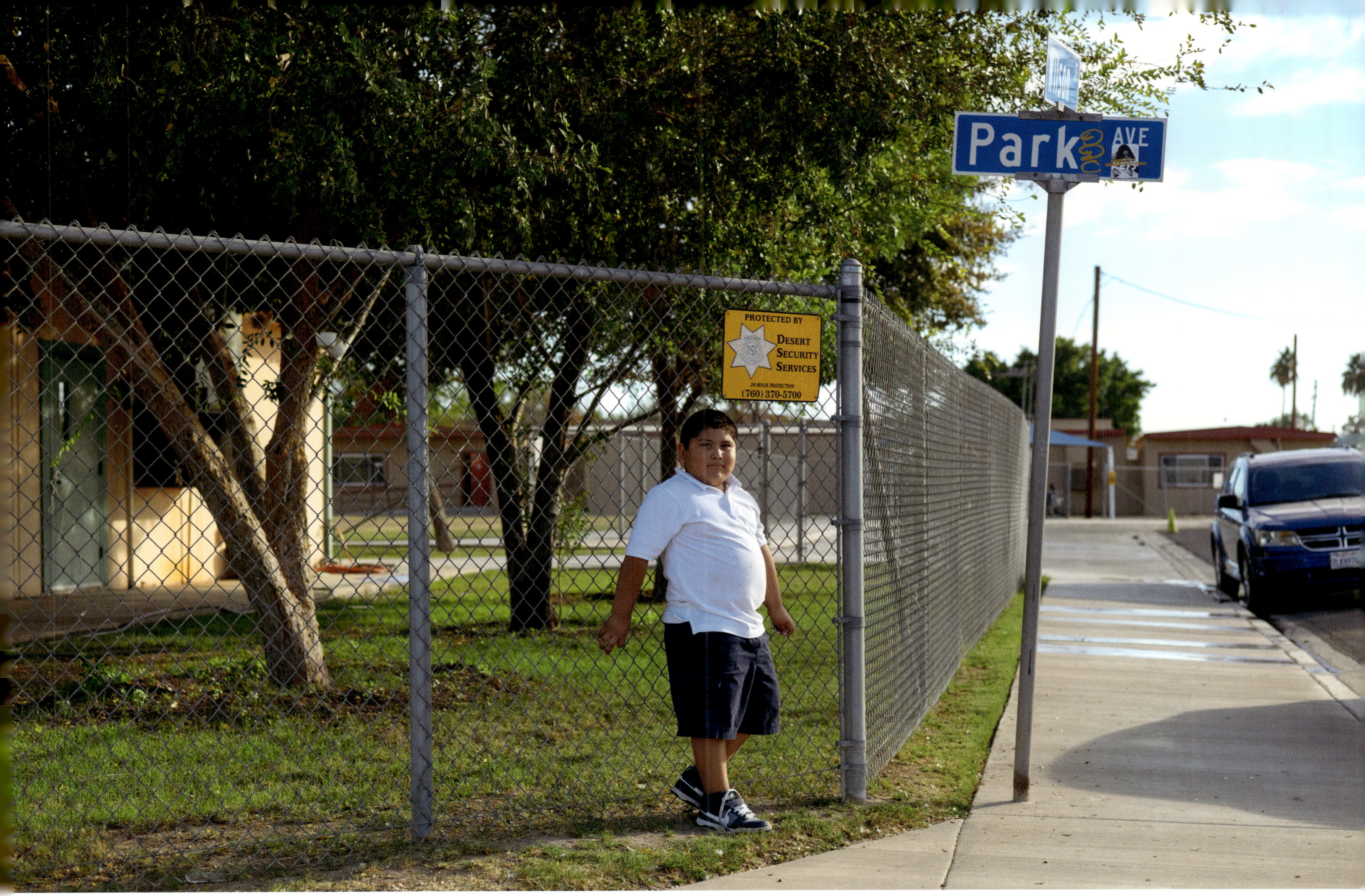

Nente, El Centro

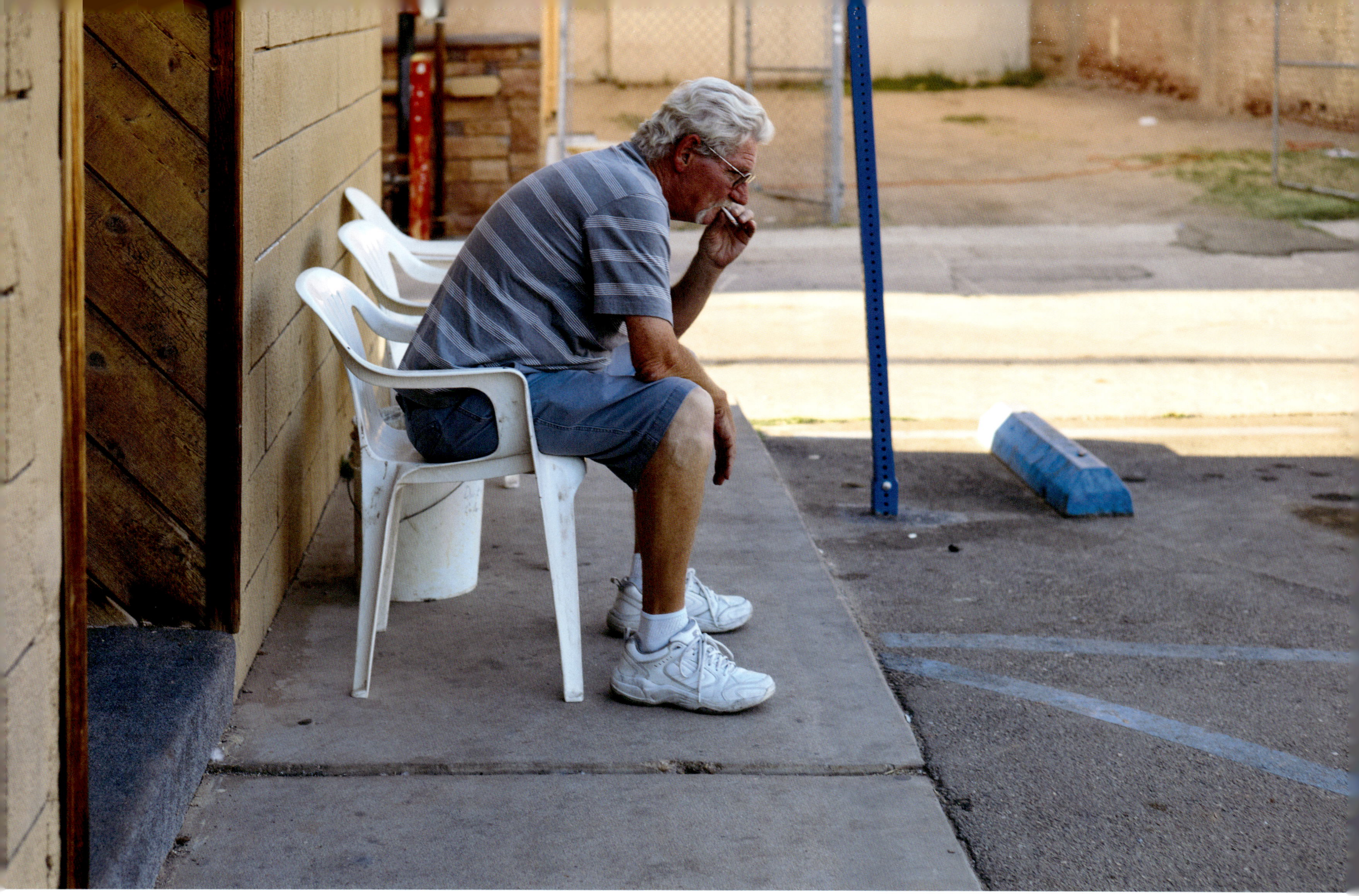

Veteran at Amercian Legion, Brawley

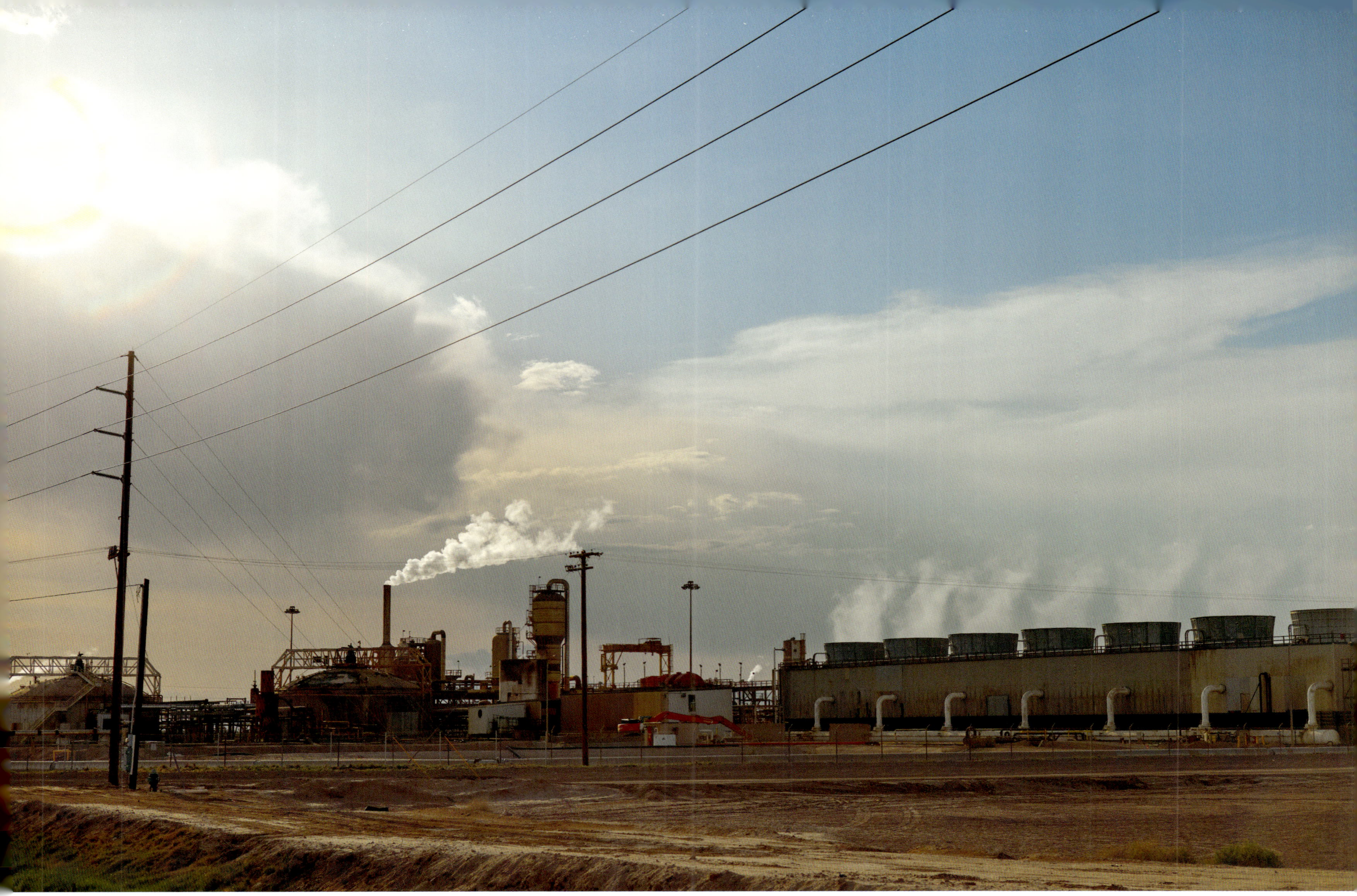

CalEnergy Geothermal Powerplant, Calipatria

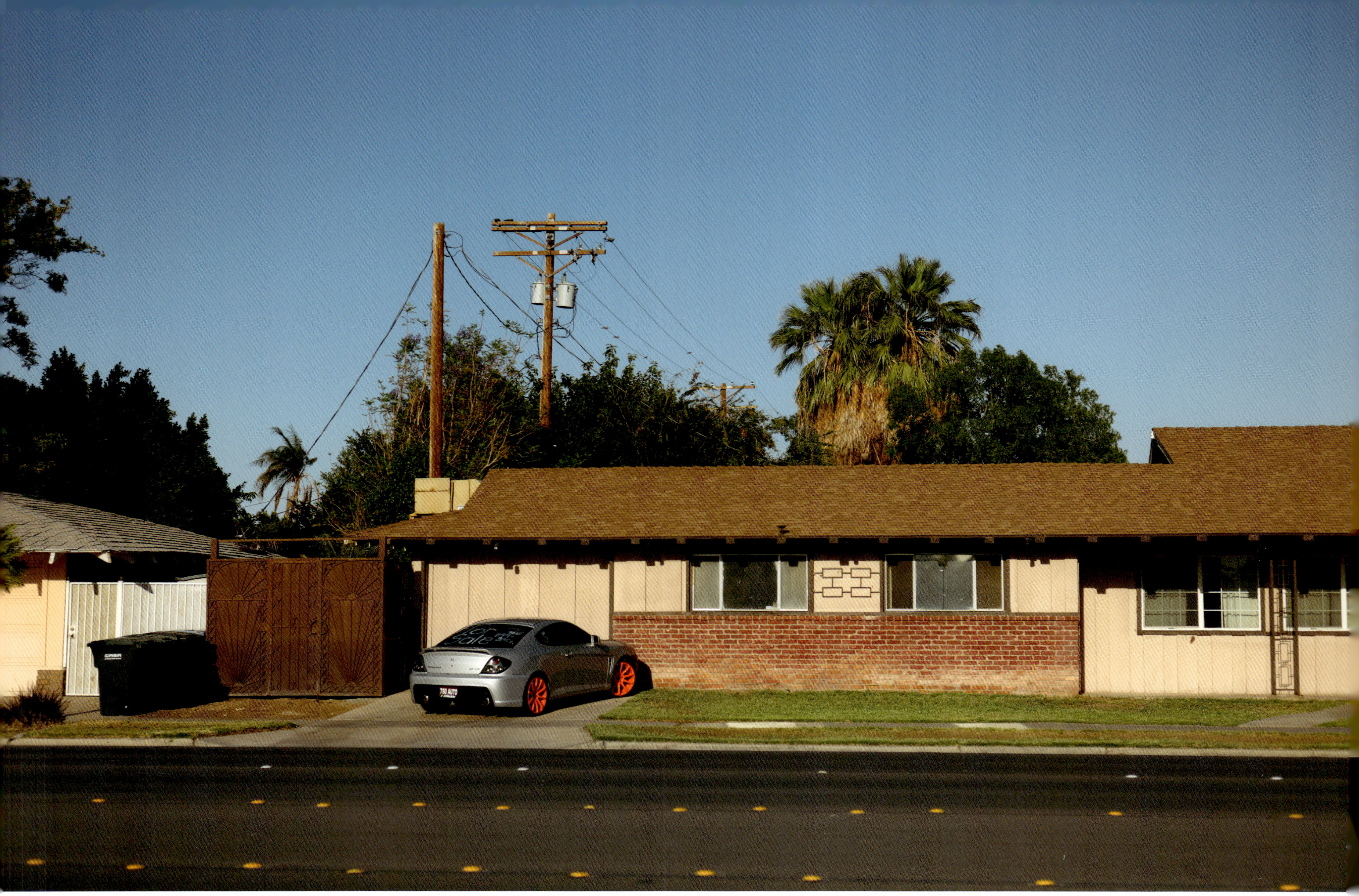

South 8th Street, El Centro

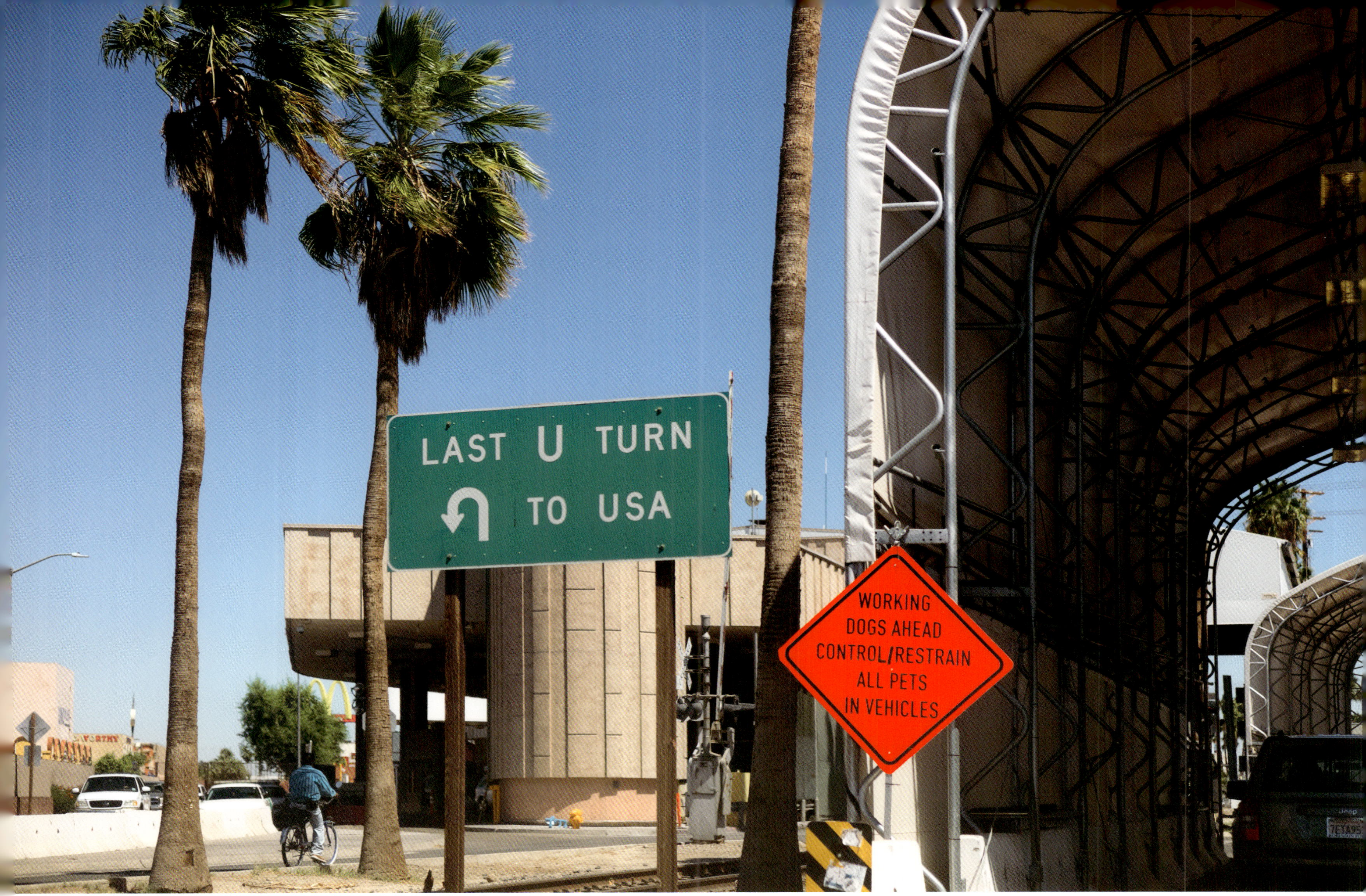

Mexican Border, Calexico

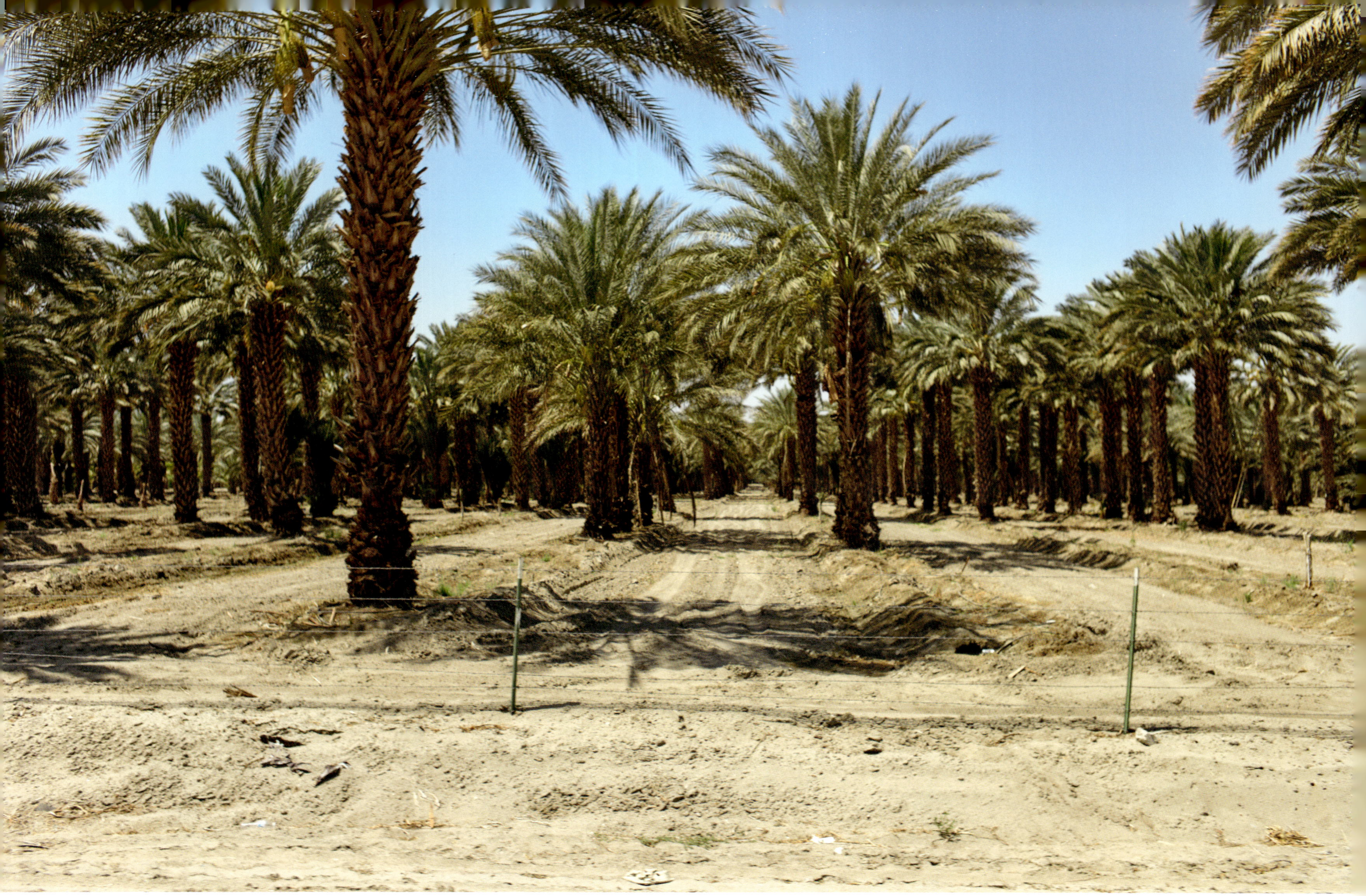

Palm tree farming, Date City

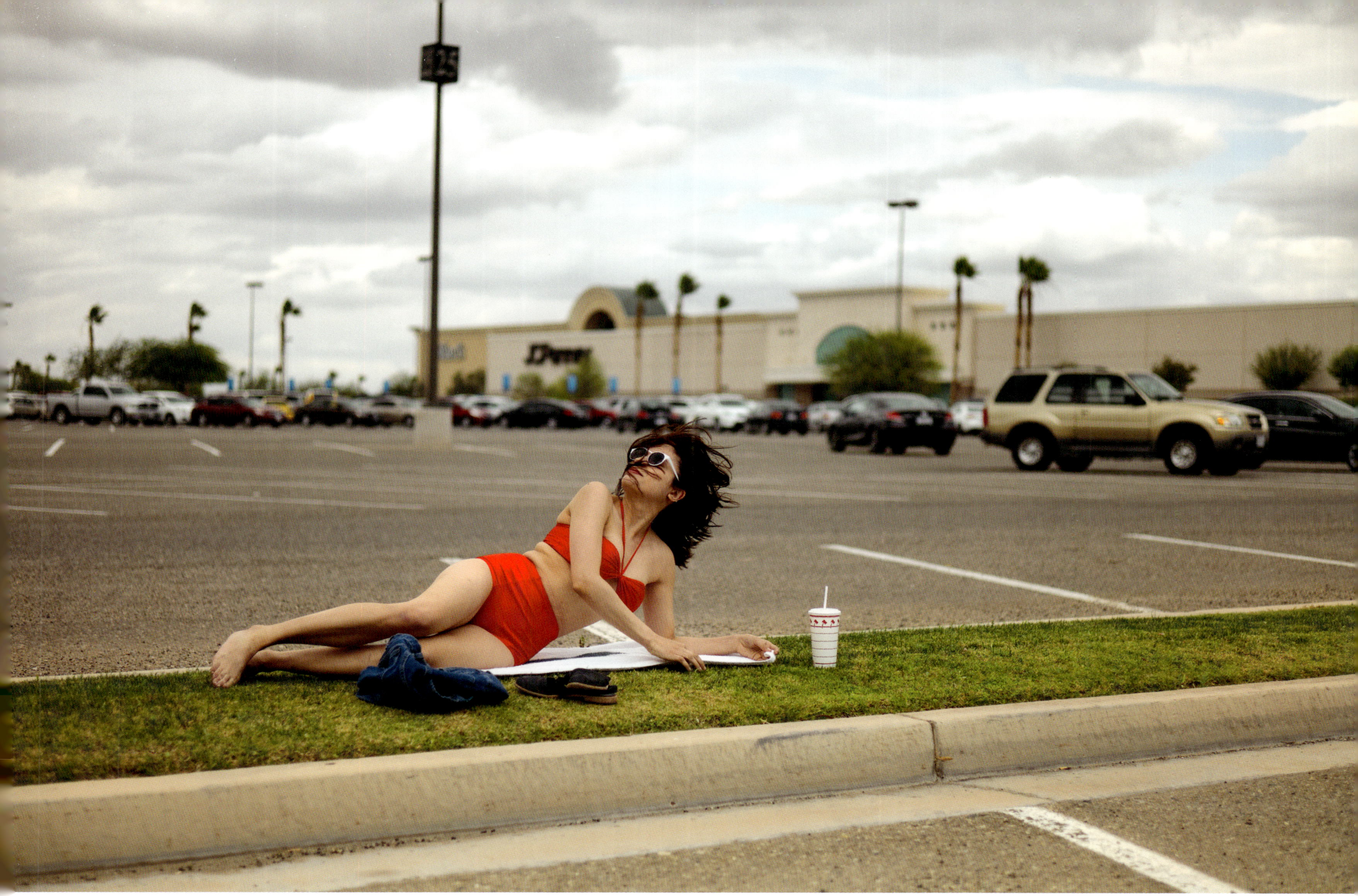

Stefanie at the Imperial Valley Mall, Salvation Mountain

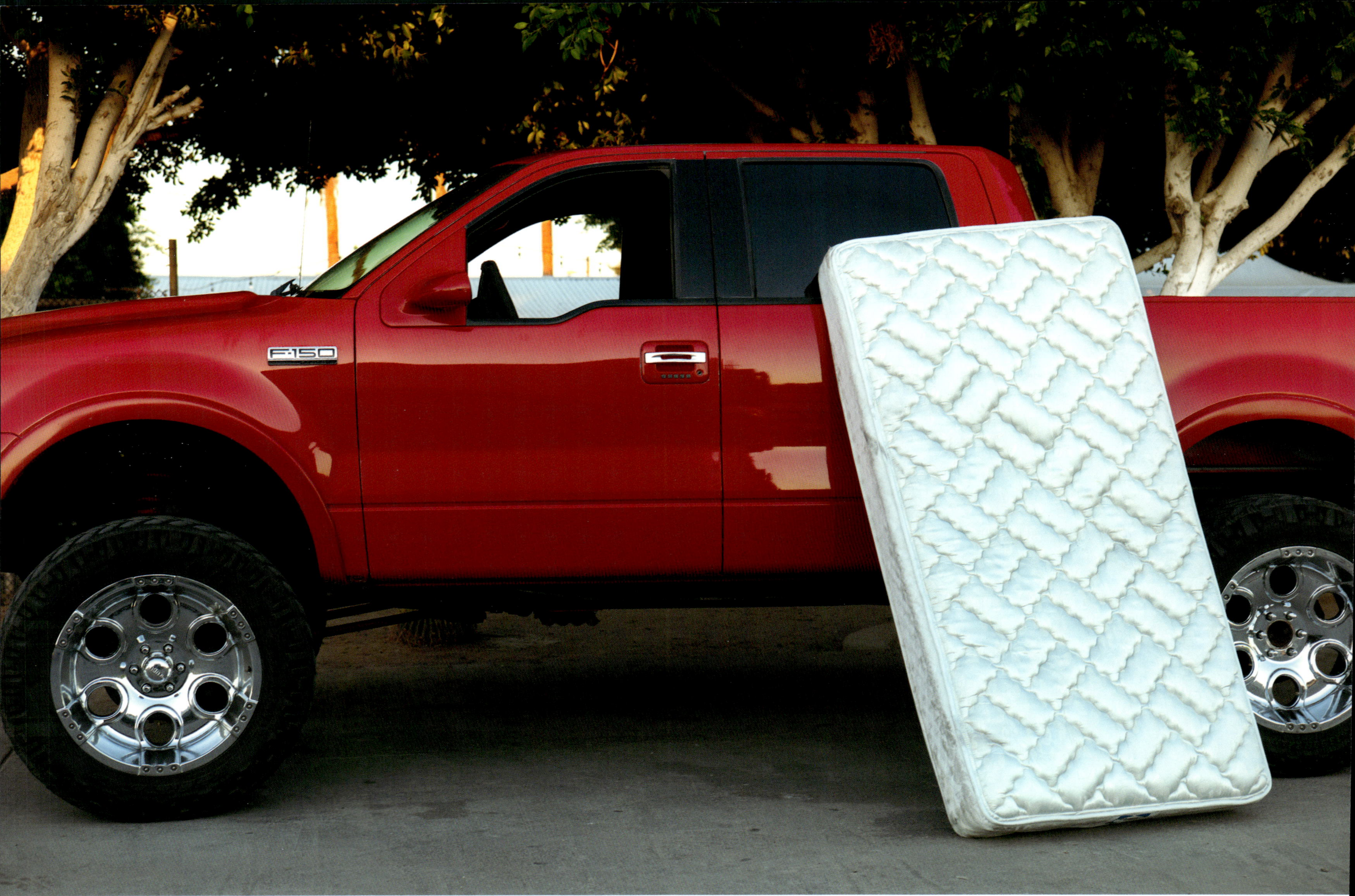

Truck at Los Cabos Tacos, Calexico

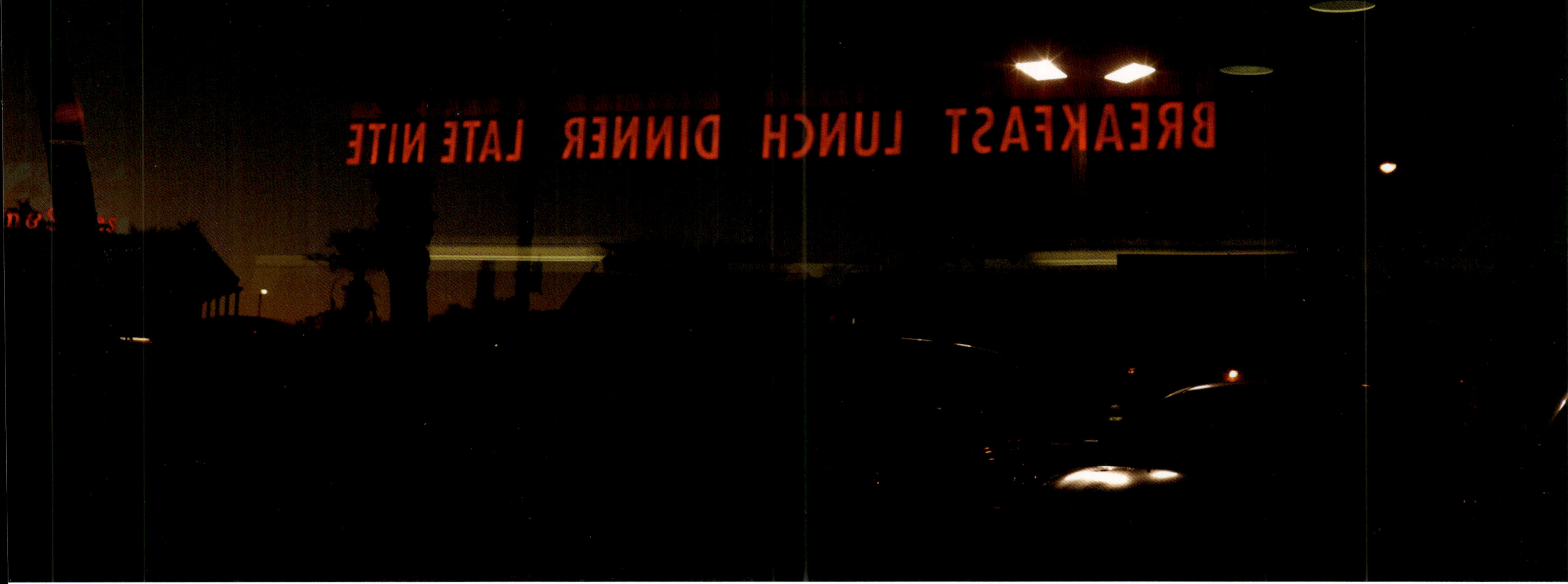

Denny's, El Centro

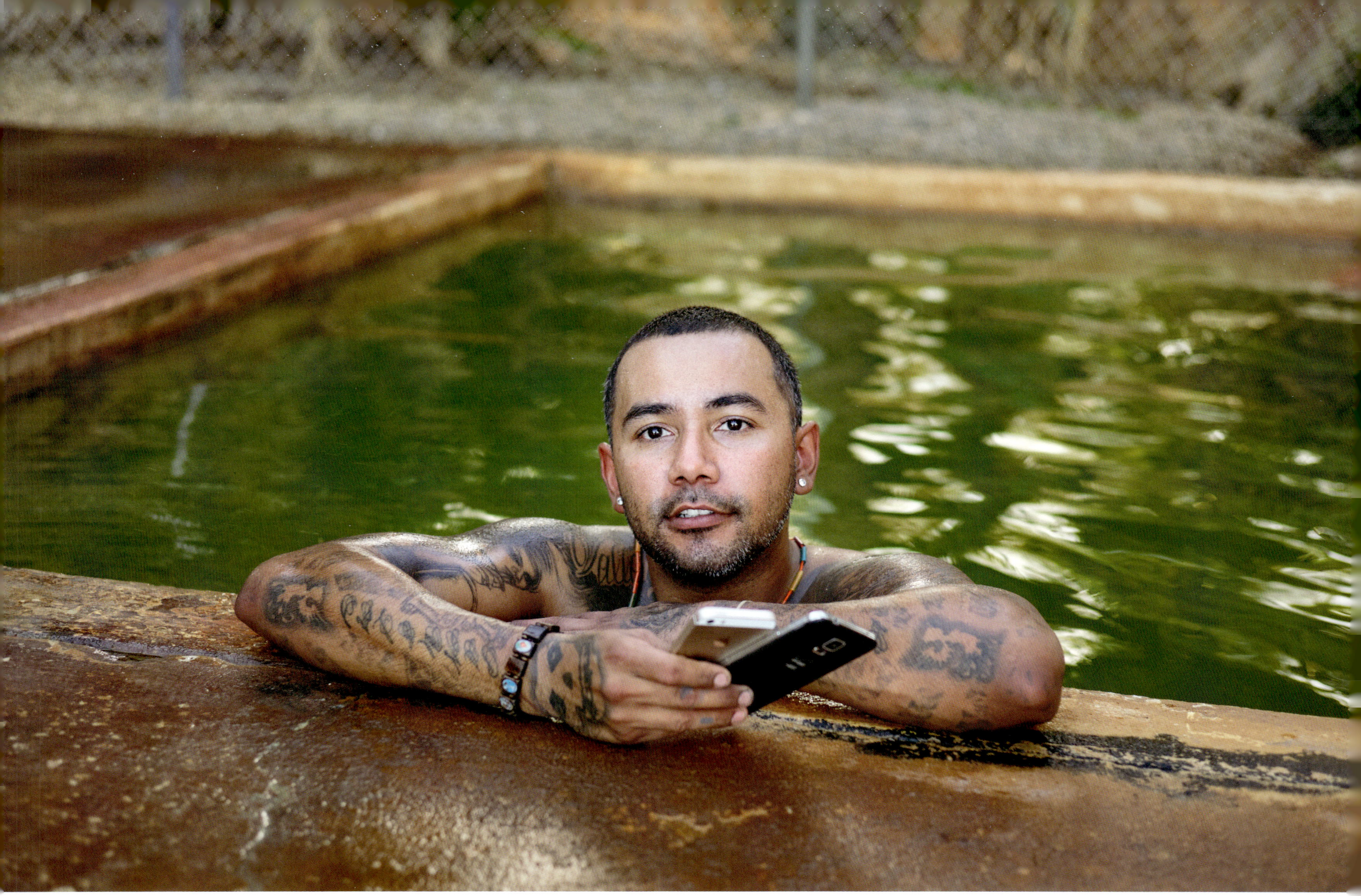

Joey in the thermal pool, BLM Hot springs

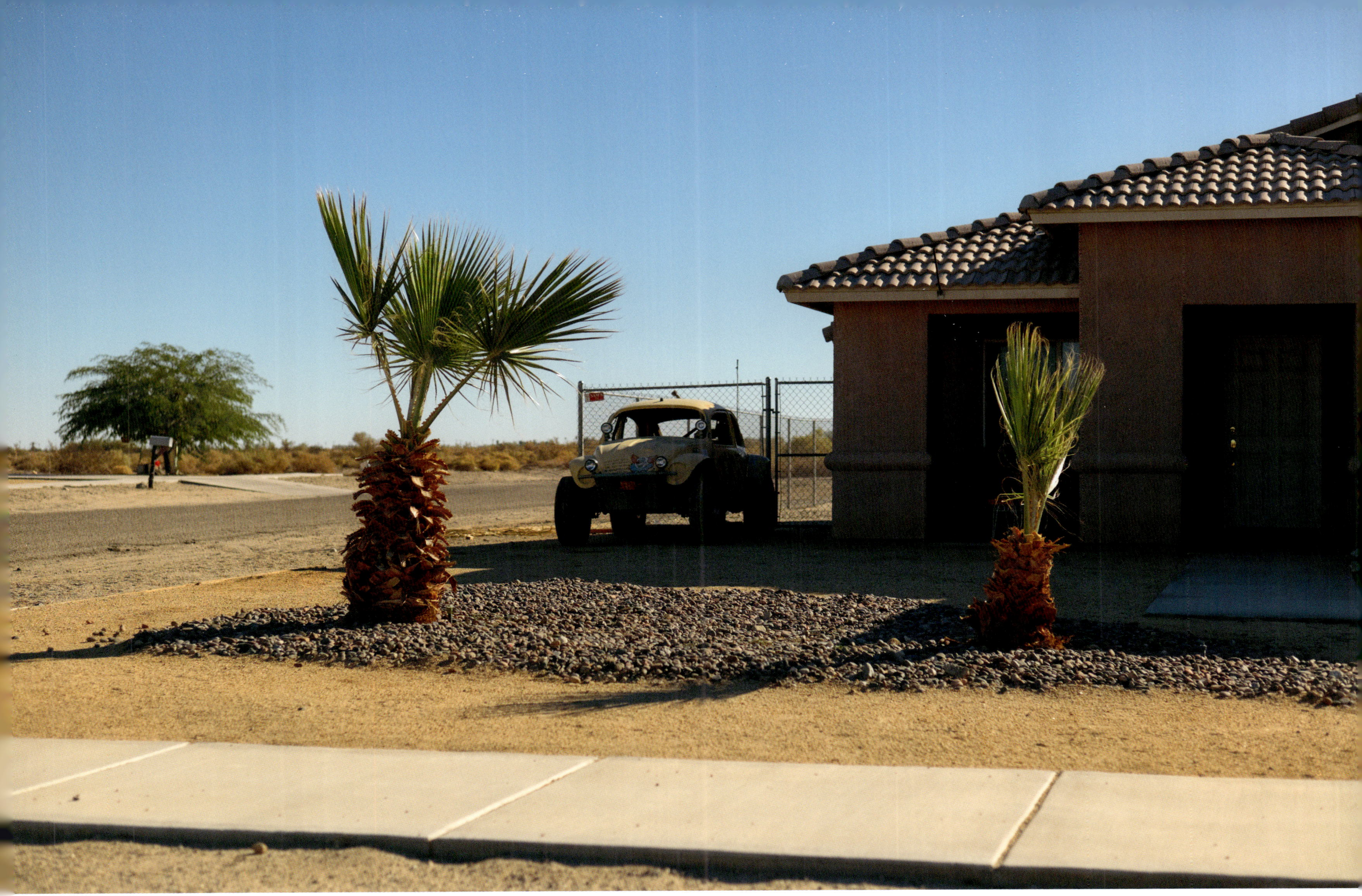

Malibu Avenue, Desert Shores

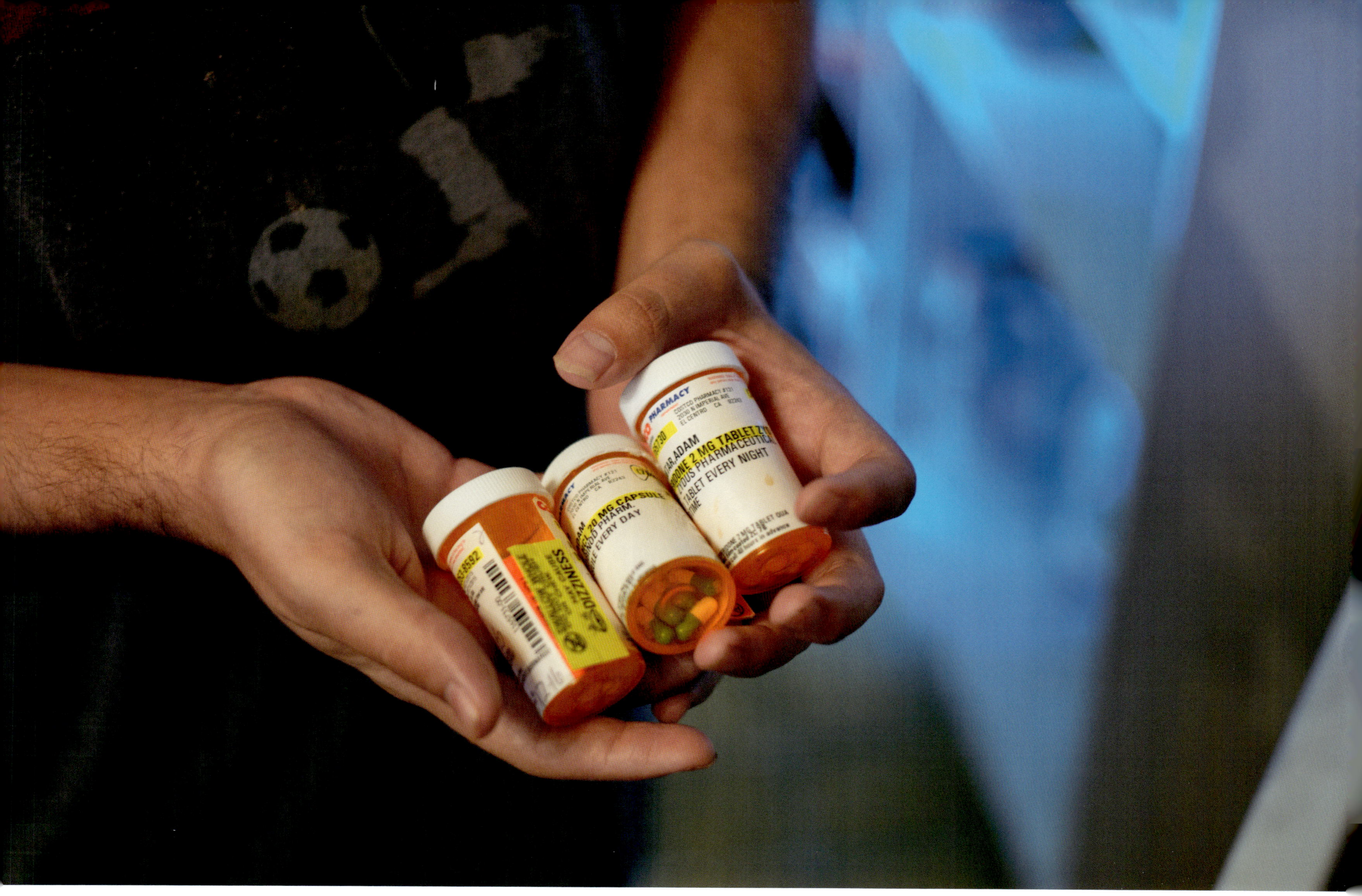

Adam's medication, El Centro

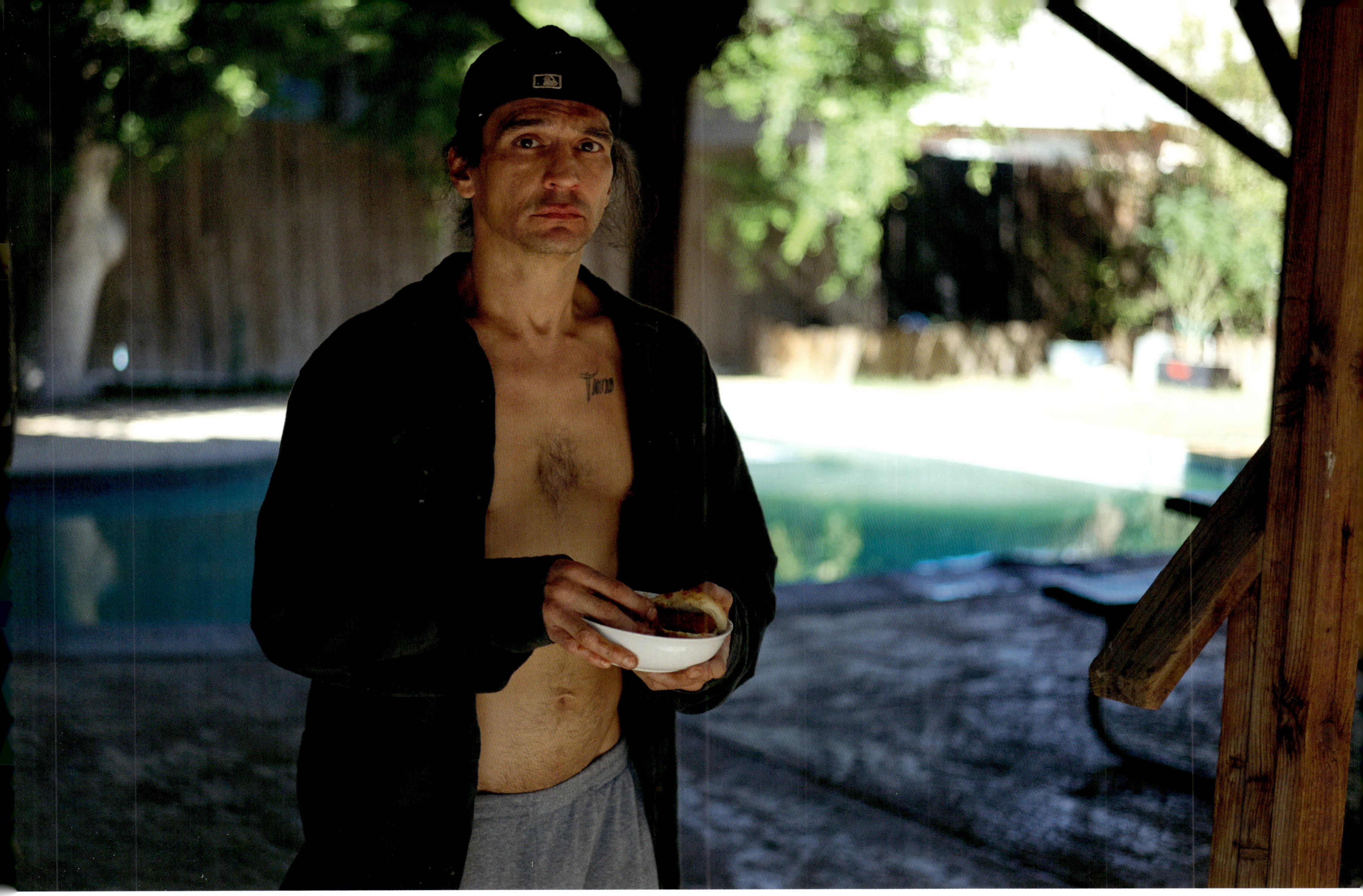

Timmy, El Centro

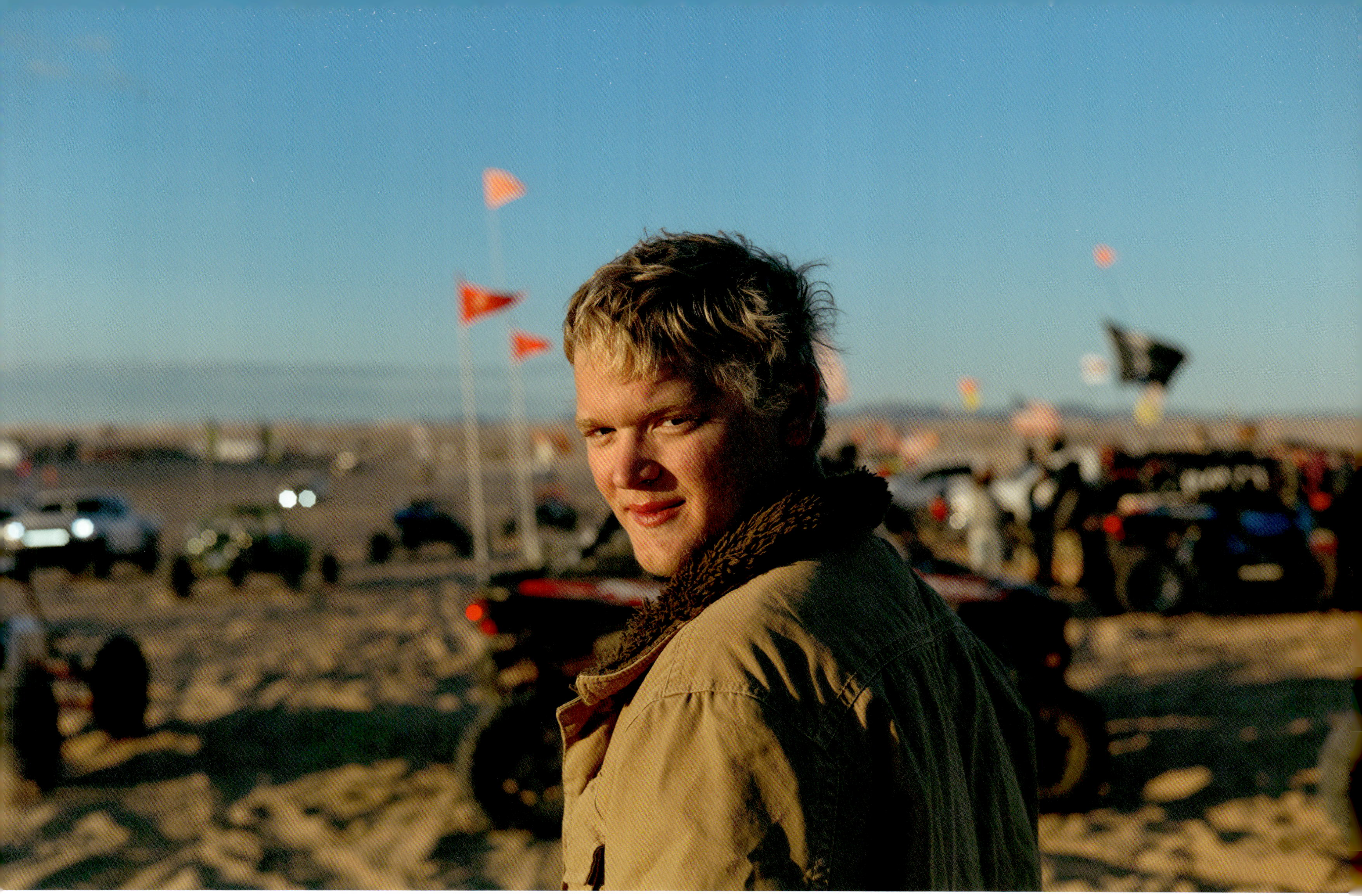

Isaac, Oldsmobile Hill

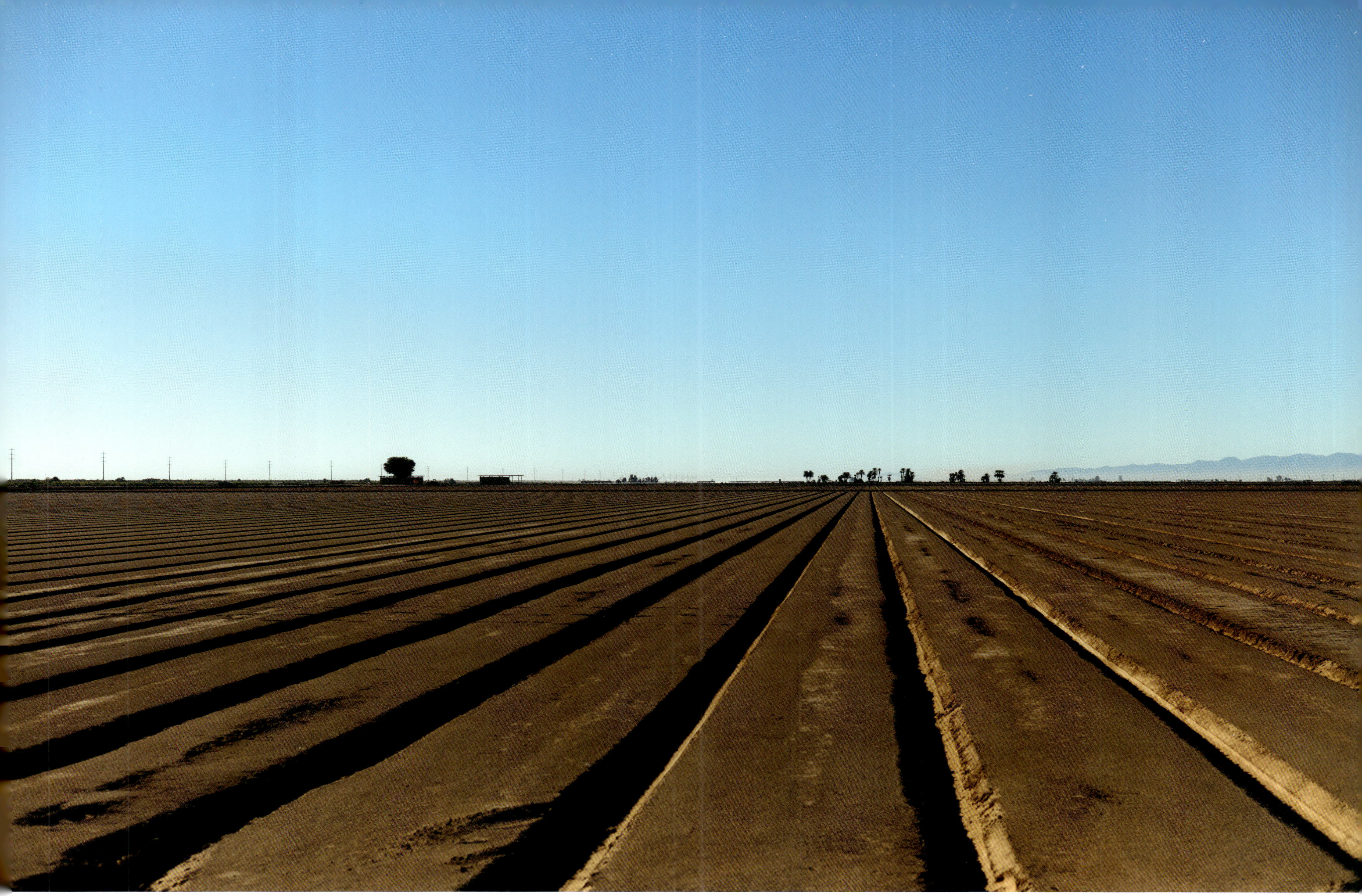

Topsoil prepared for seeding, Westmorland

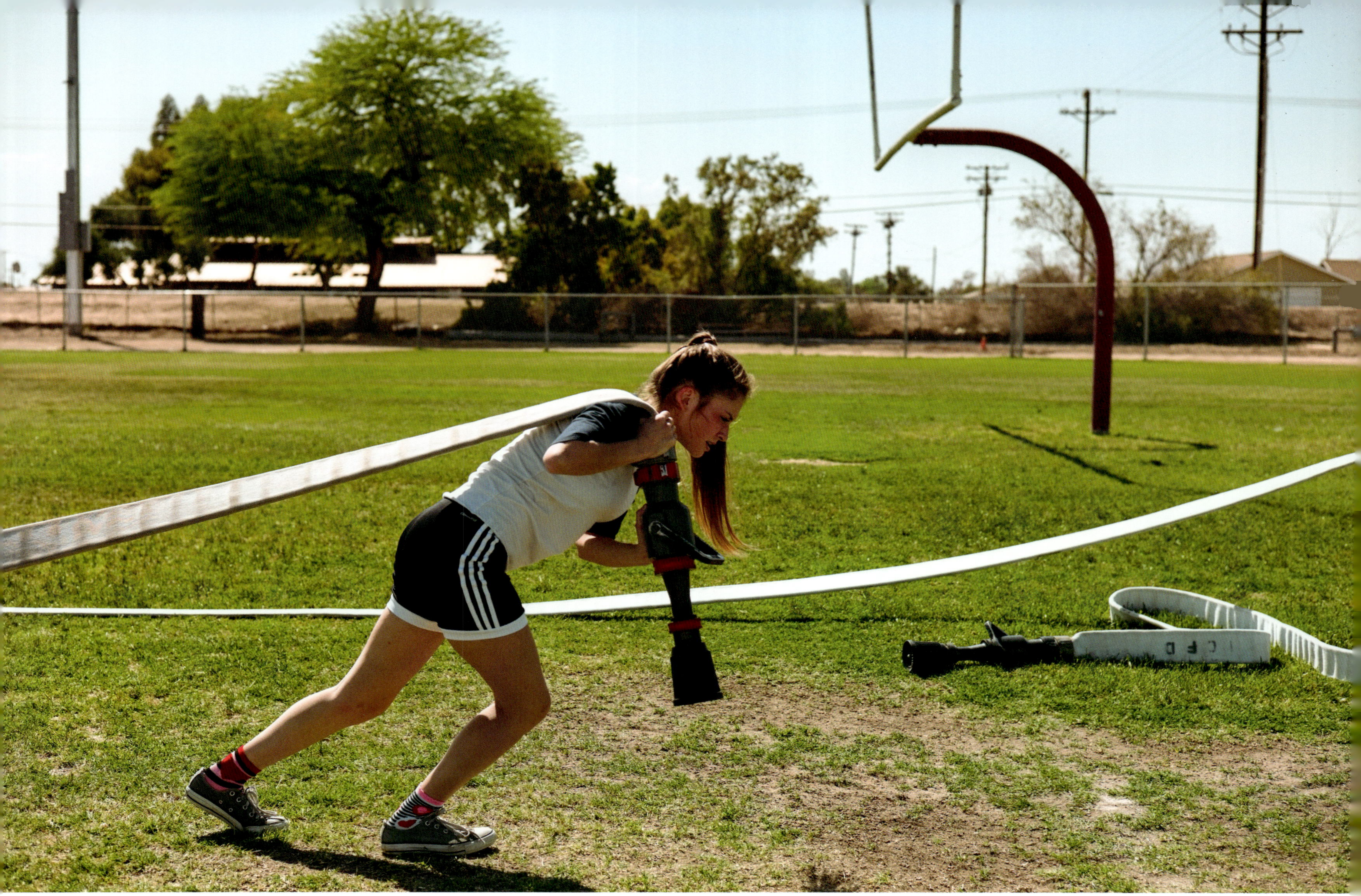

Sandra at Central Union High School, El Centro

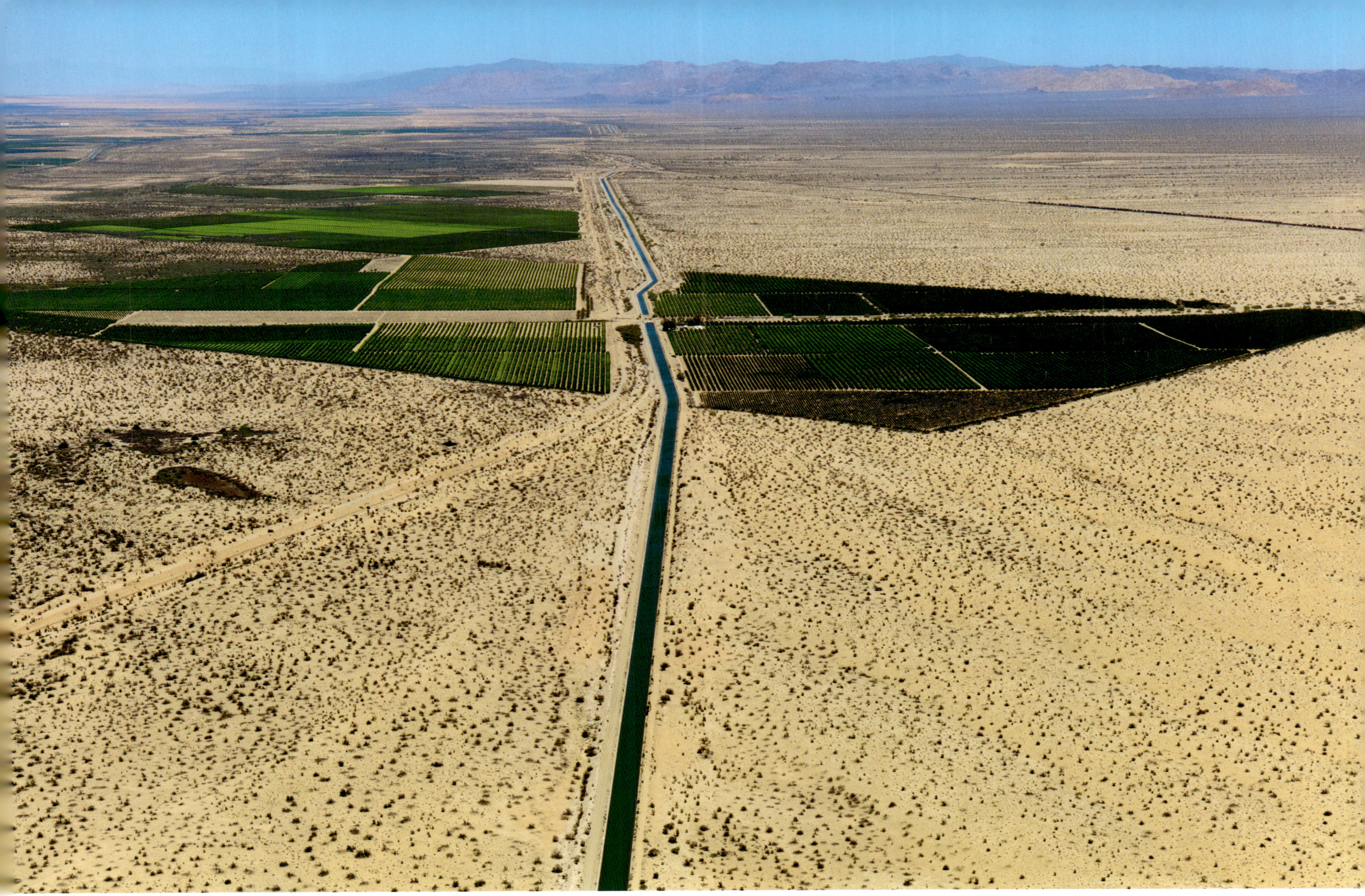

Coachella Canal, Tortuga

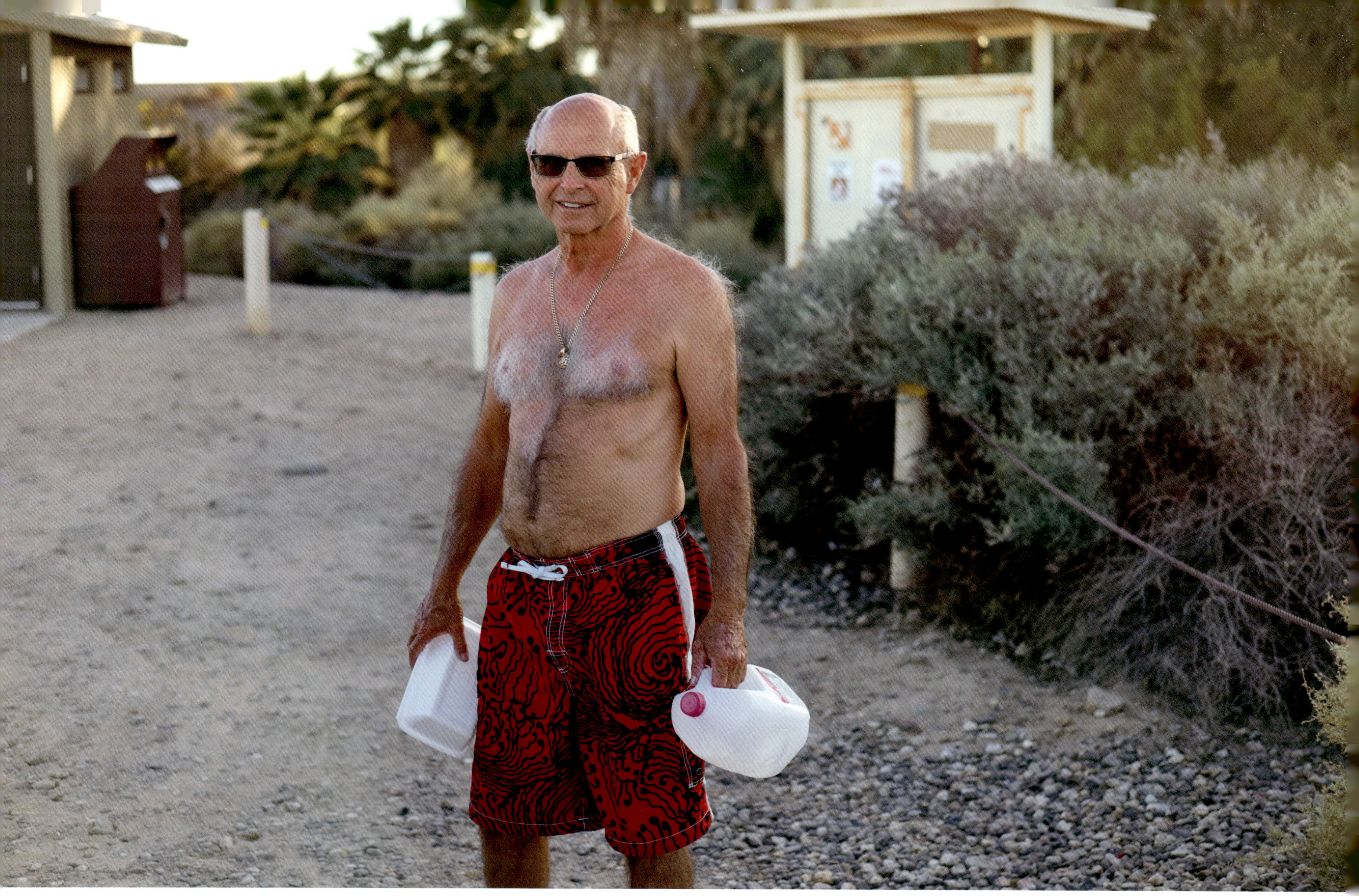

Jim at the Long Term Vehicle Area, Holtvile

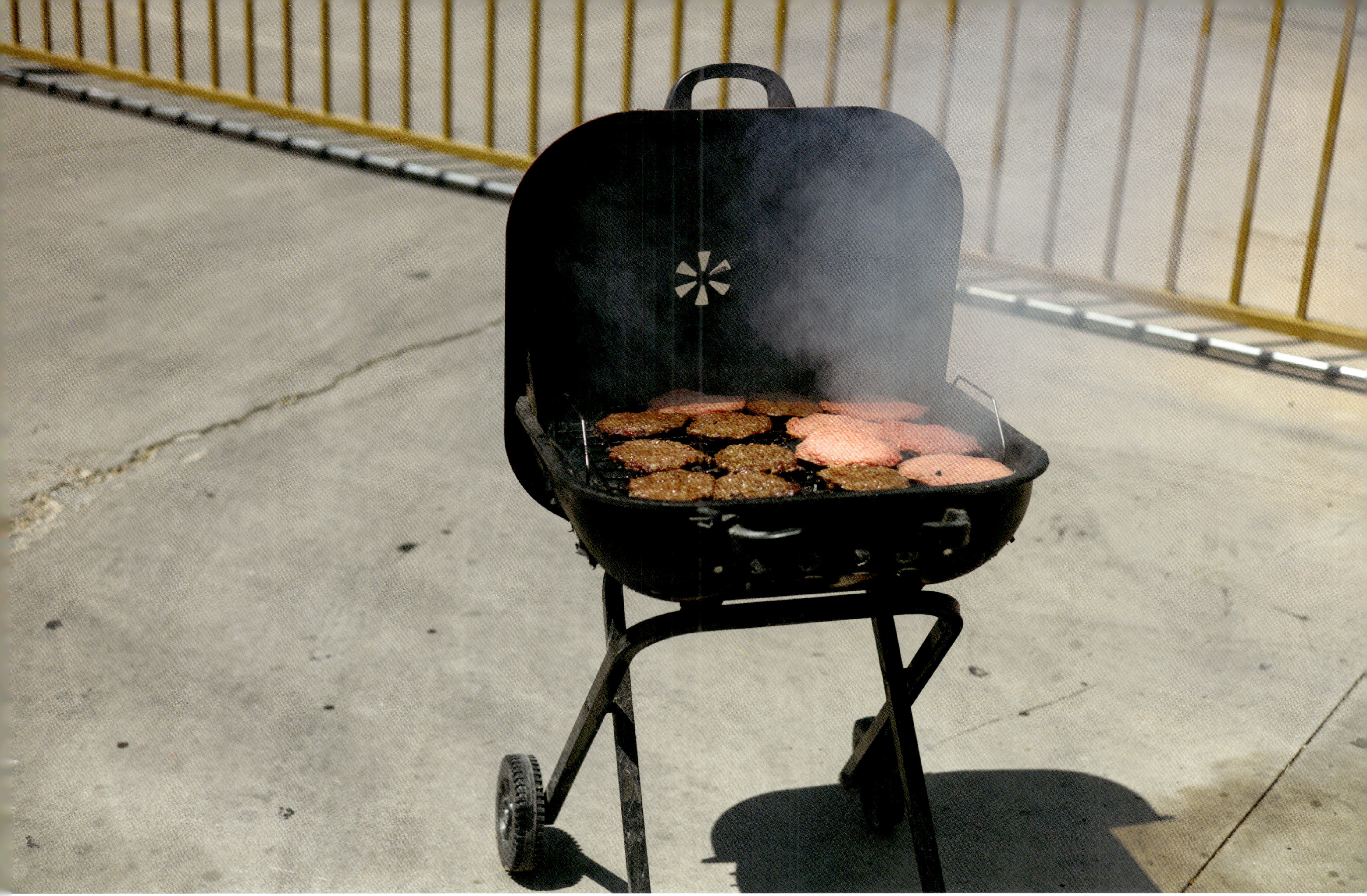

Barbecque at Our Lady of Guadeloupe Church, El Centro

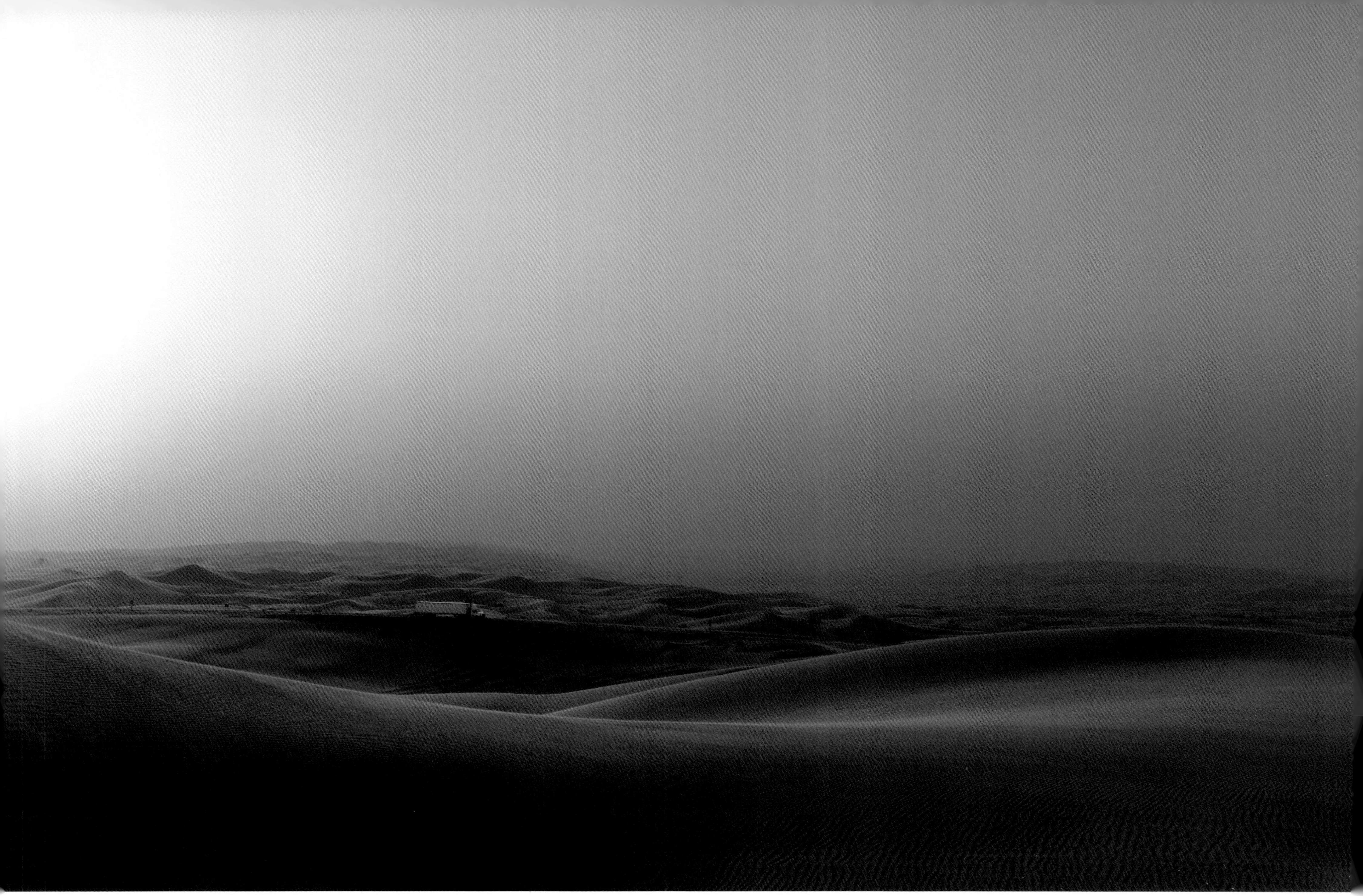

Cooling truck, Algodones Dunes

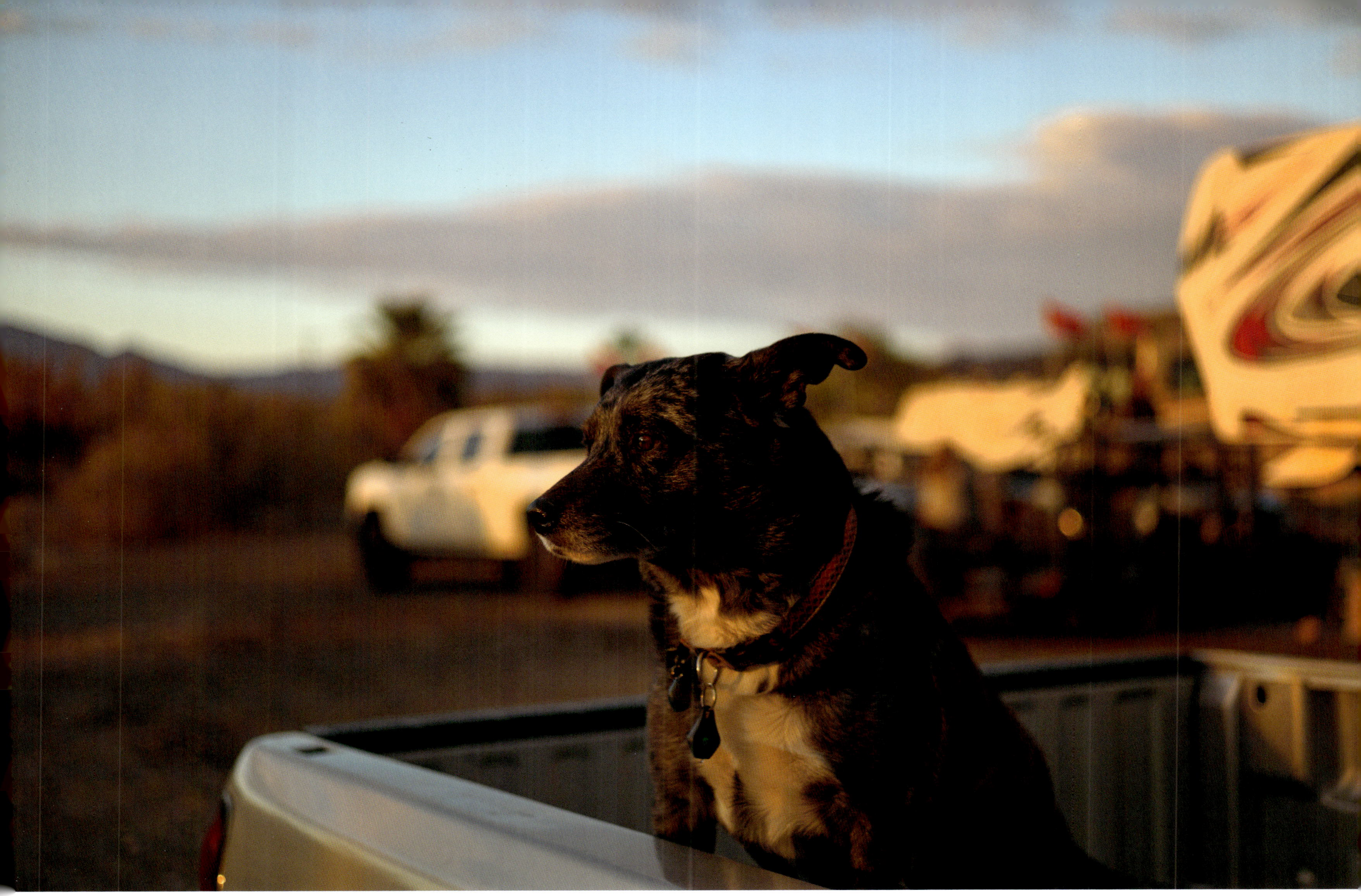

Ross' Dog, Chocolate Mountains

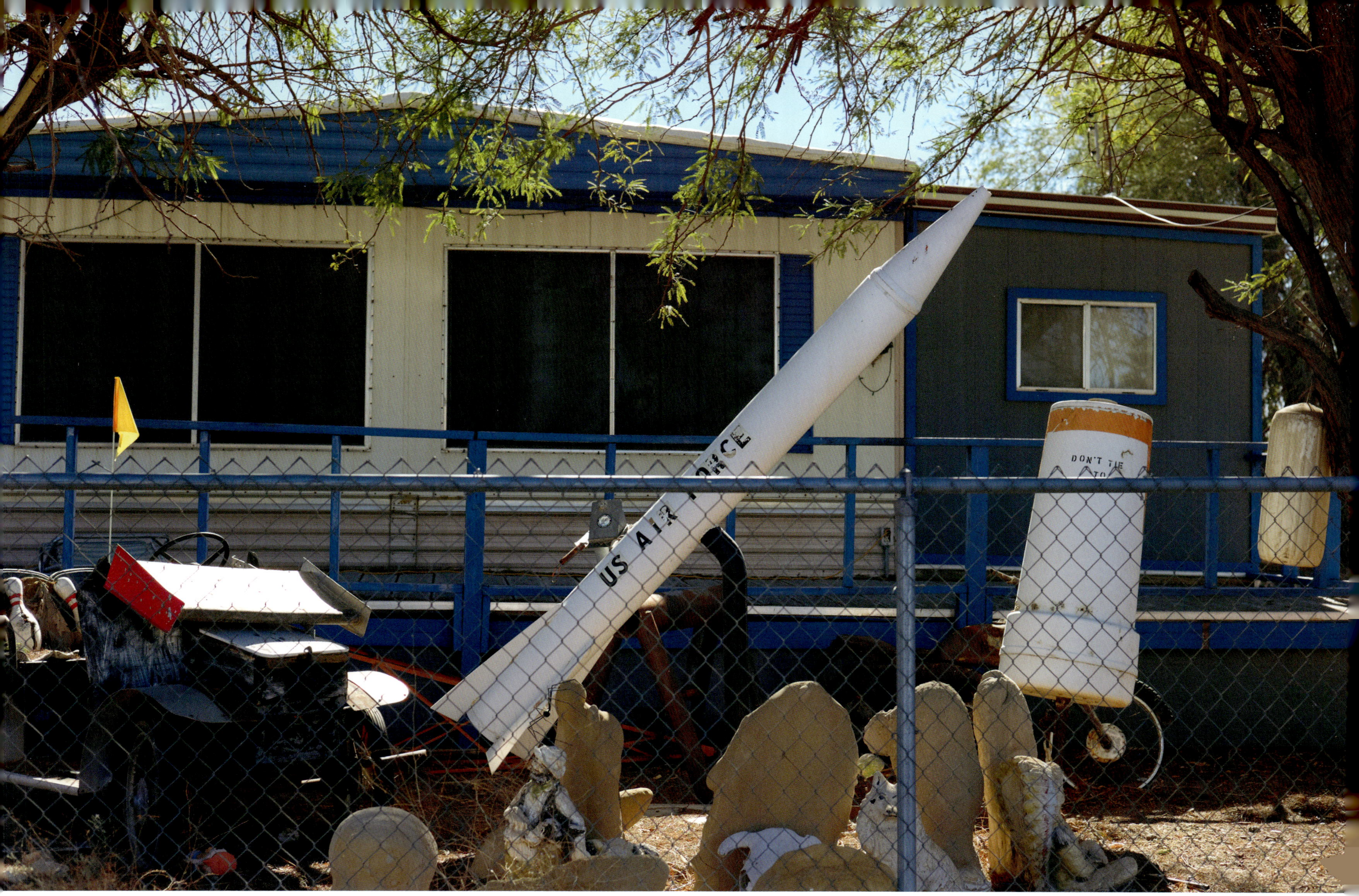

Veterans yard, Desert Shores

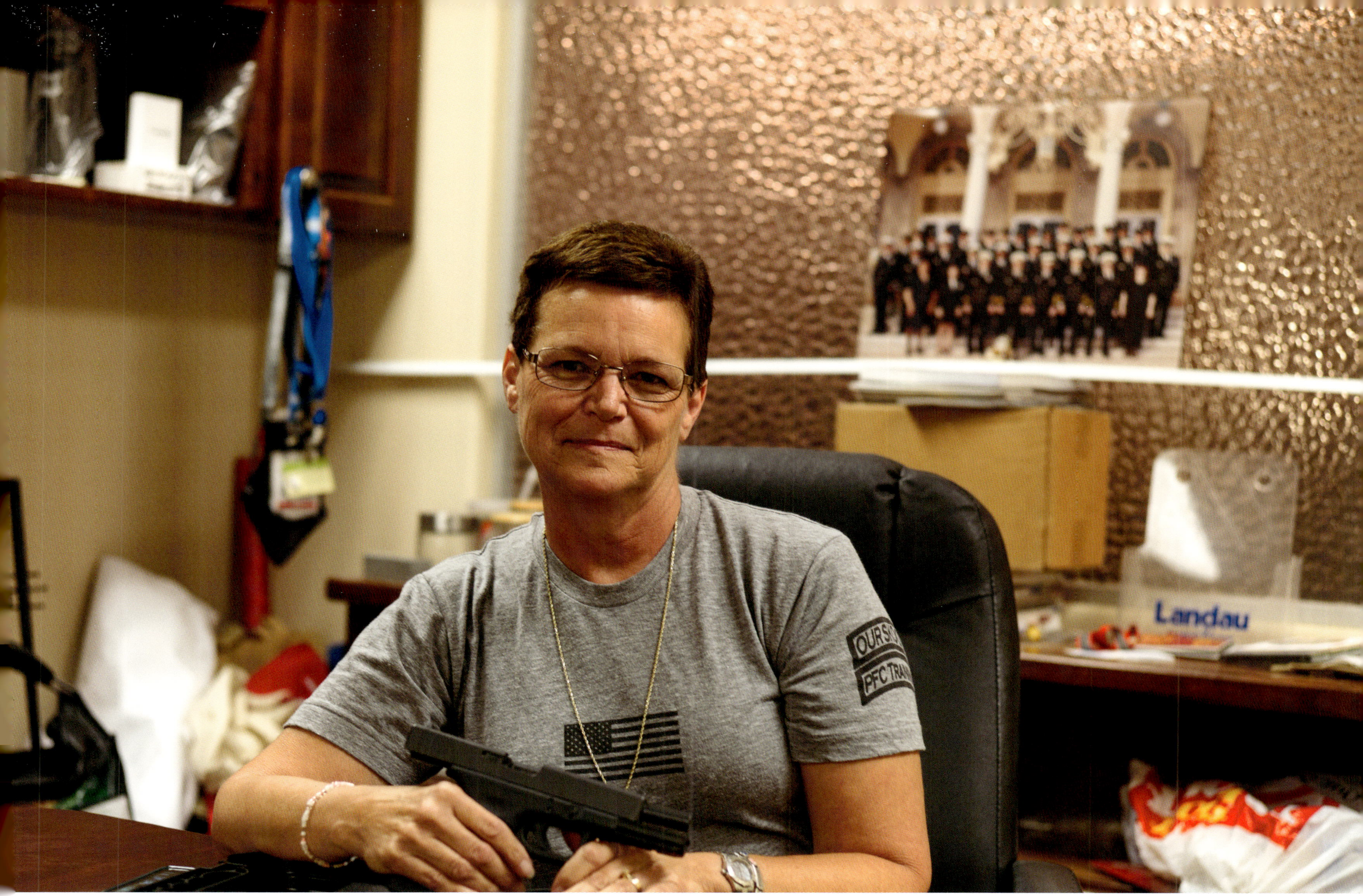

Karen at Border Tactile Indoor Range, El Centro

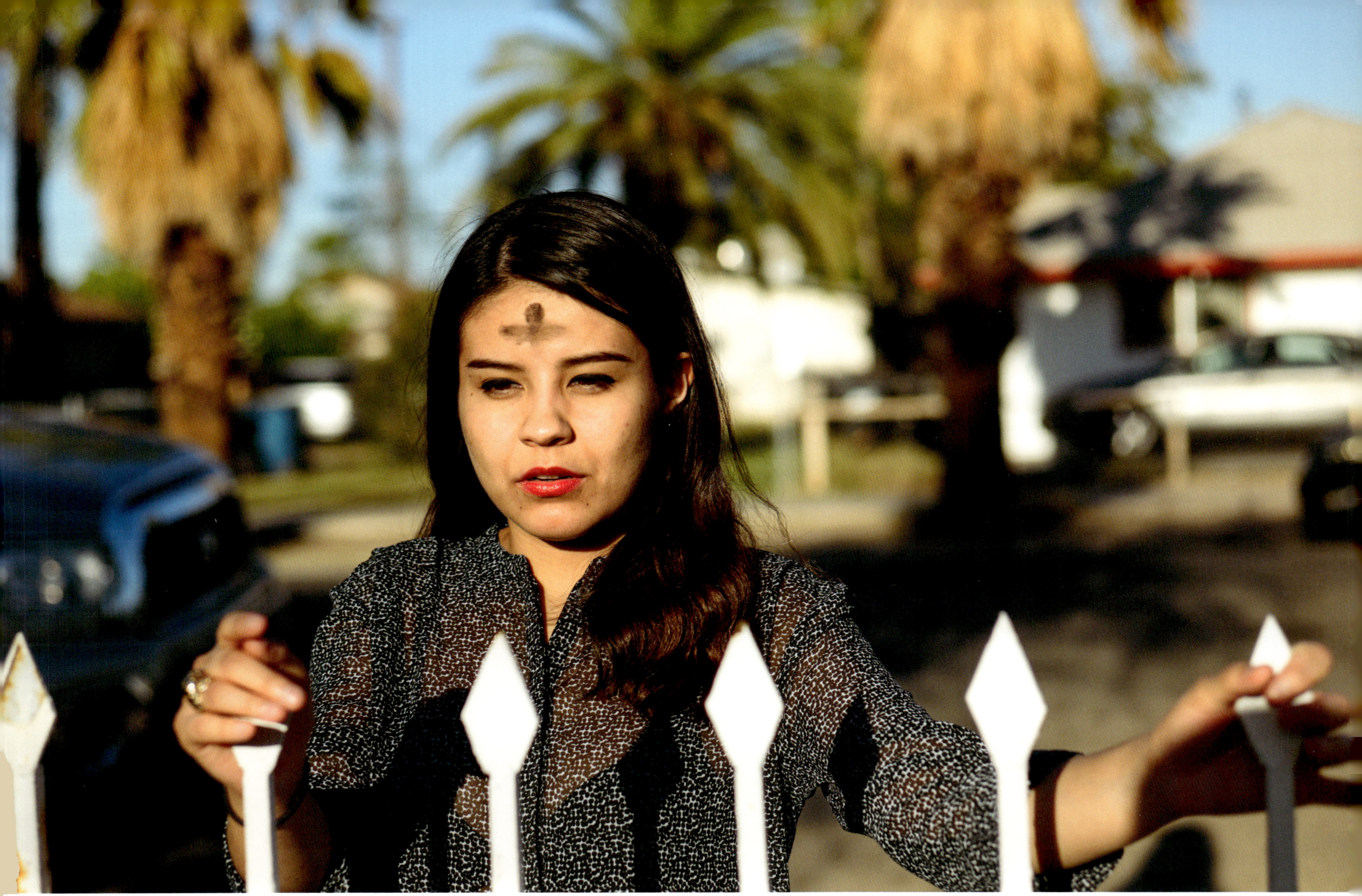

Carla on Ash Wedenesday, Calexico

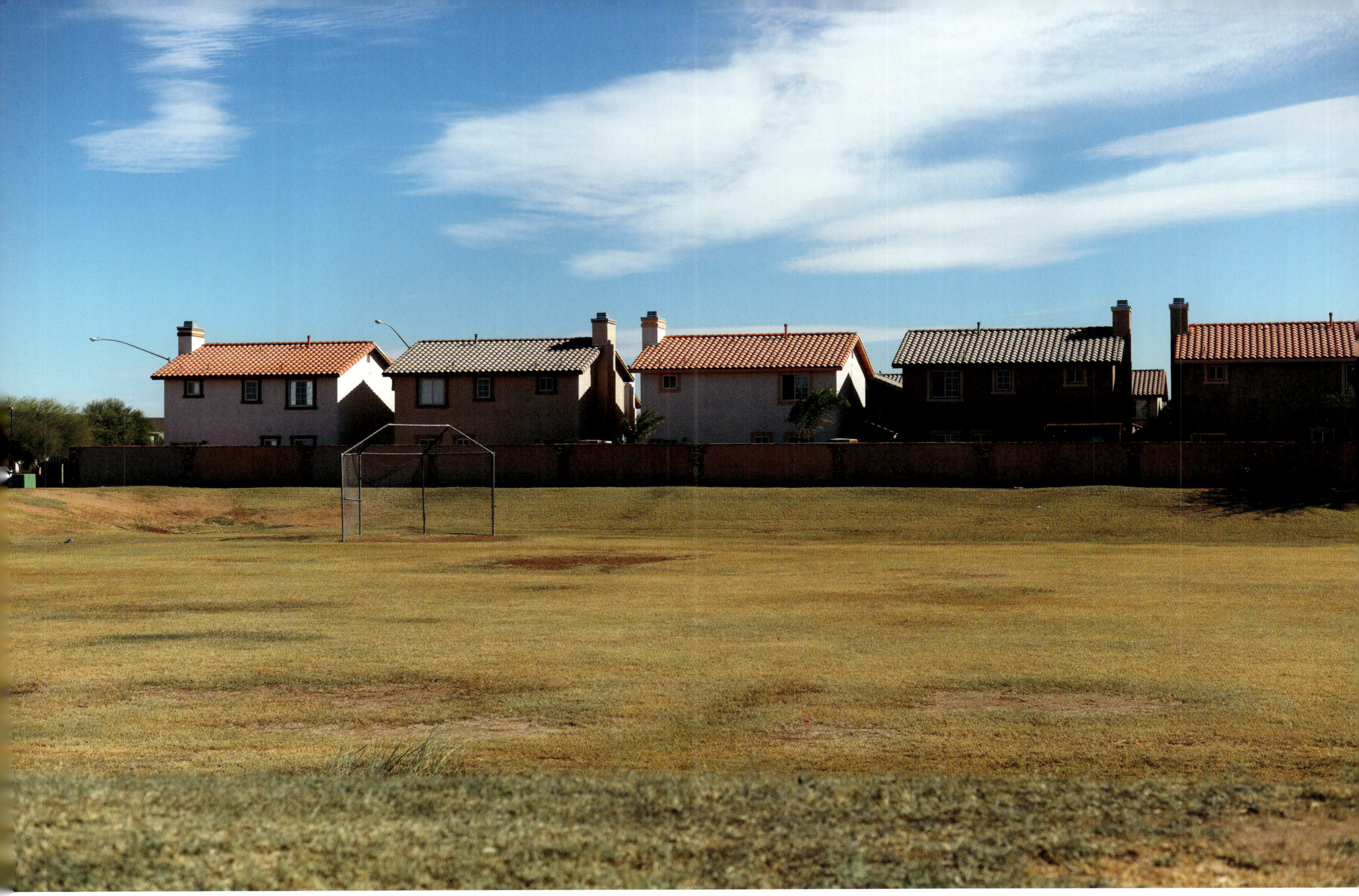

Gated Homes, Calexico

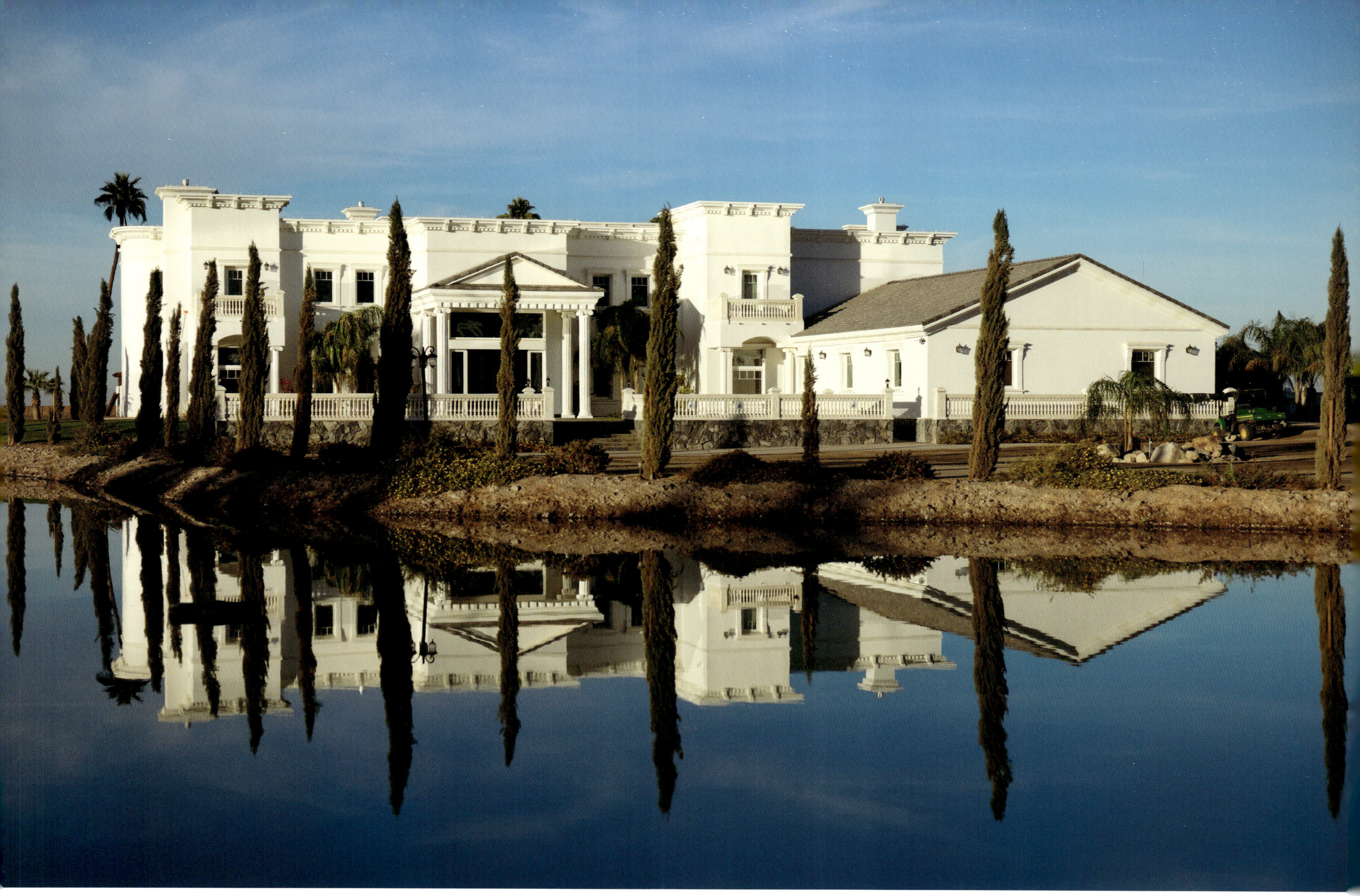

Mansion, Holtville

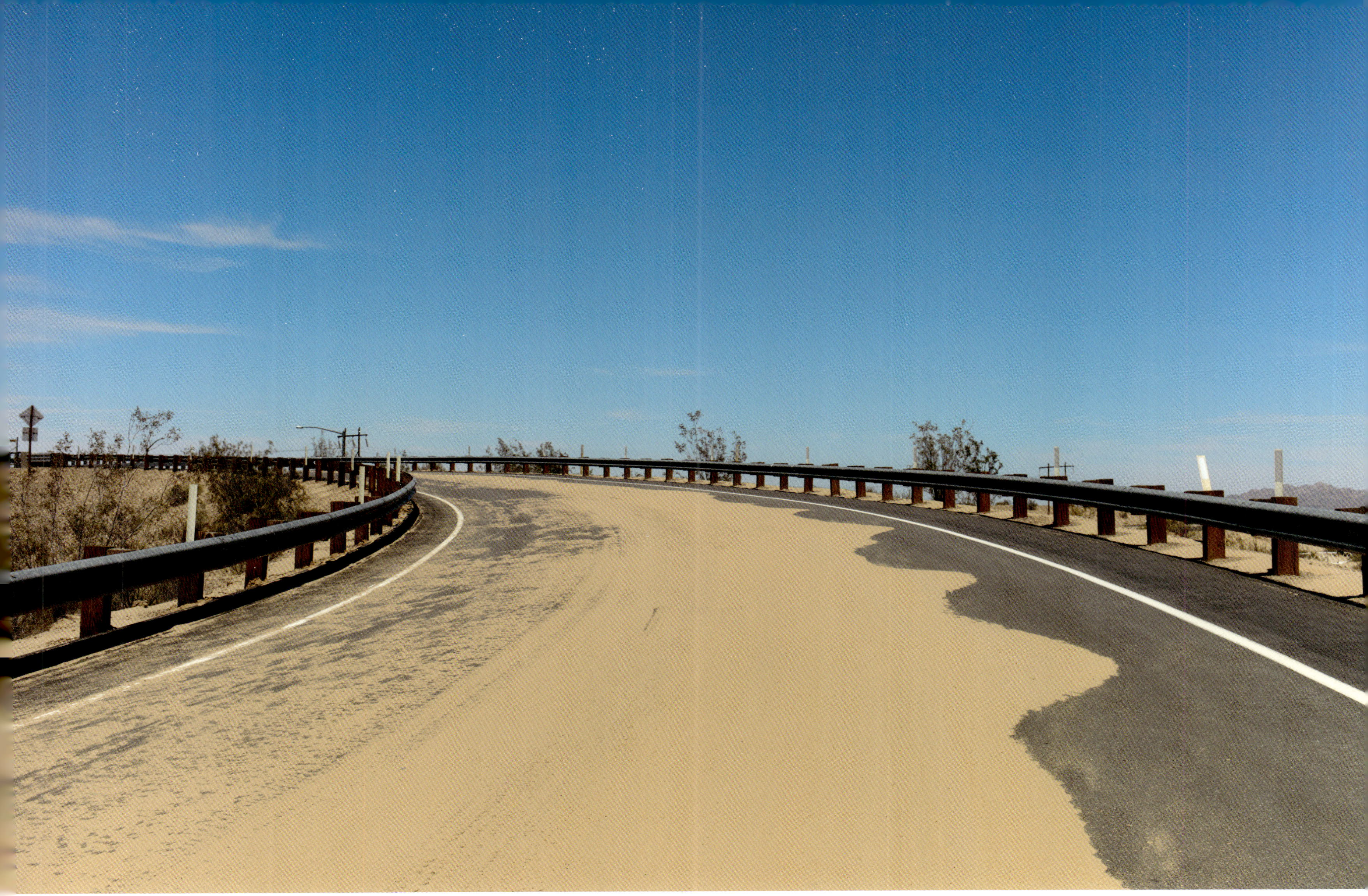

Bridge crossing Interstate 8, Buttercup Sand Dunes

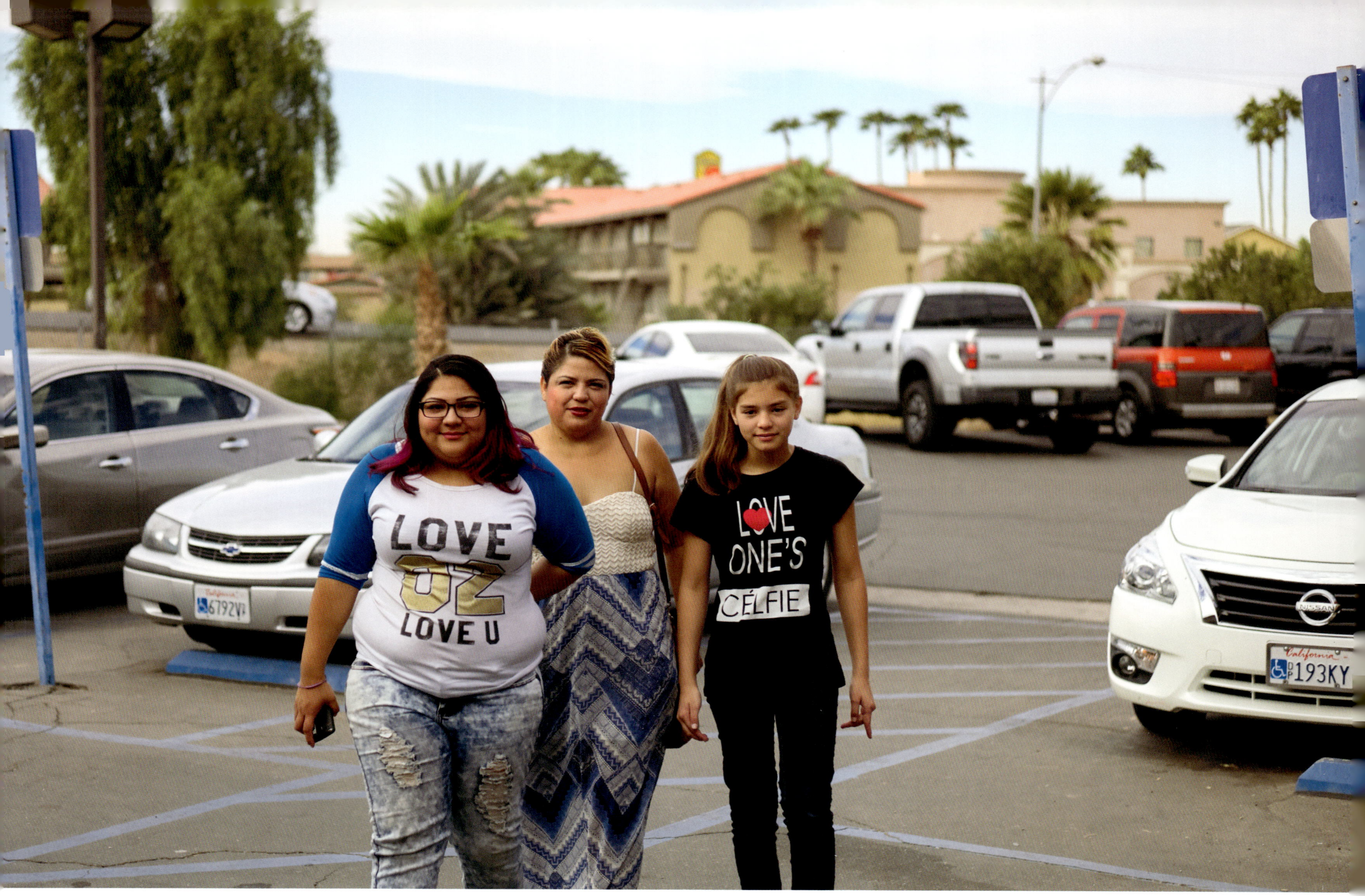

Quality Inn car park, El Centro

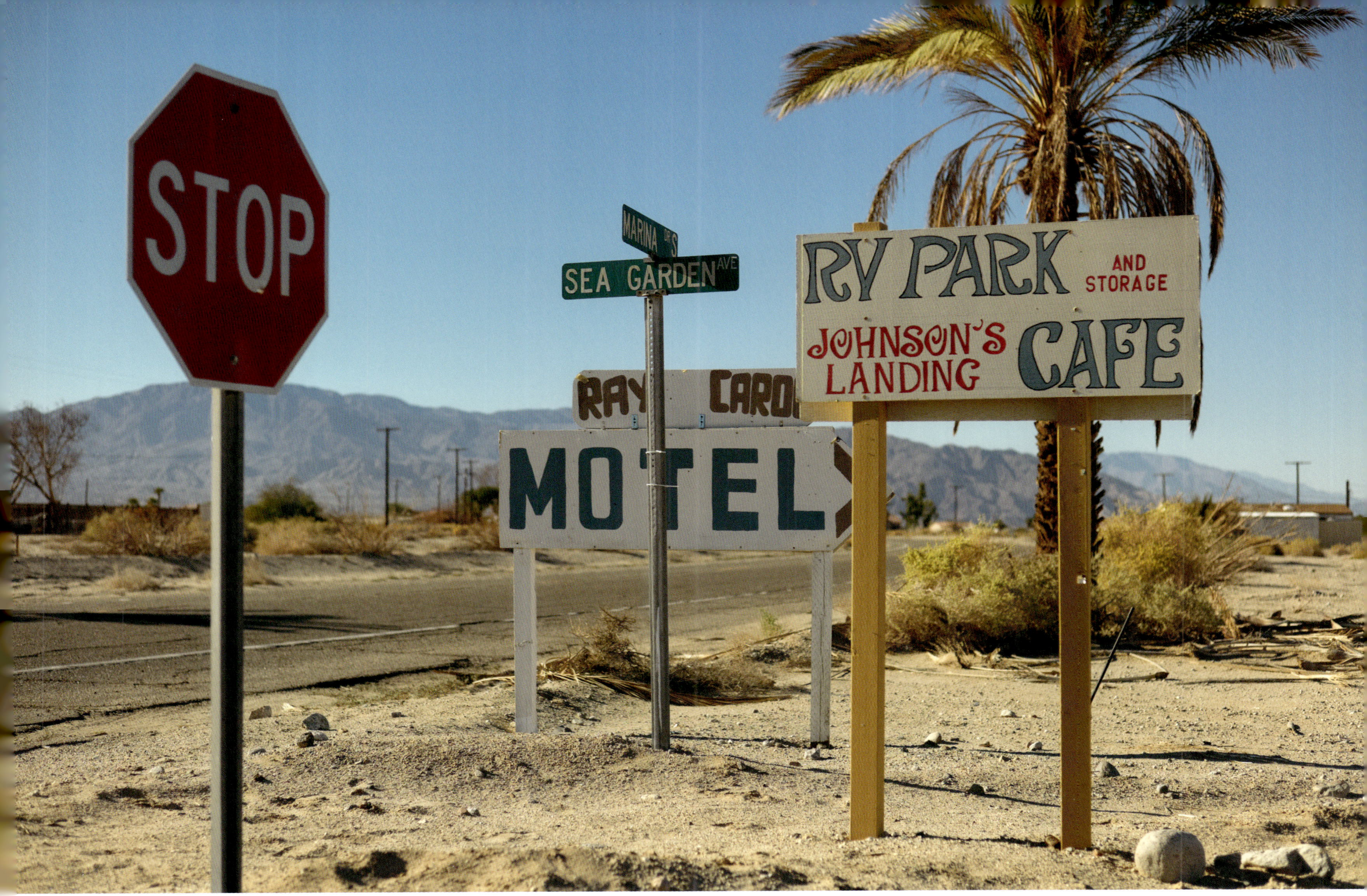

Marina Drive, Salton City

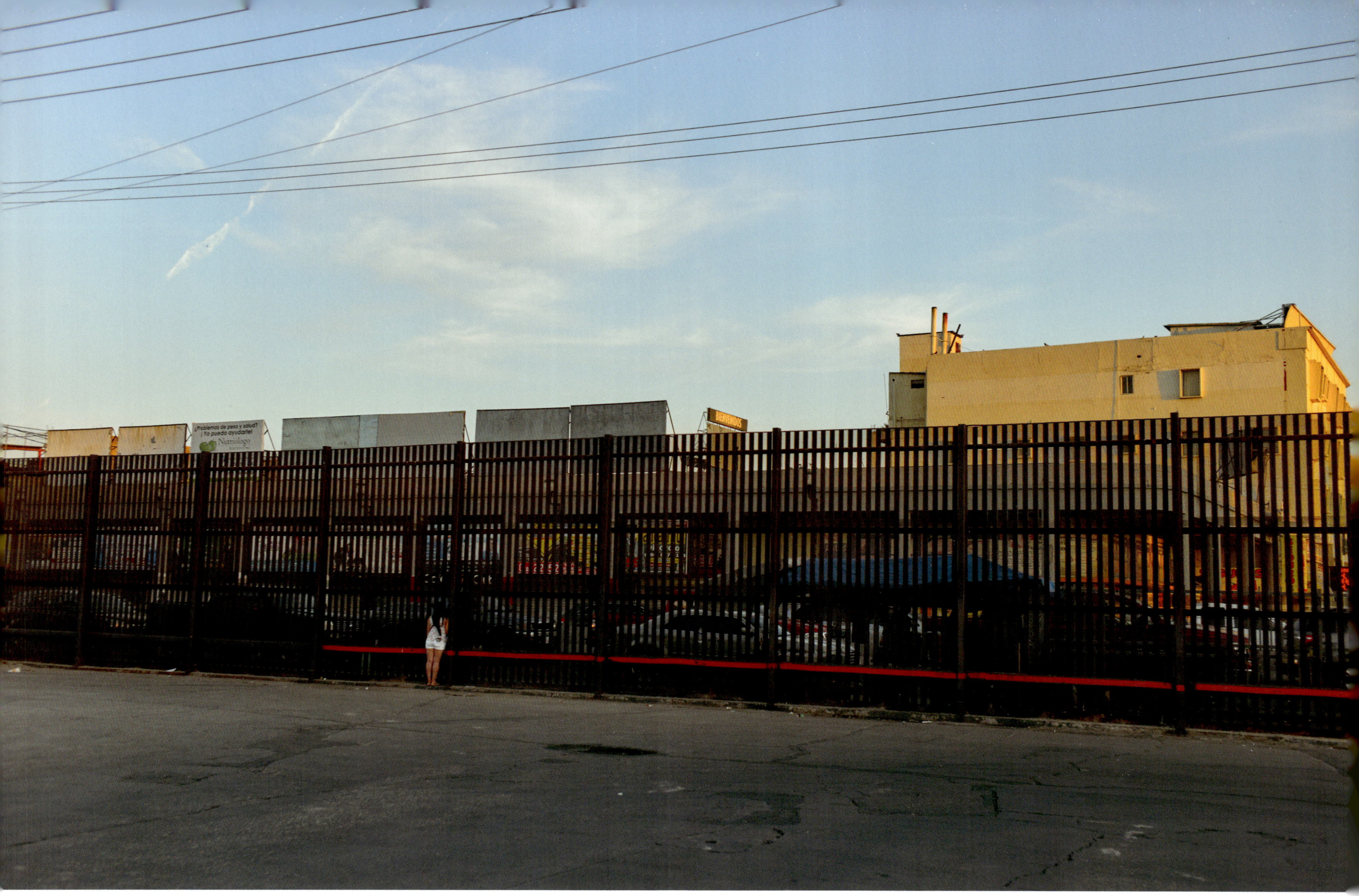

Amata and Manuel at the border fence, Calexico

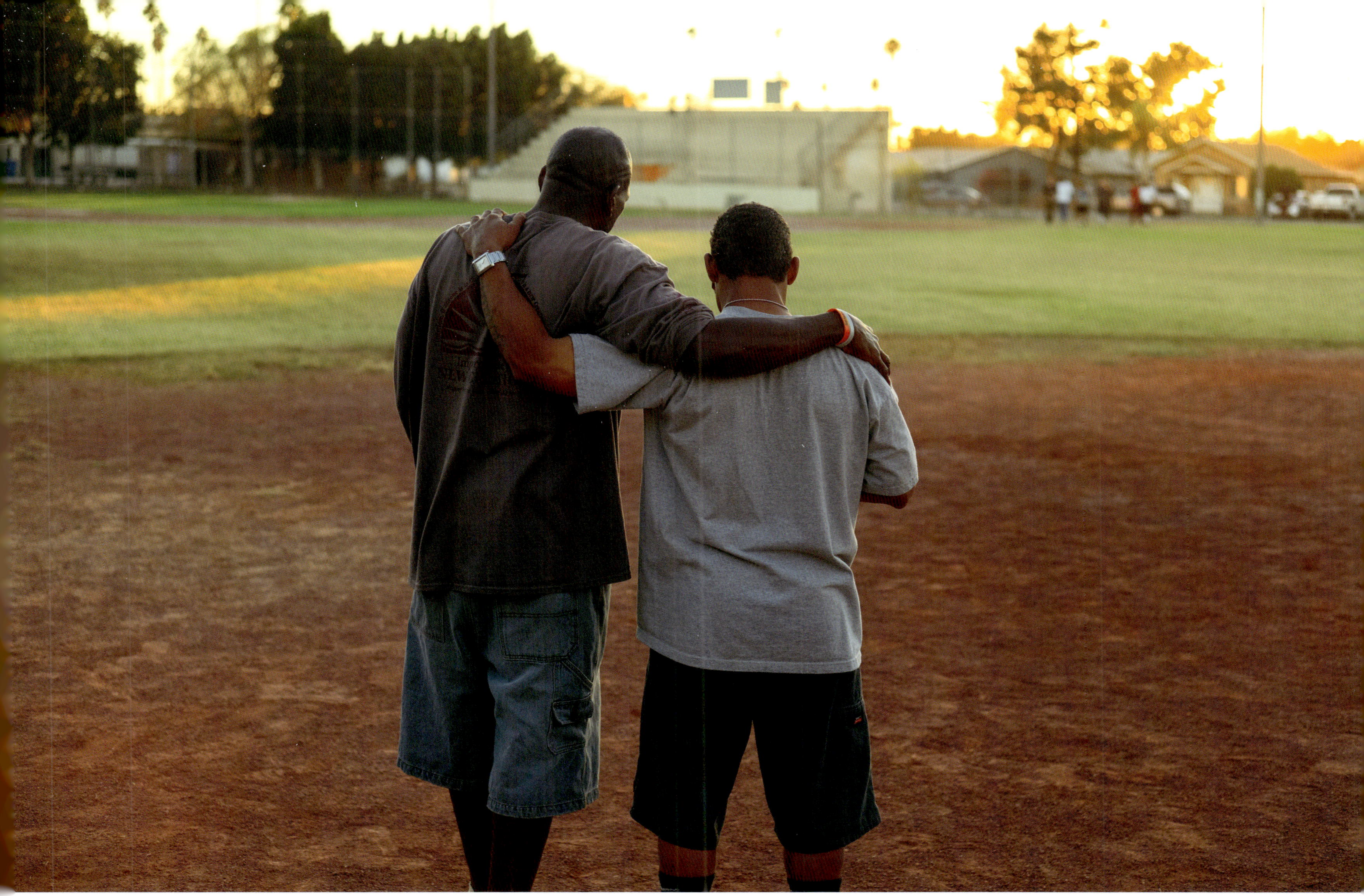

Luis and Frank in the Recreation Park, Holtville

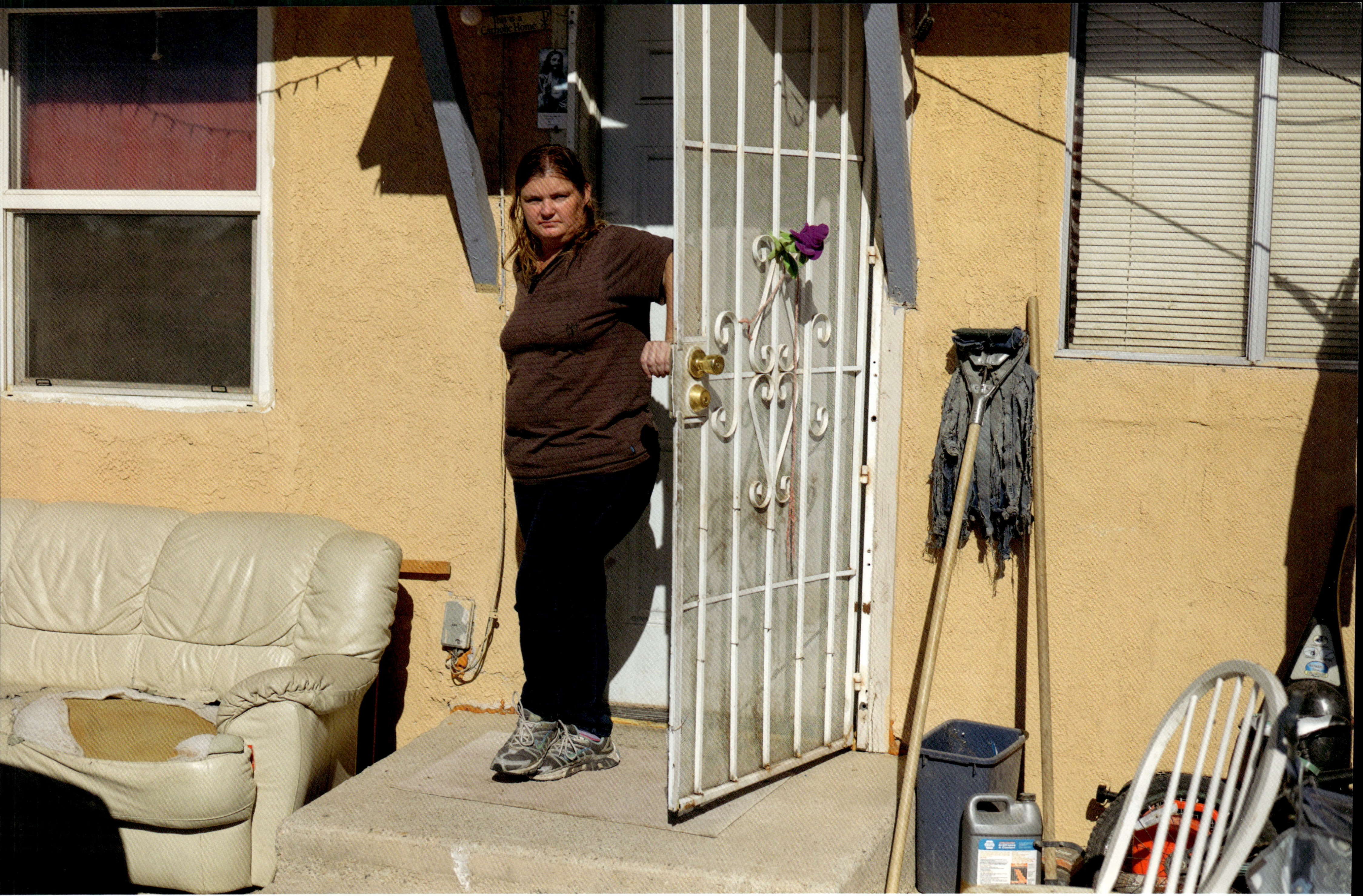

Katie, Calipatria

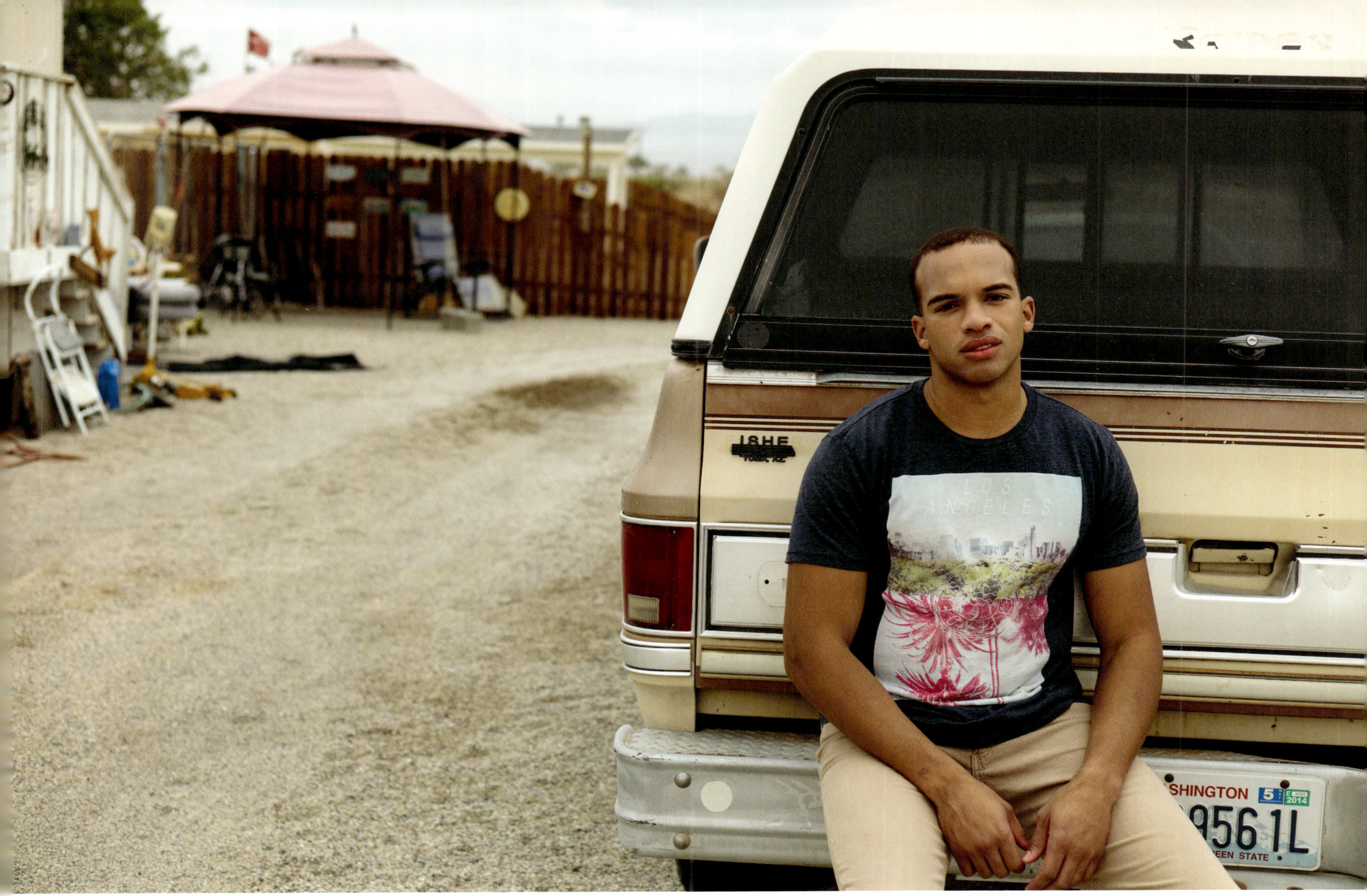

Iraq War veteran Adrian, Salton Sea Beach

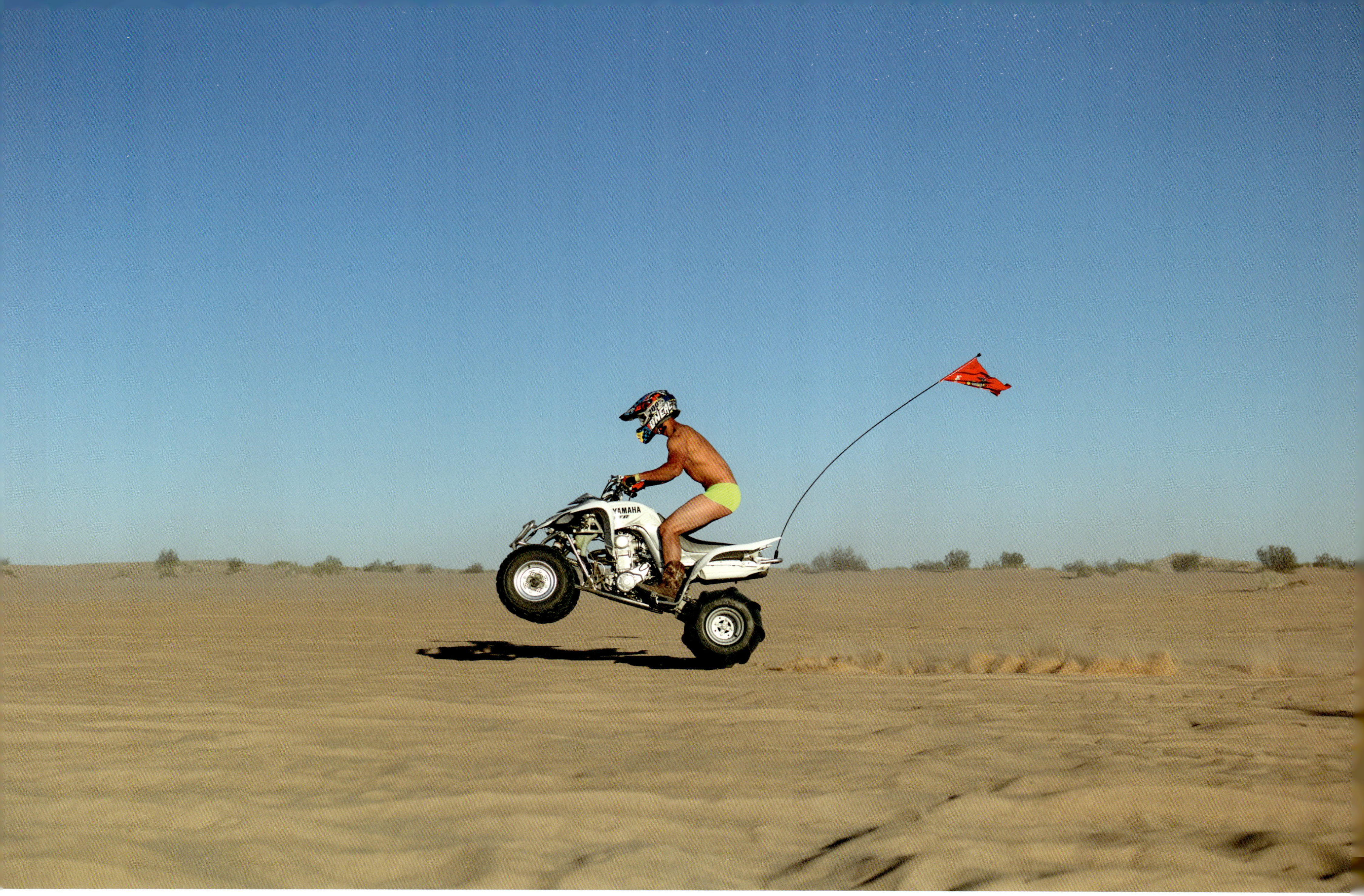

Prustin on Thanksgiving, Glamis

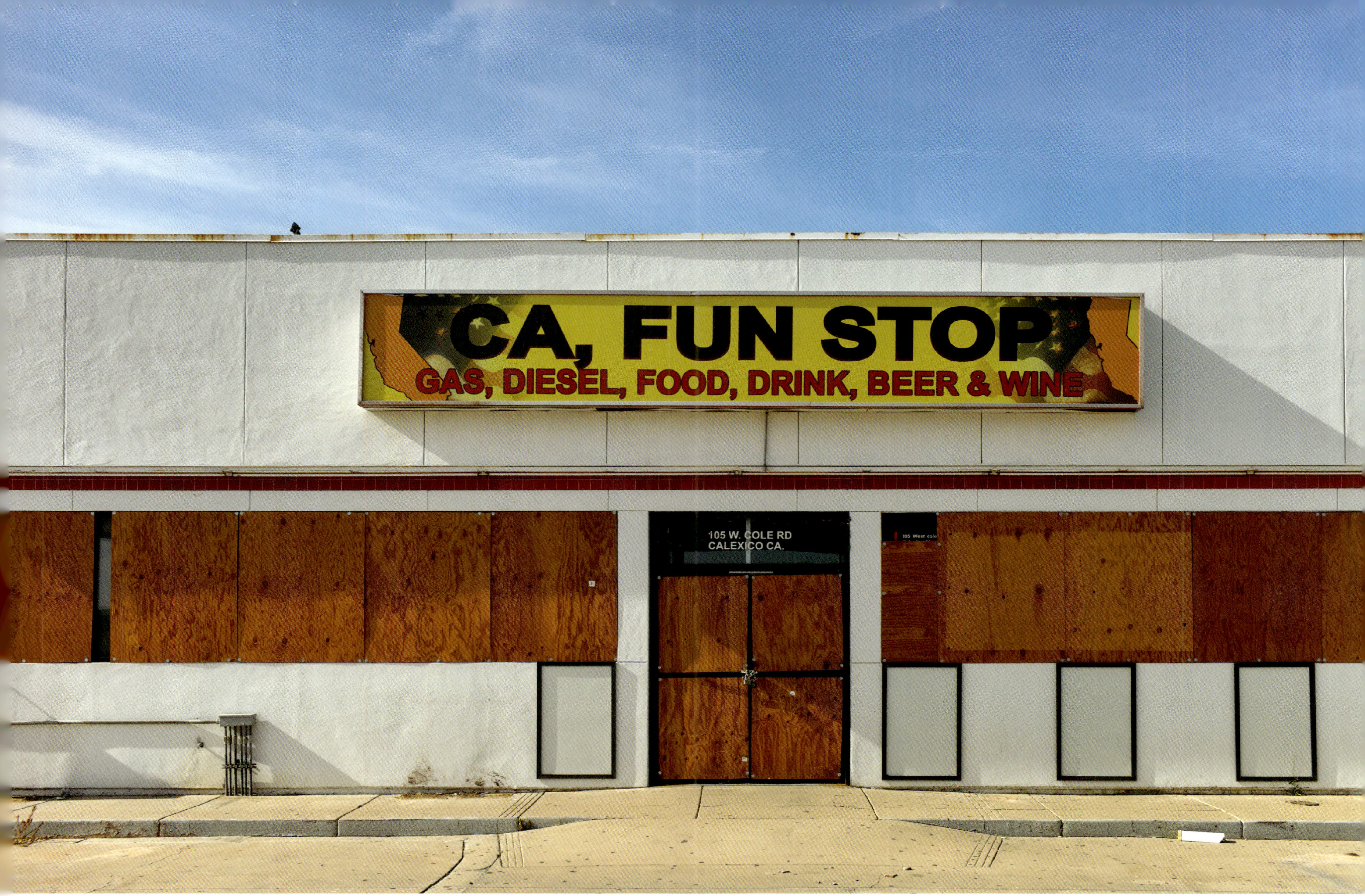

Closed down rest area, Calexico

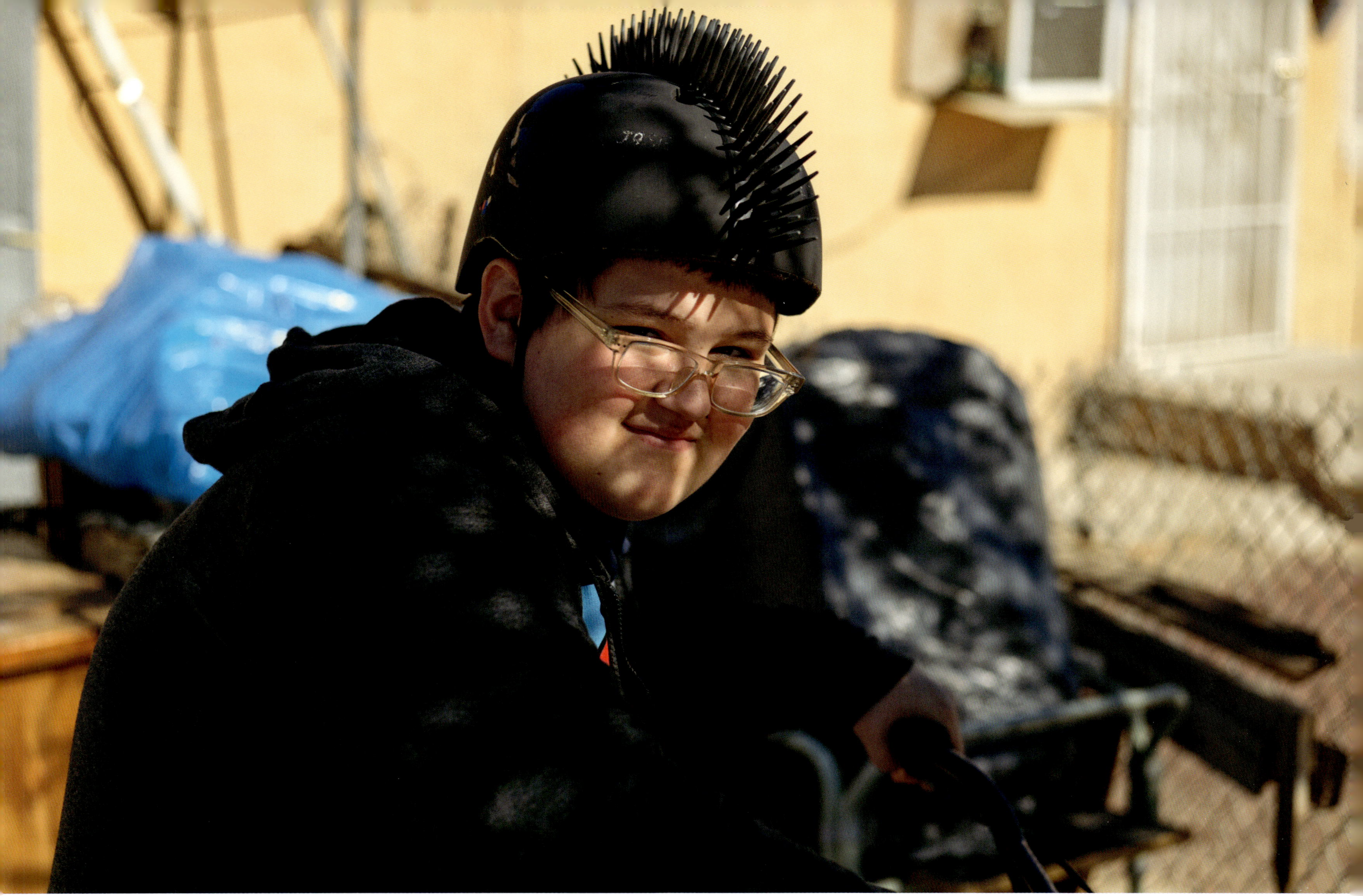

José, Calipatria

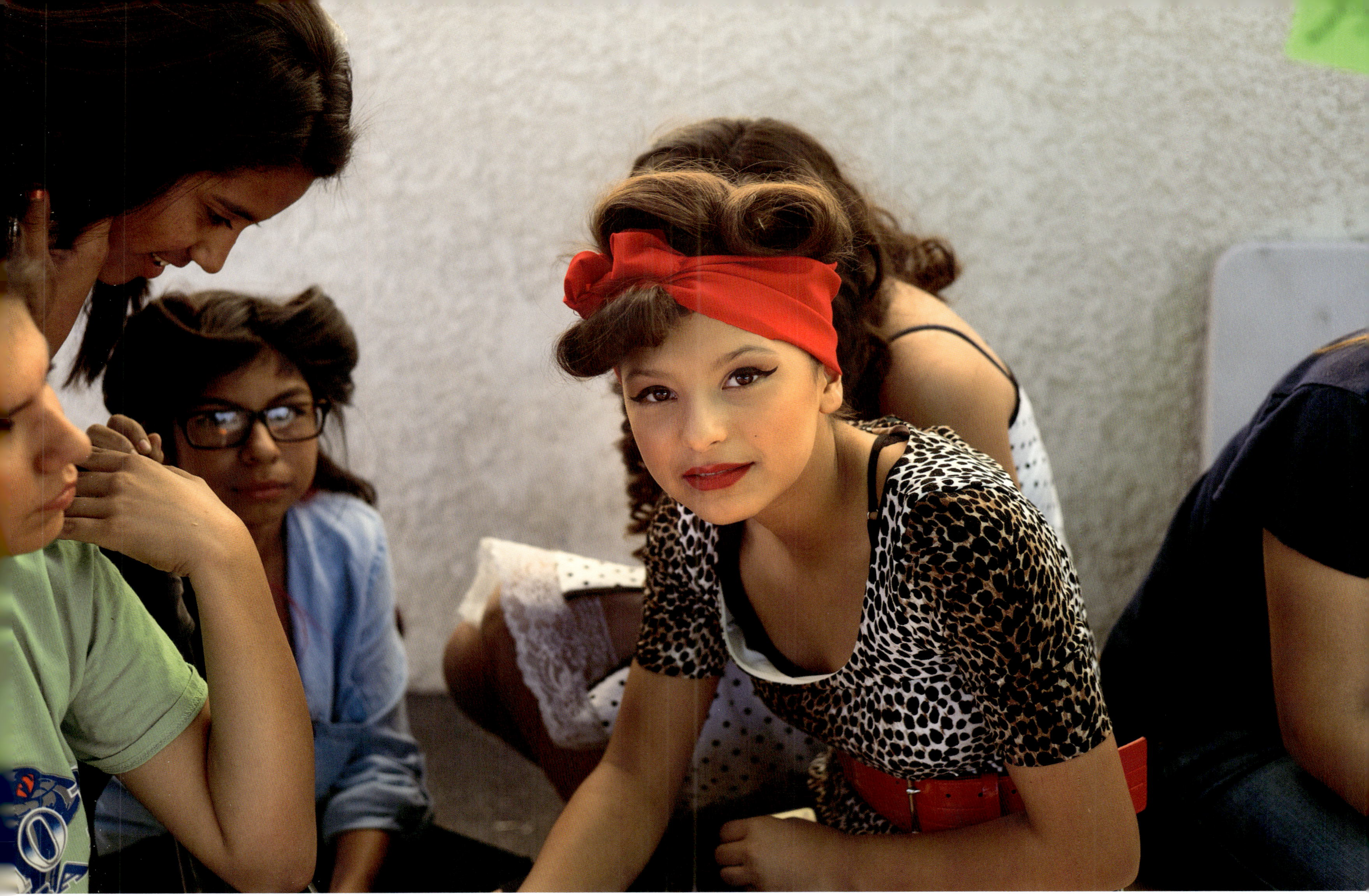

Heli at the Pin-up contest, El Centro

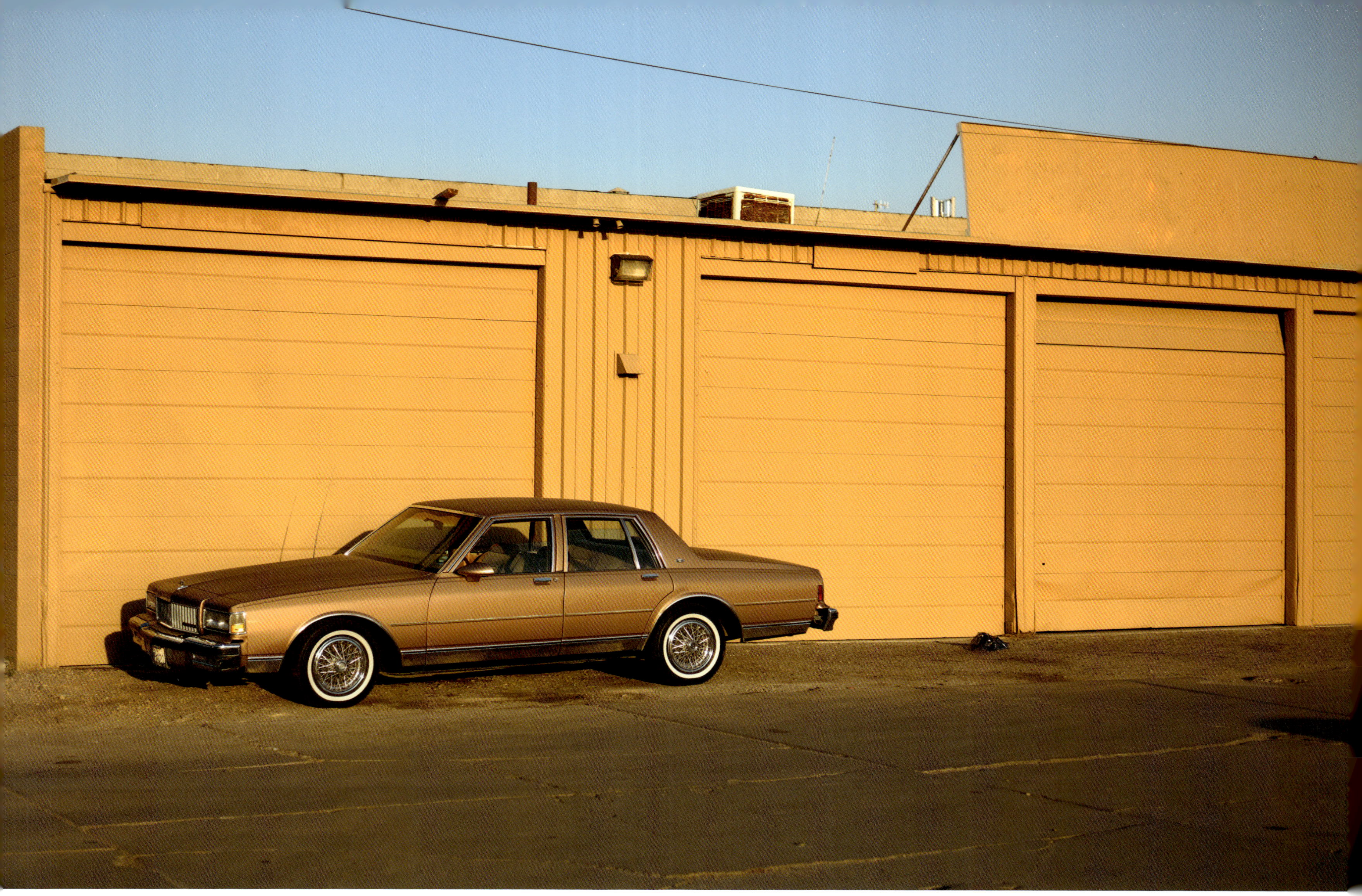

West State Street, El Centro

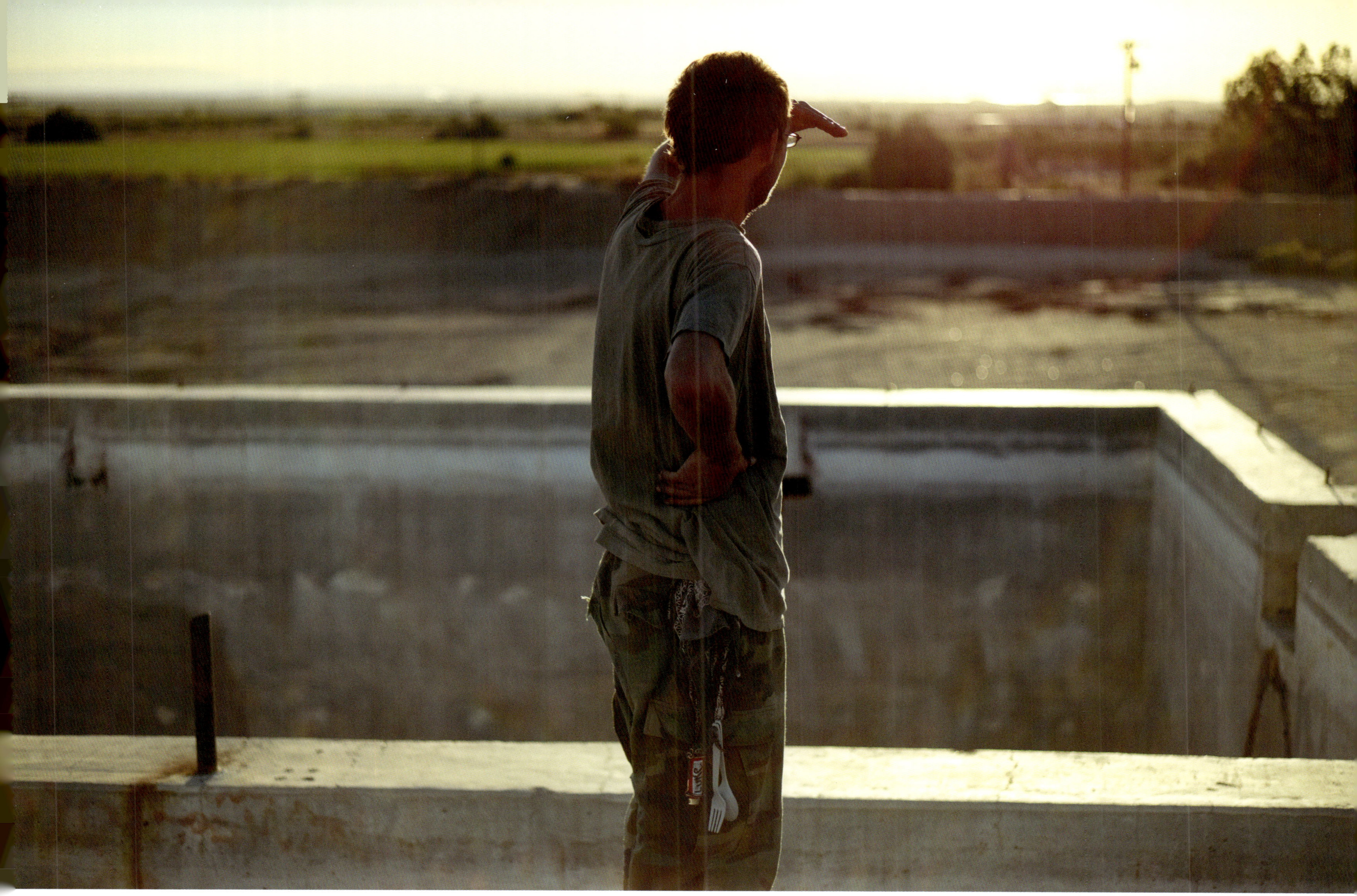

Alabama at the castle, between Niland and Slab City

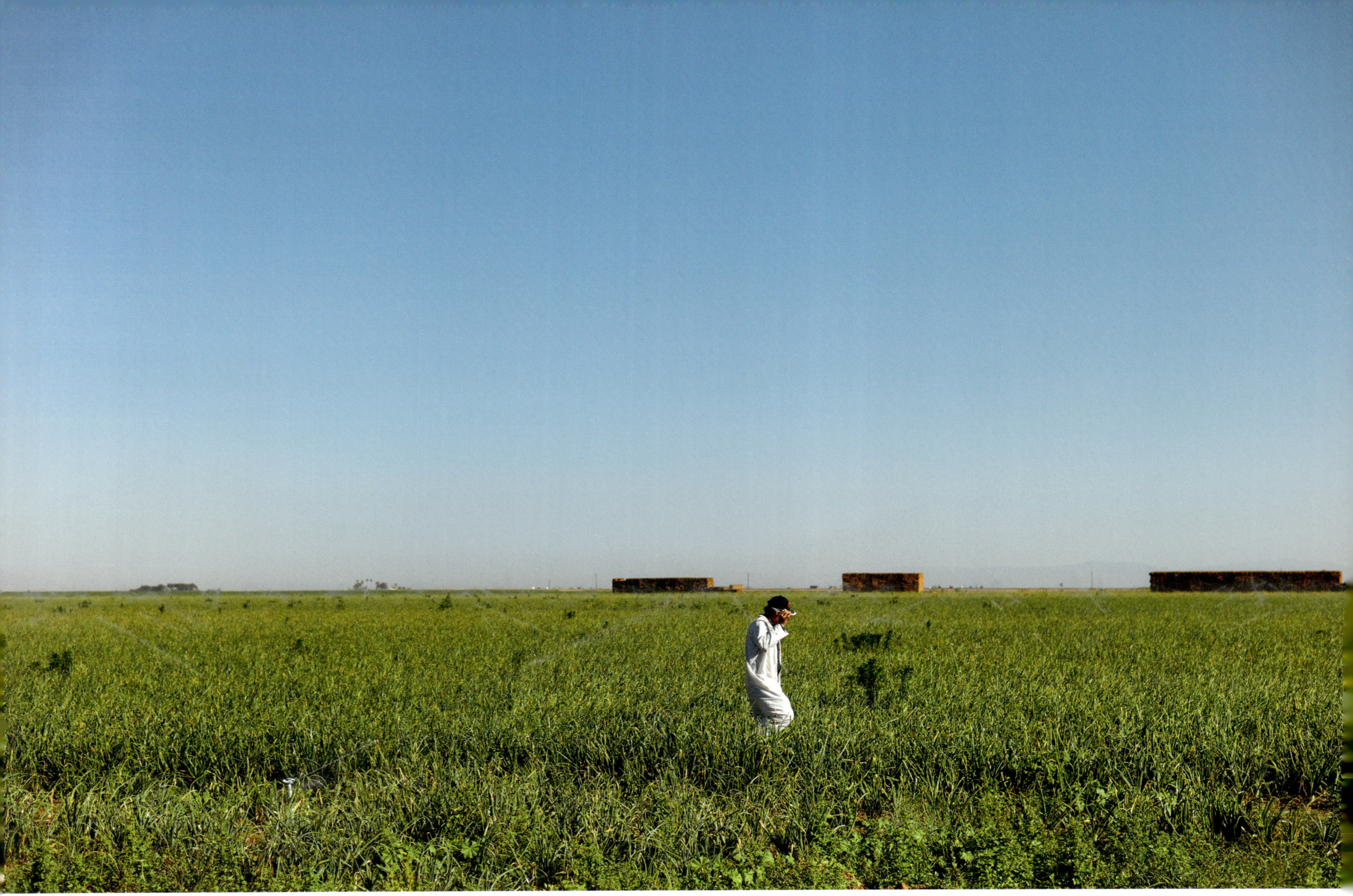

Farm worker in the fields, Watermans Corner

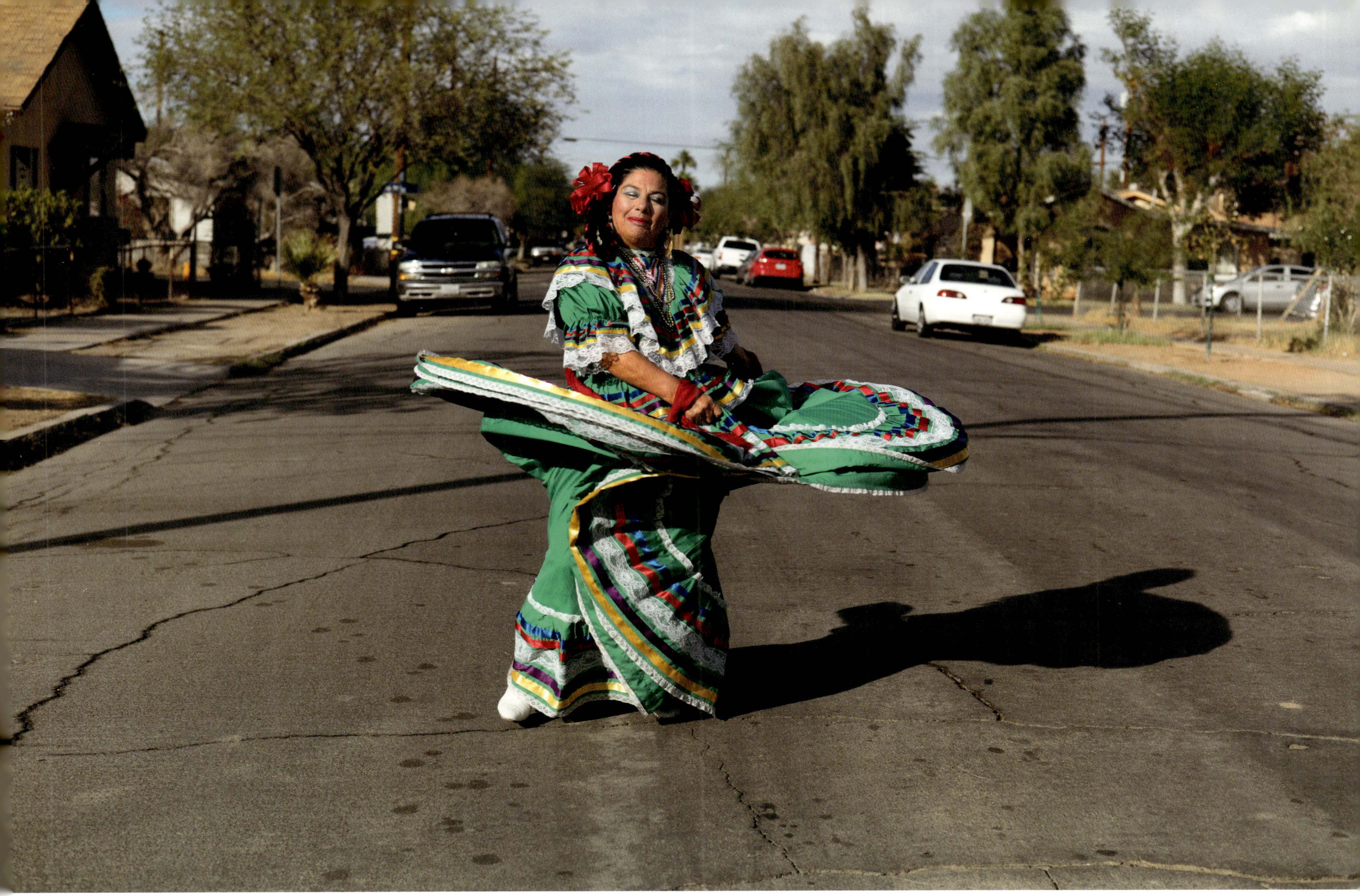

Maria del Carmen, El Centro

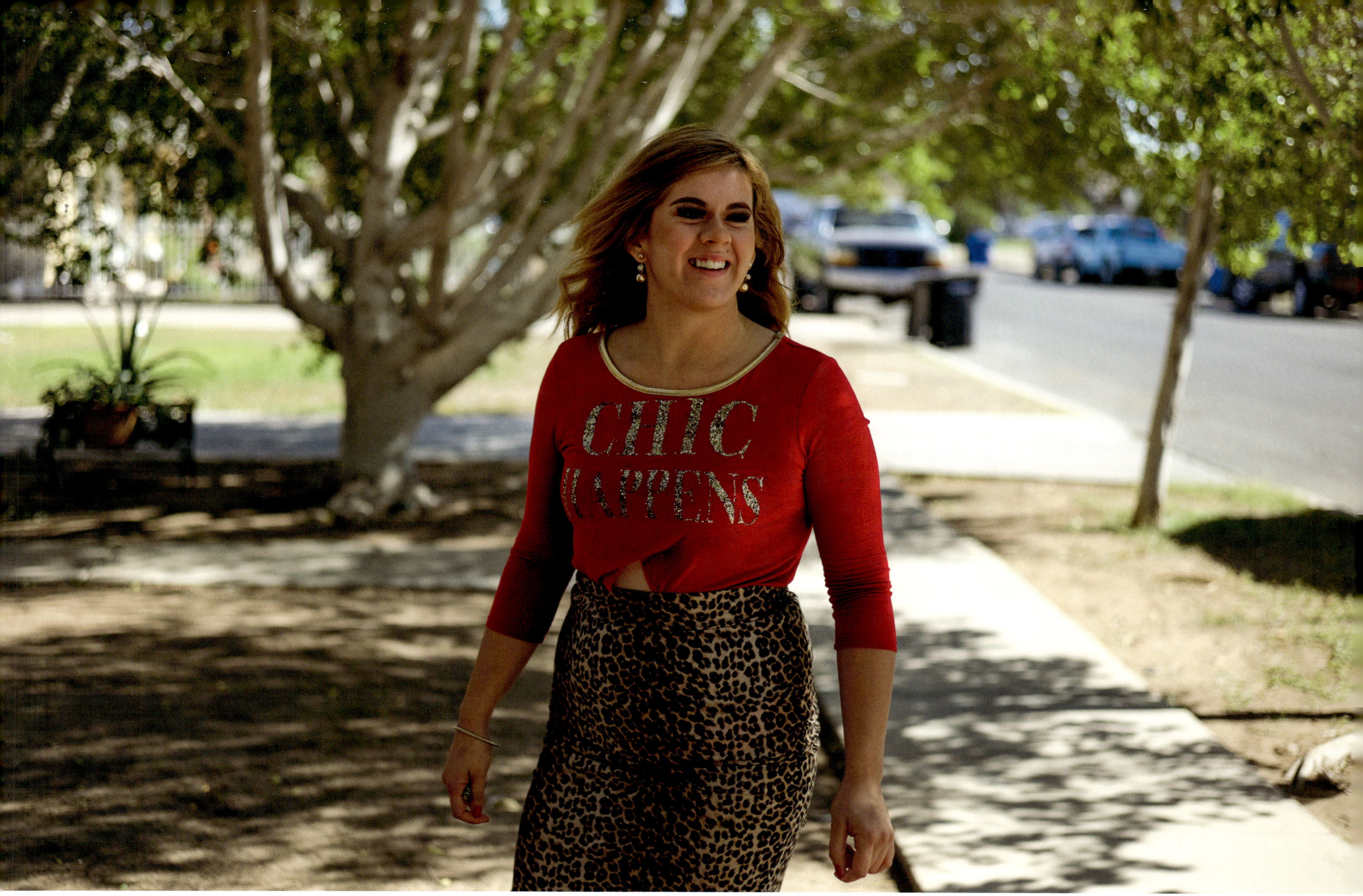

Adriana Ray, El Centro

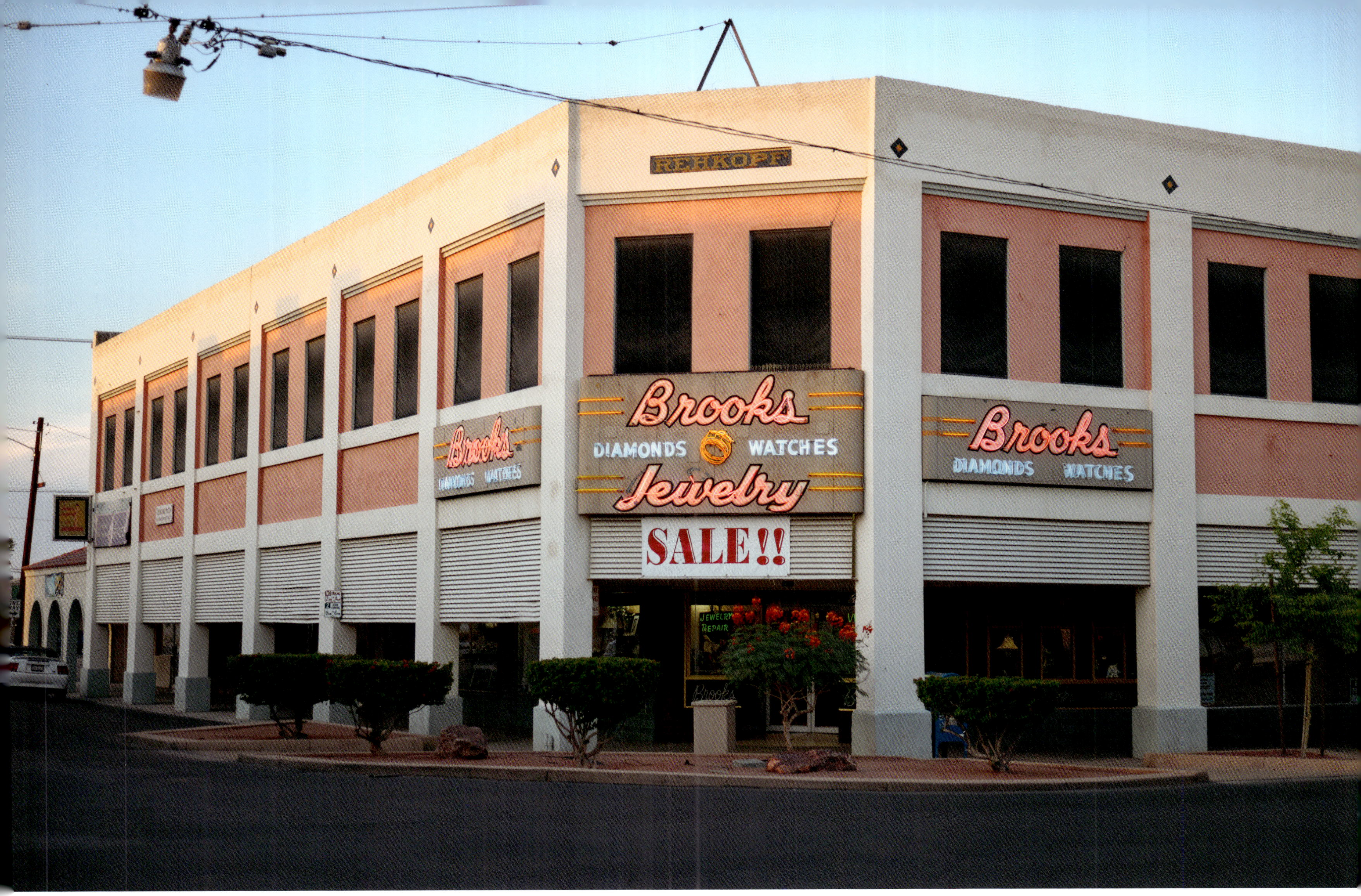

Main Street, El Centro

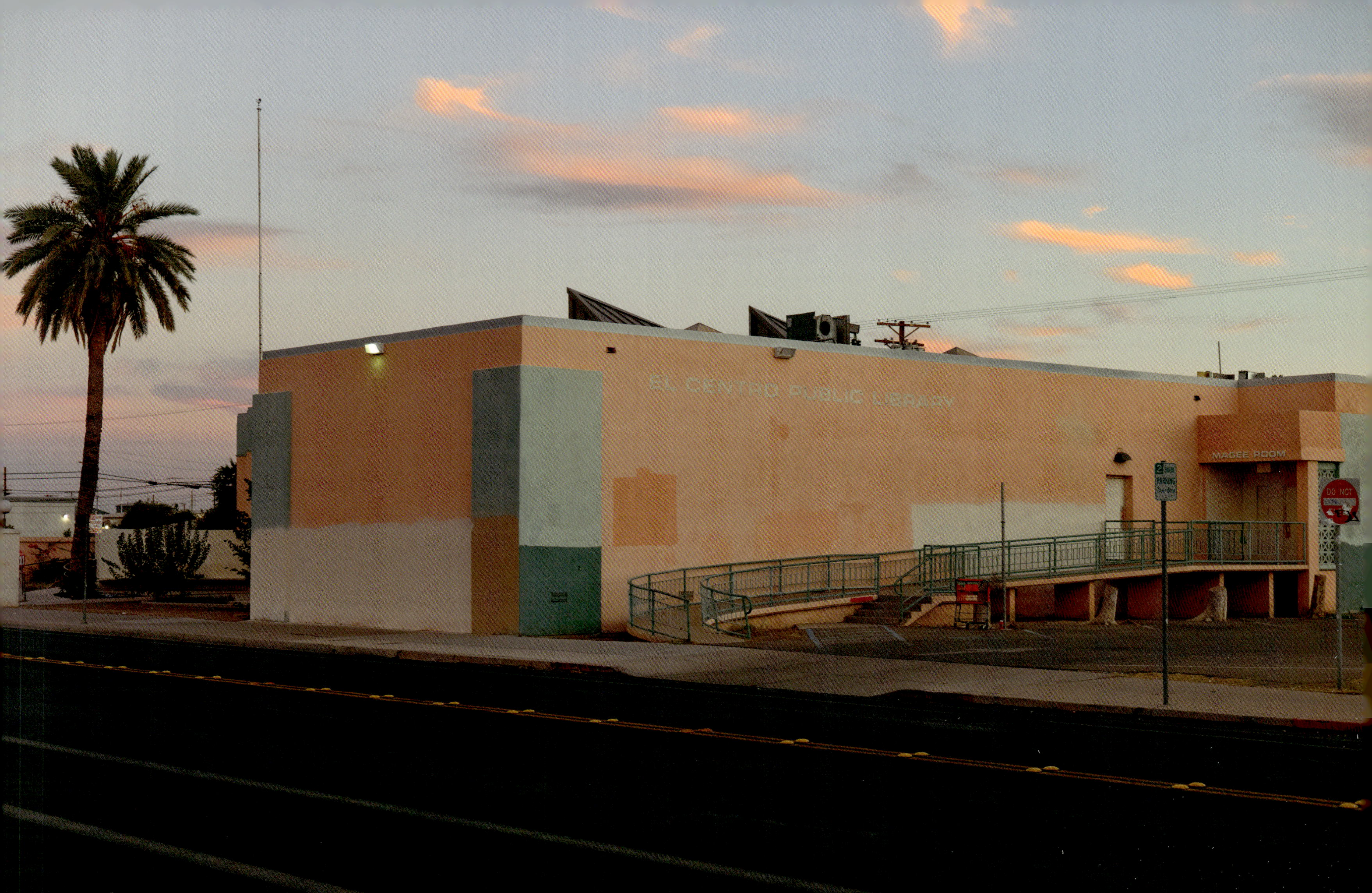

State Street, El Centro

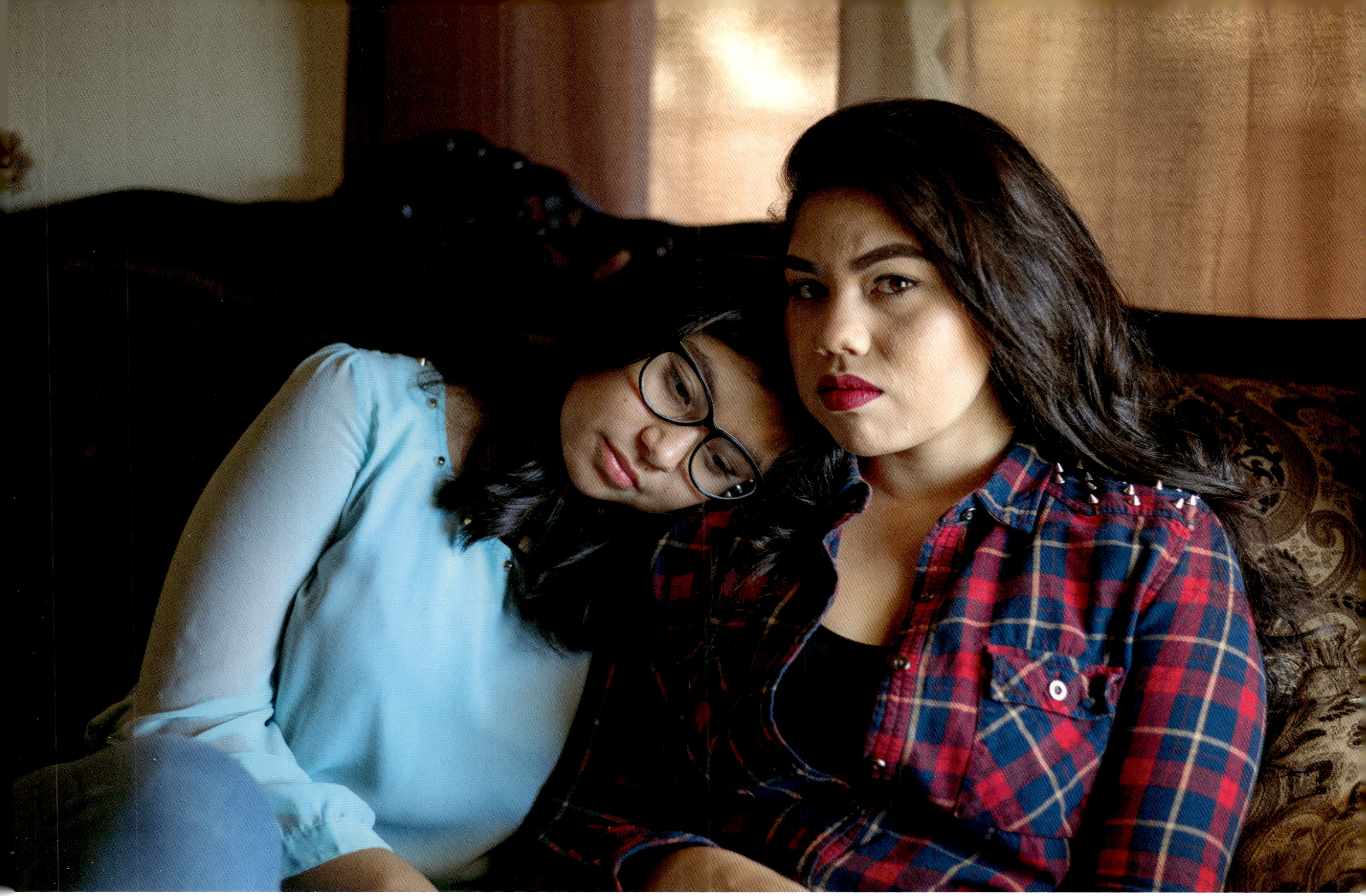

Estrella and Alejandra, Holtville

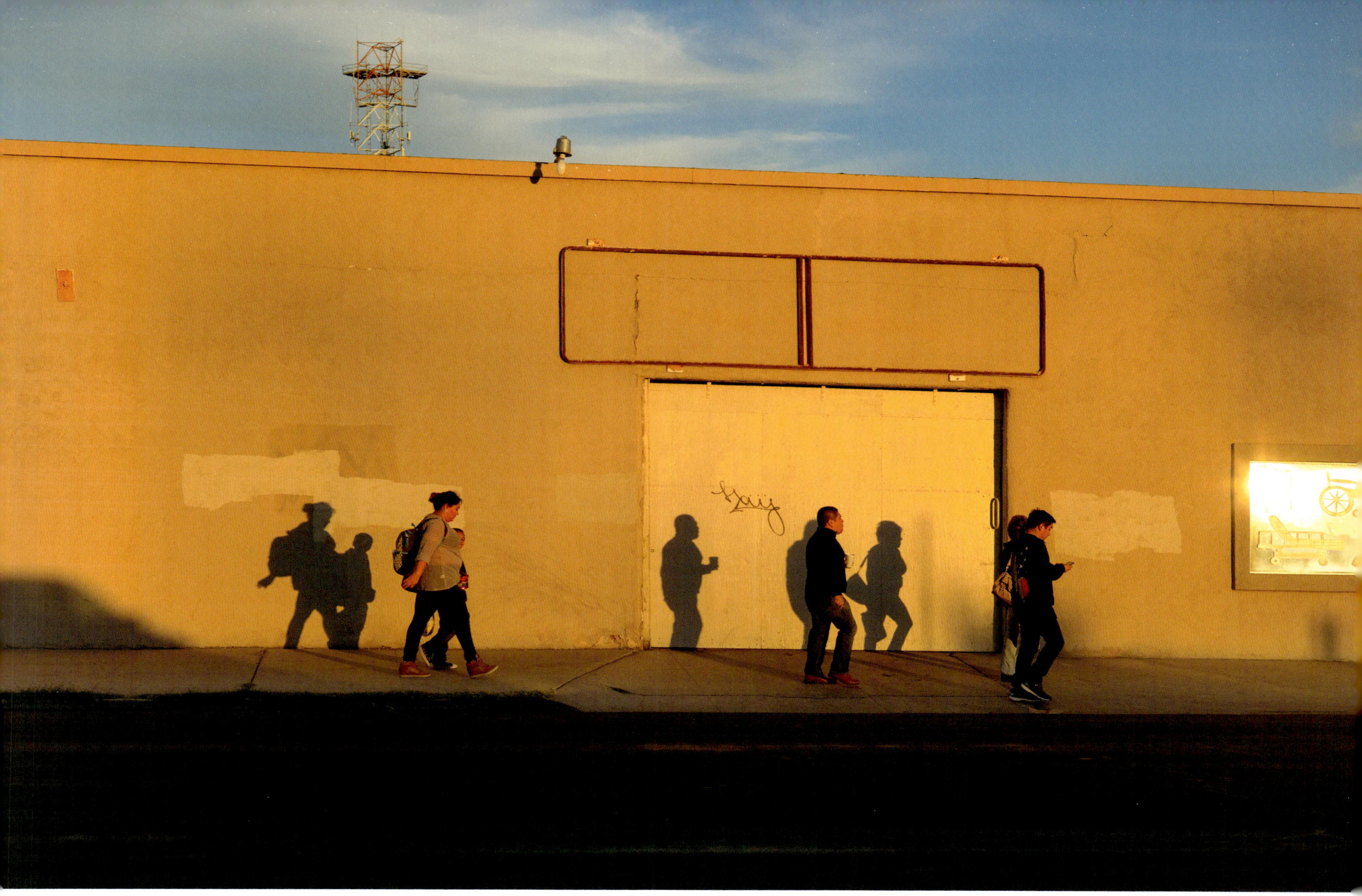

Border Park, Calexico

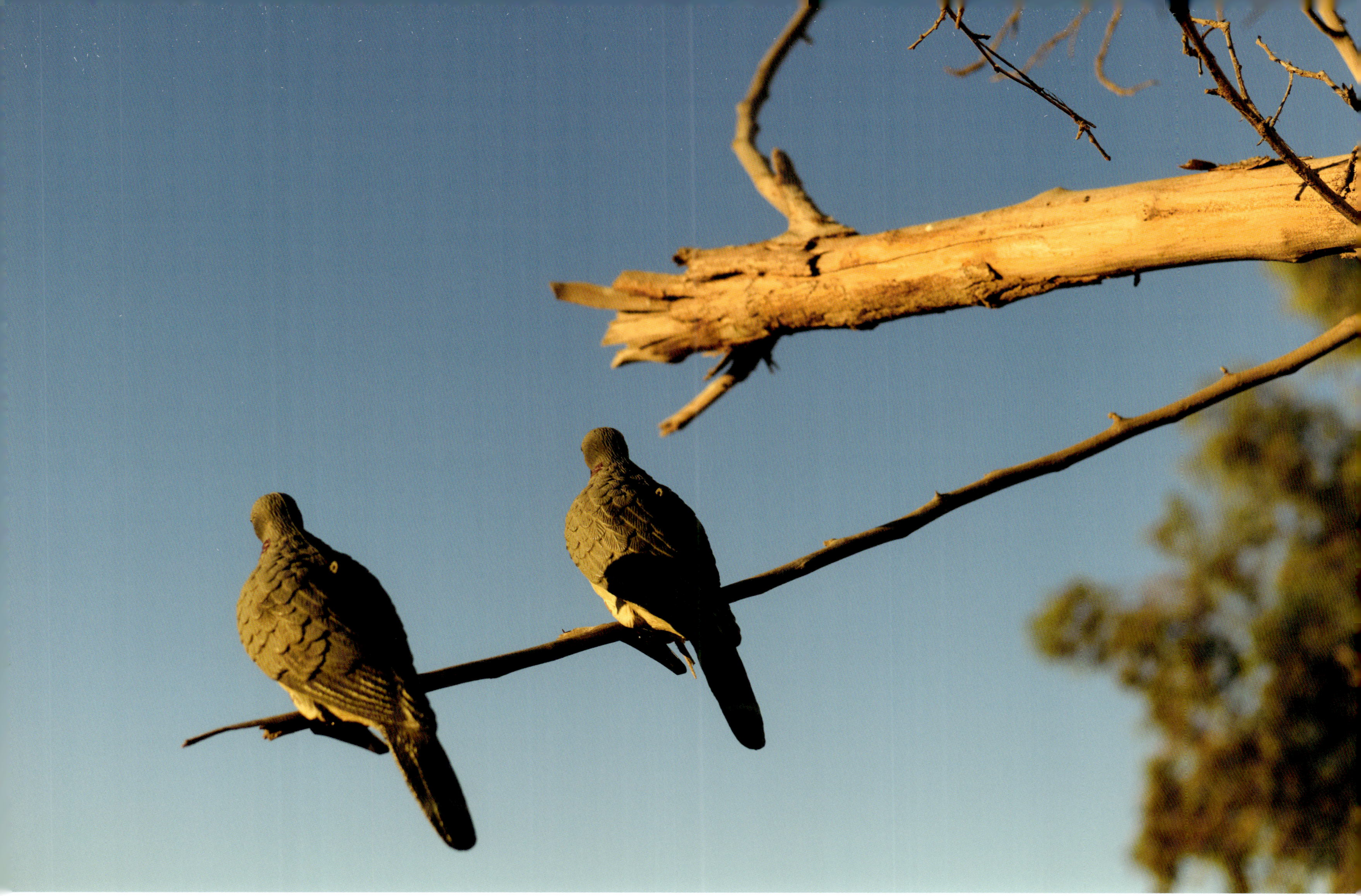

Fake pigeons, Heber

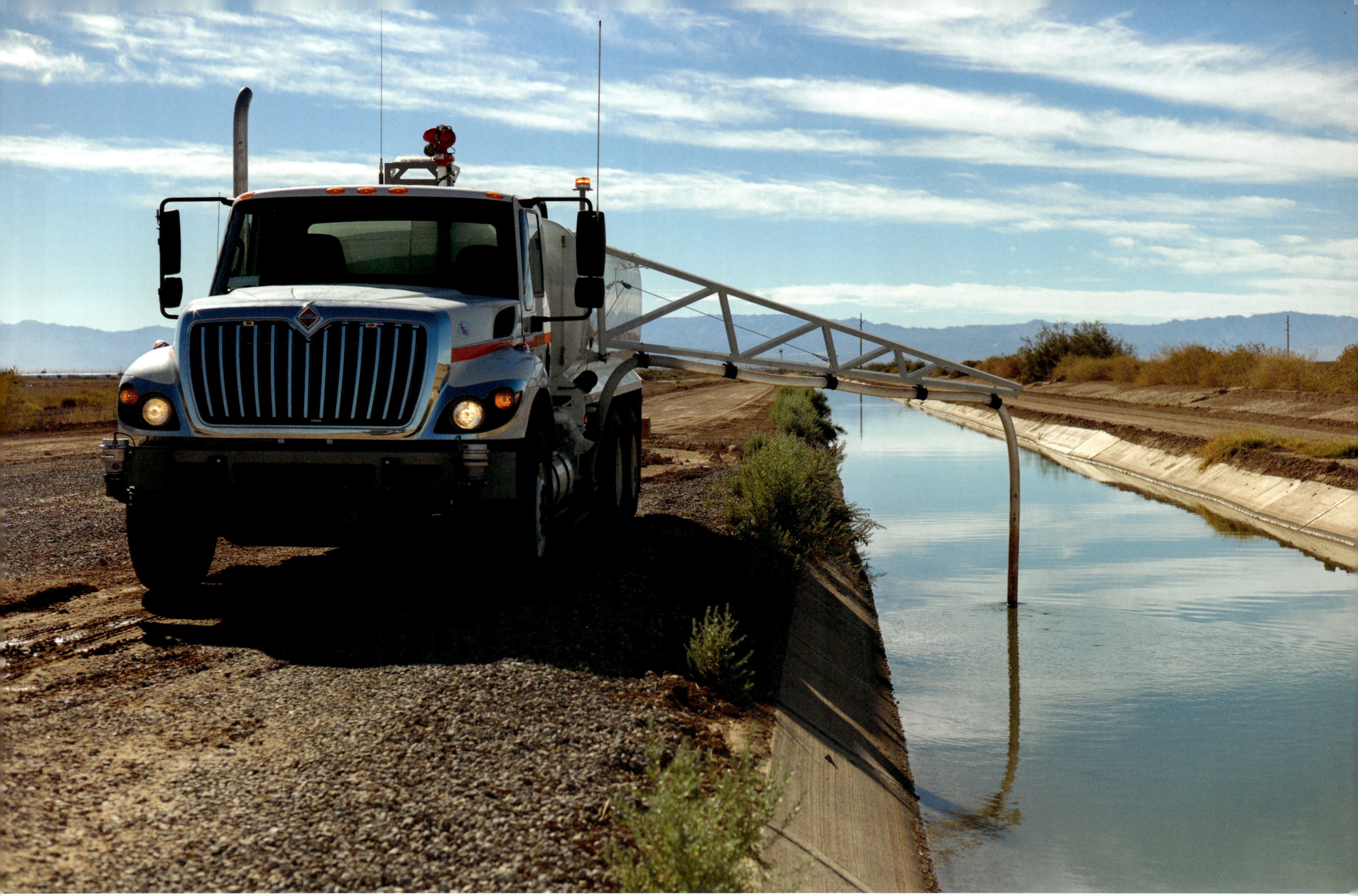

Water Tank Vehicle, Superstition

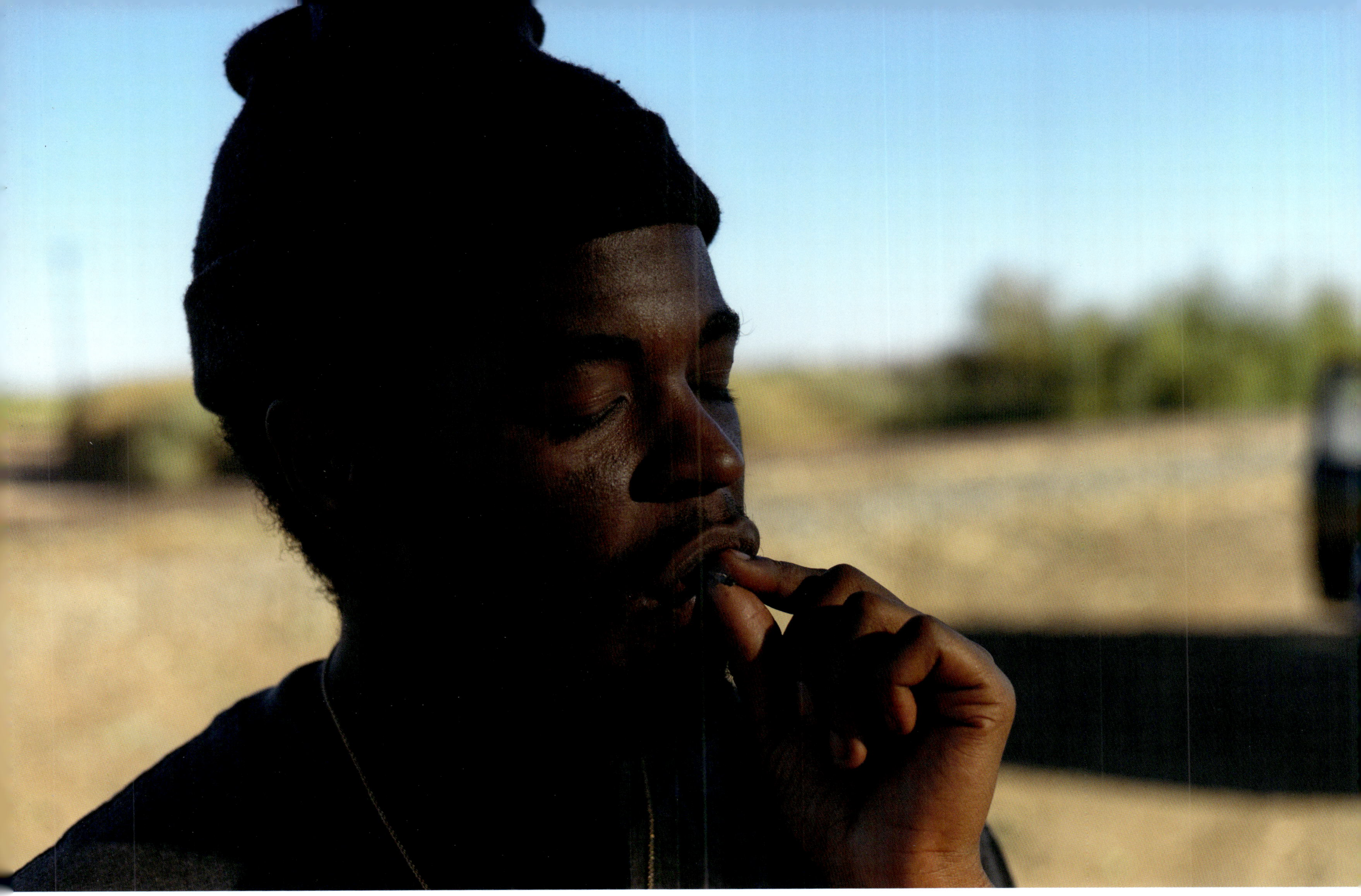

Shedon by the All-American-Canal, Heber

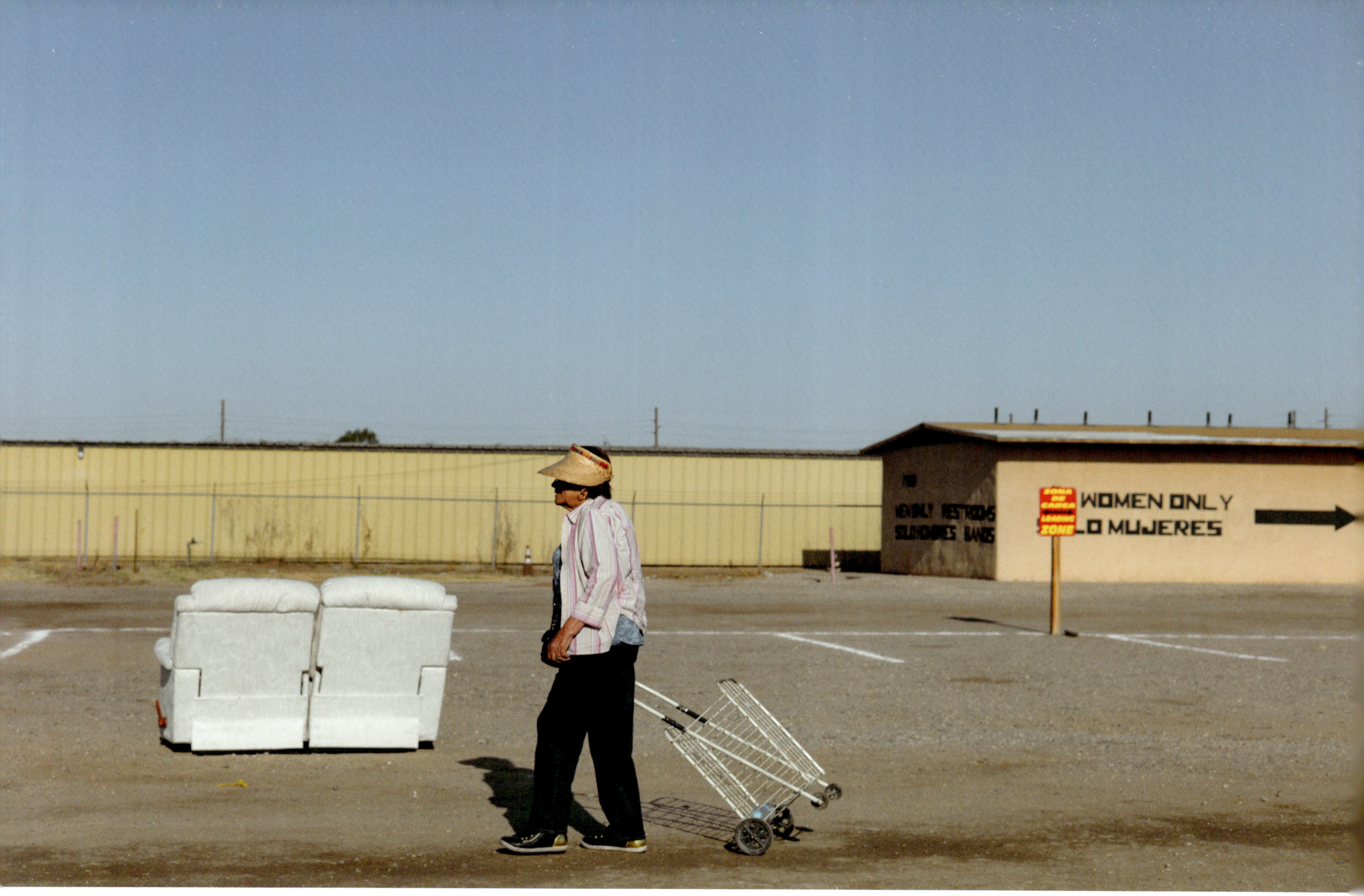

Carmen at the Santo Tomas Swap Meet, Calexico

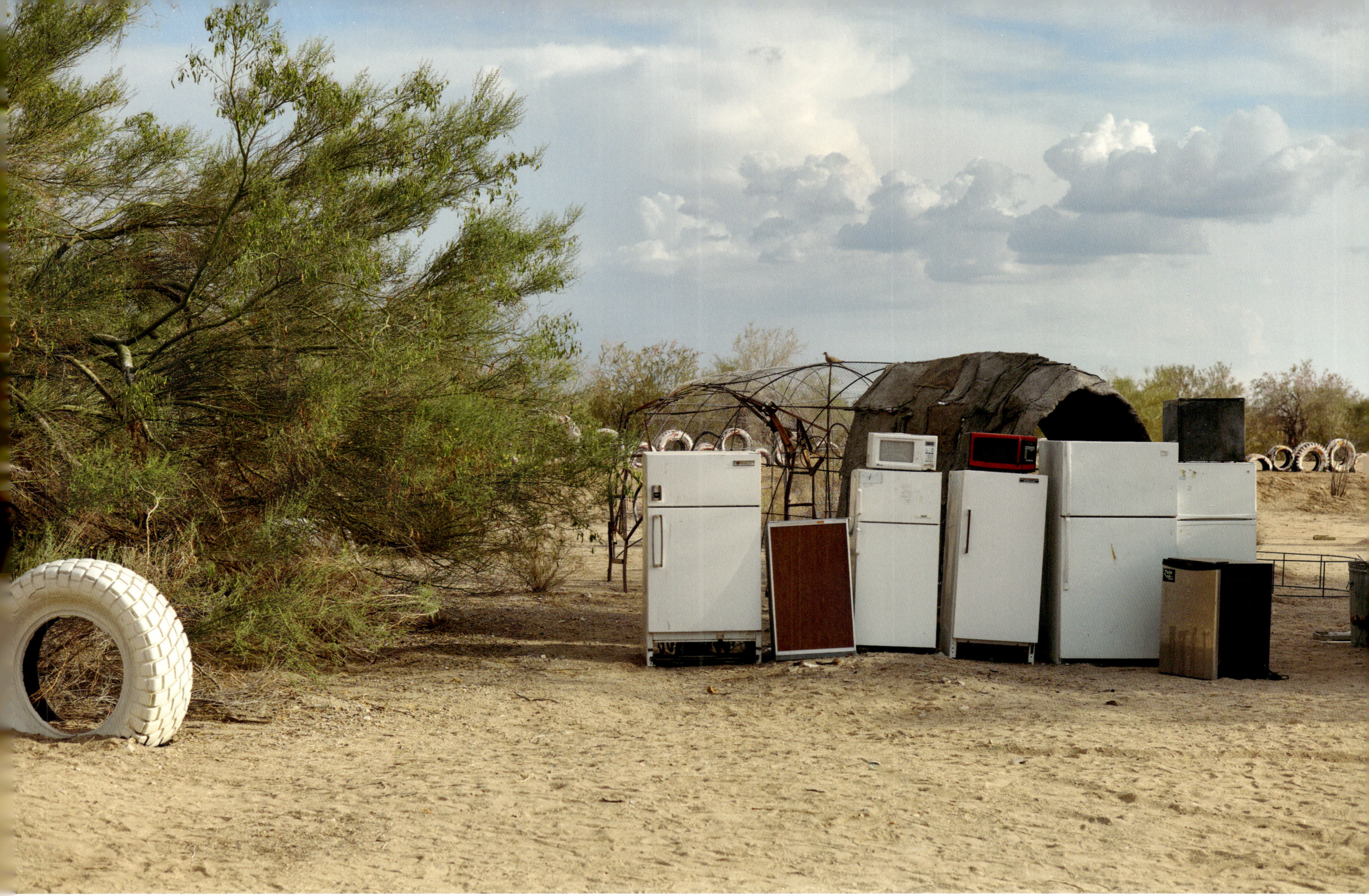

Art installation, East Jesus

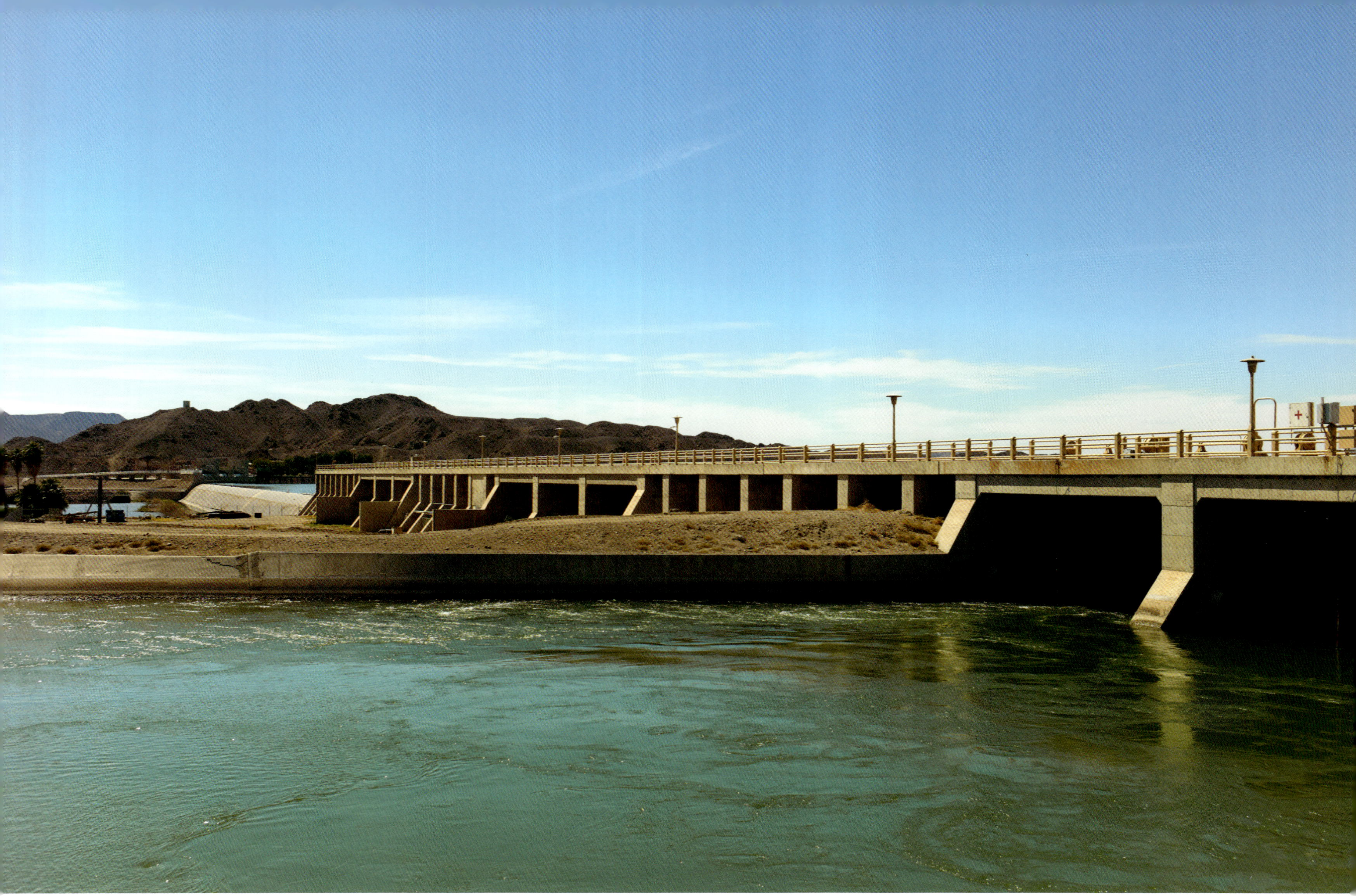

The Imperial Dam, Senator Wash

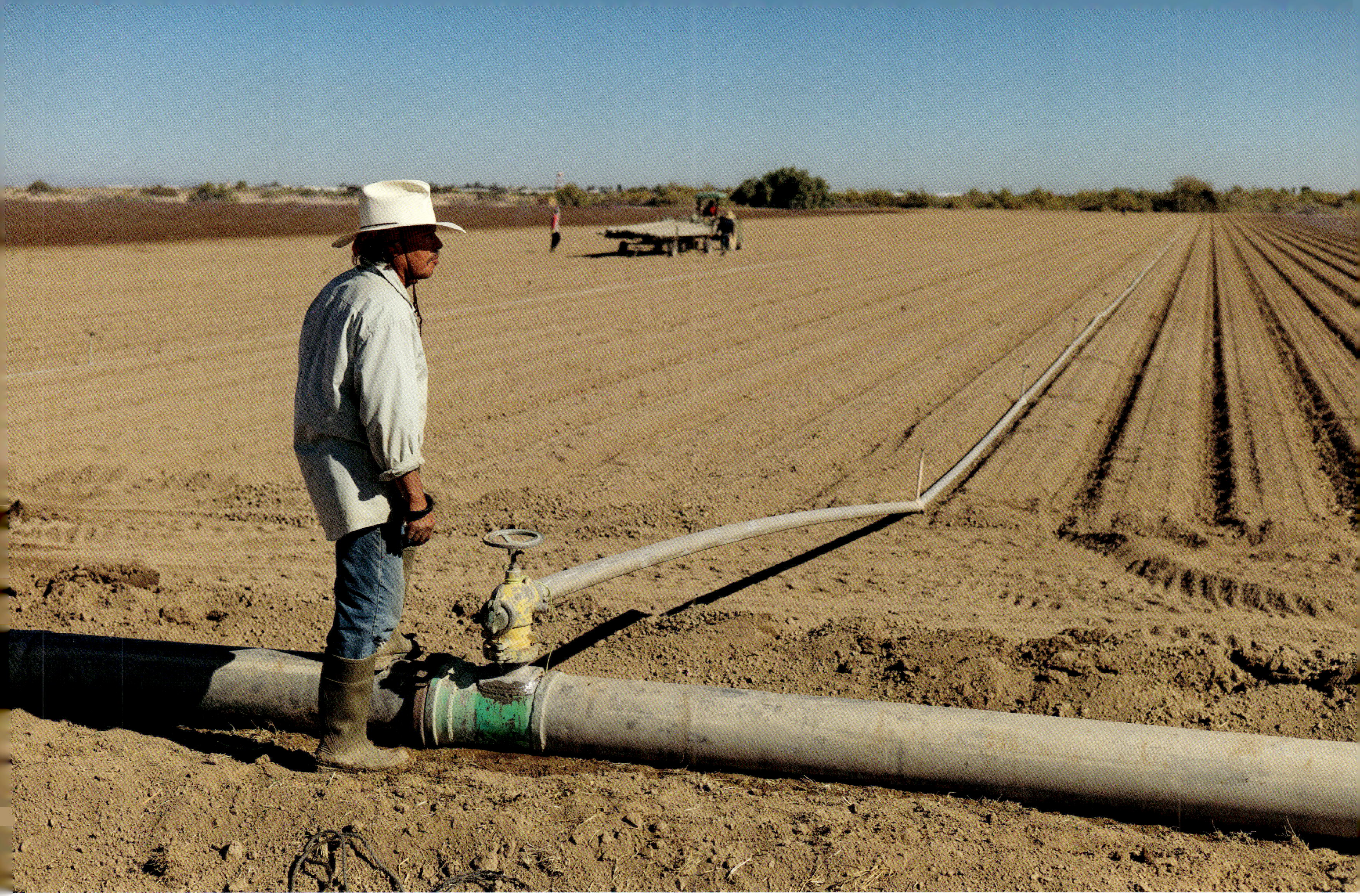

Installing irrigation pipes, near Naval Air Facility

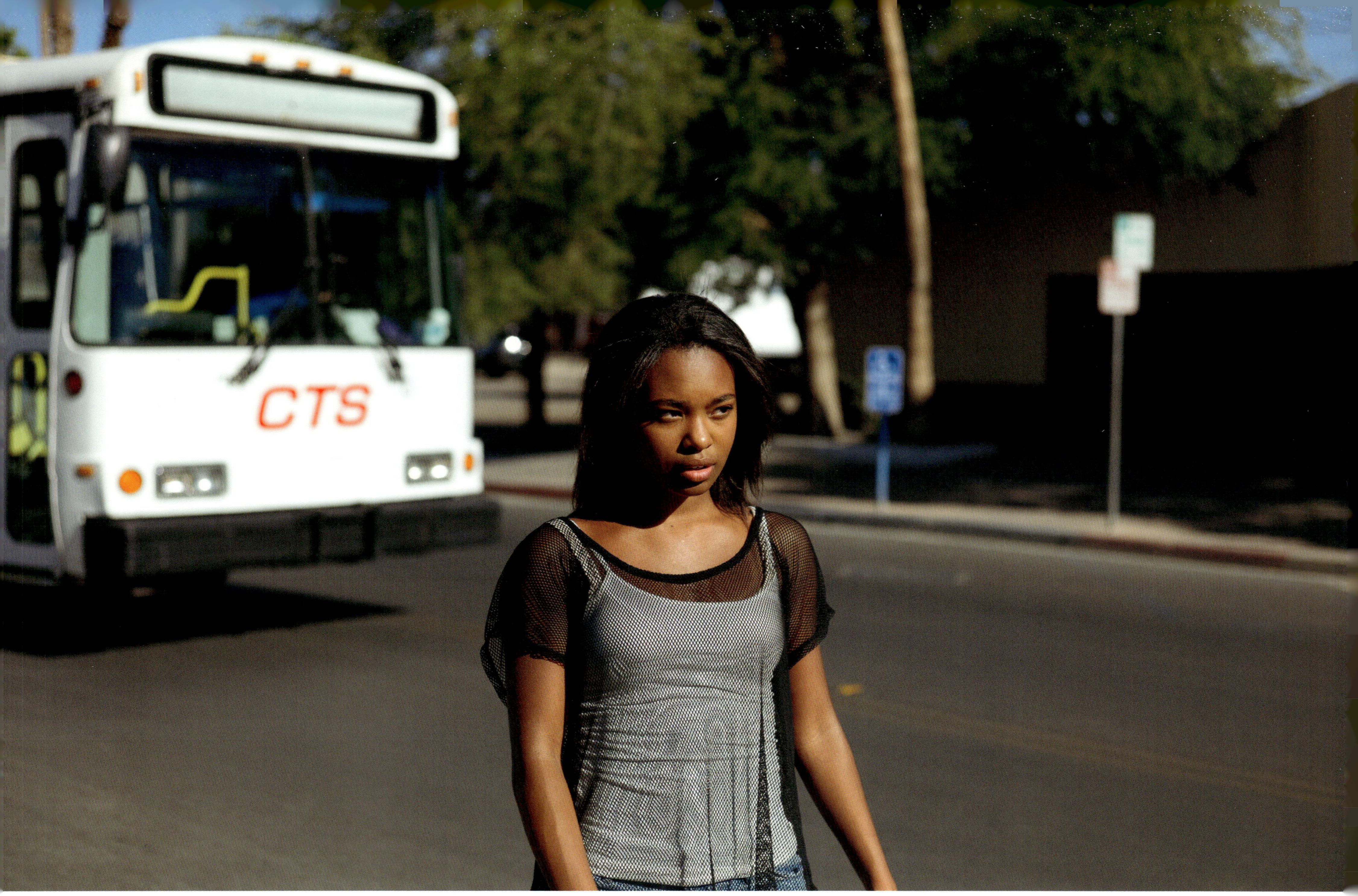

Zaria at the bus stop, Calexico

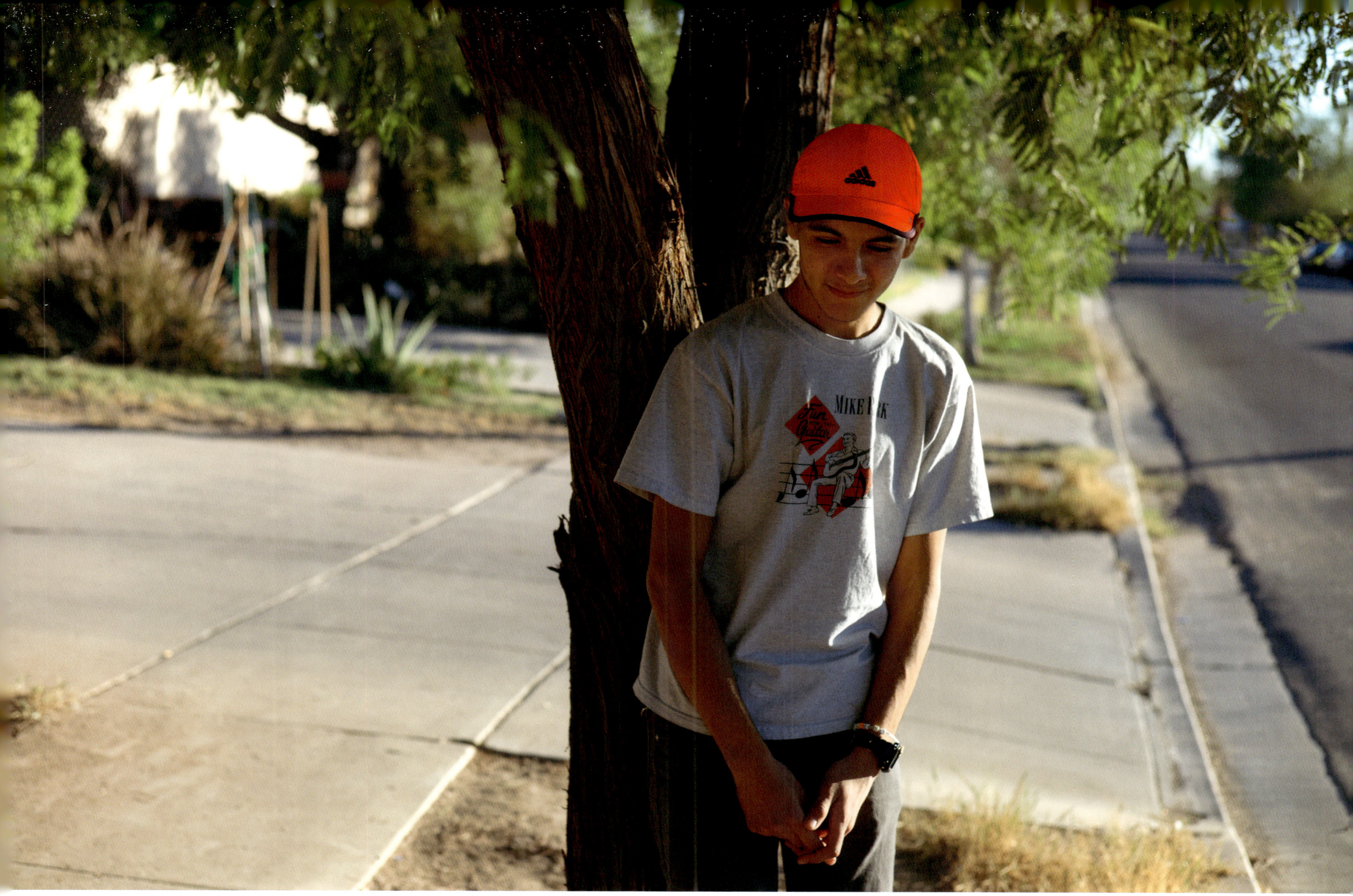

Julian, El Centro

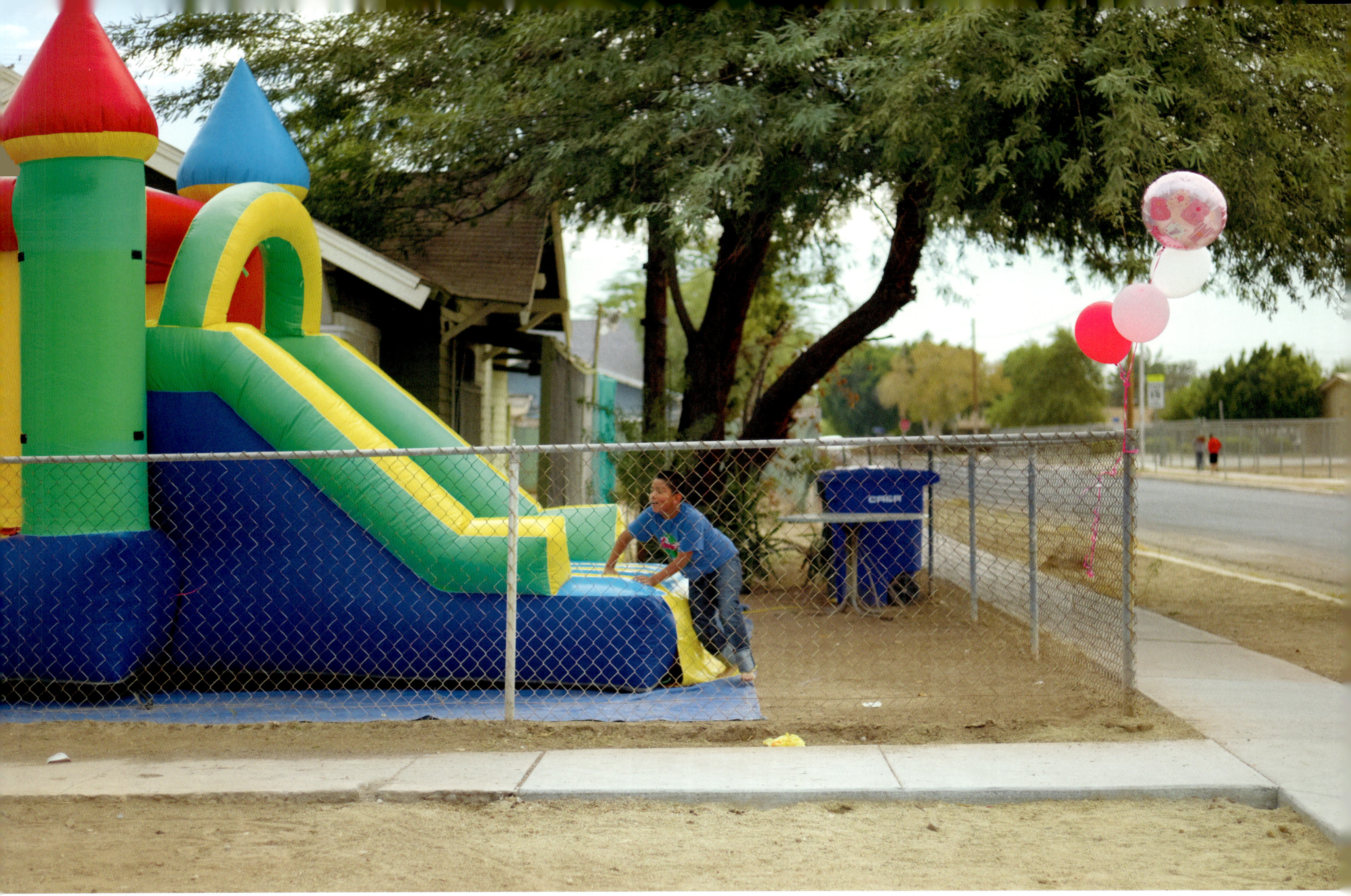

Jesus, El Centro

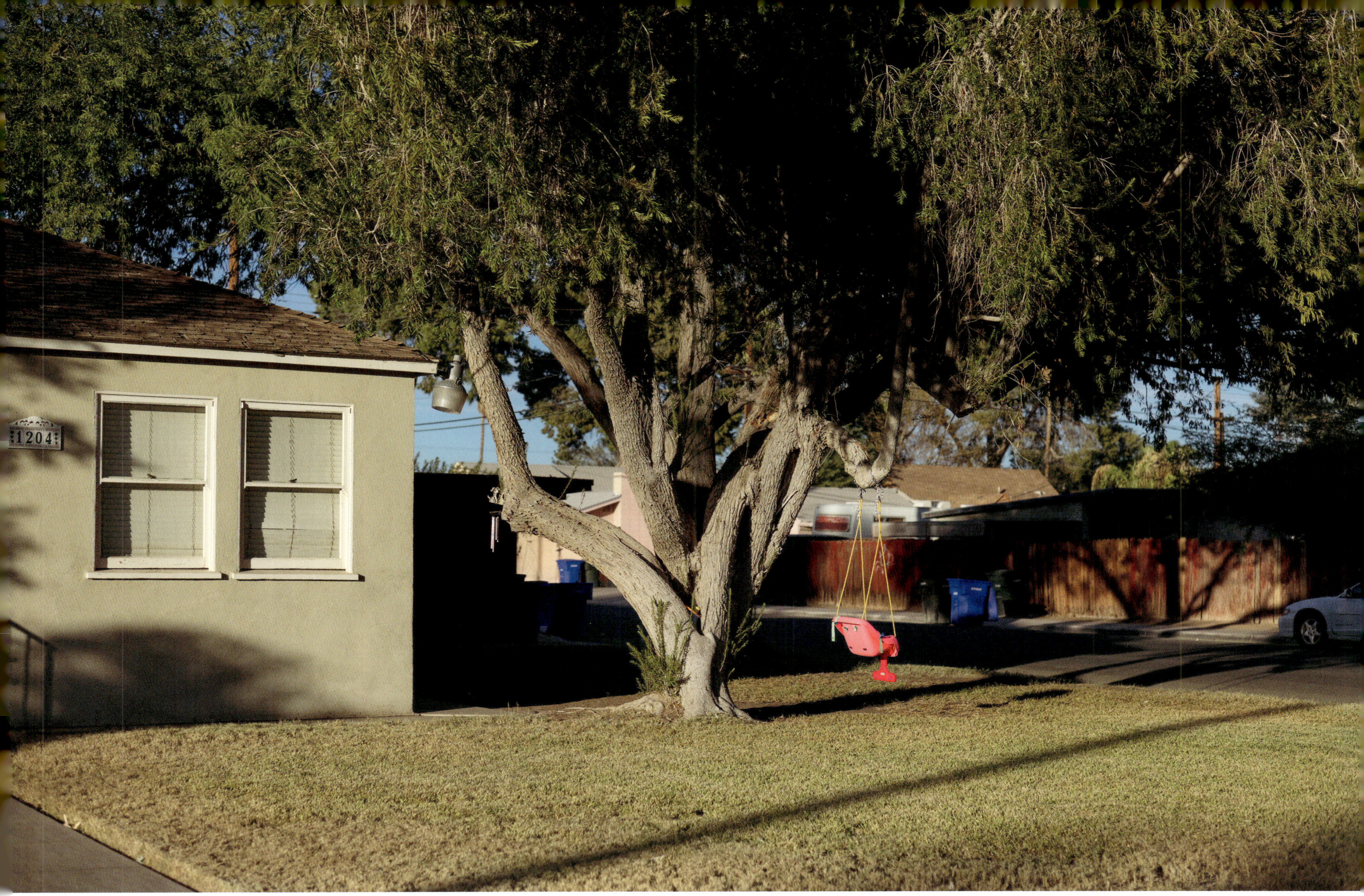

Sandalwood Drive, El Centro

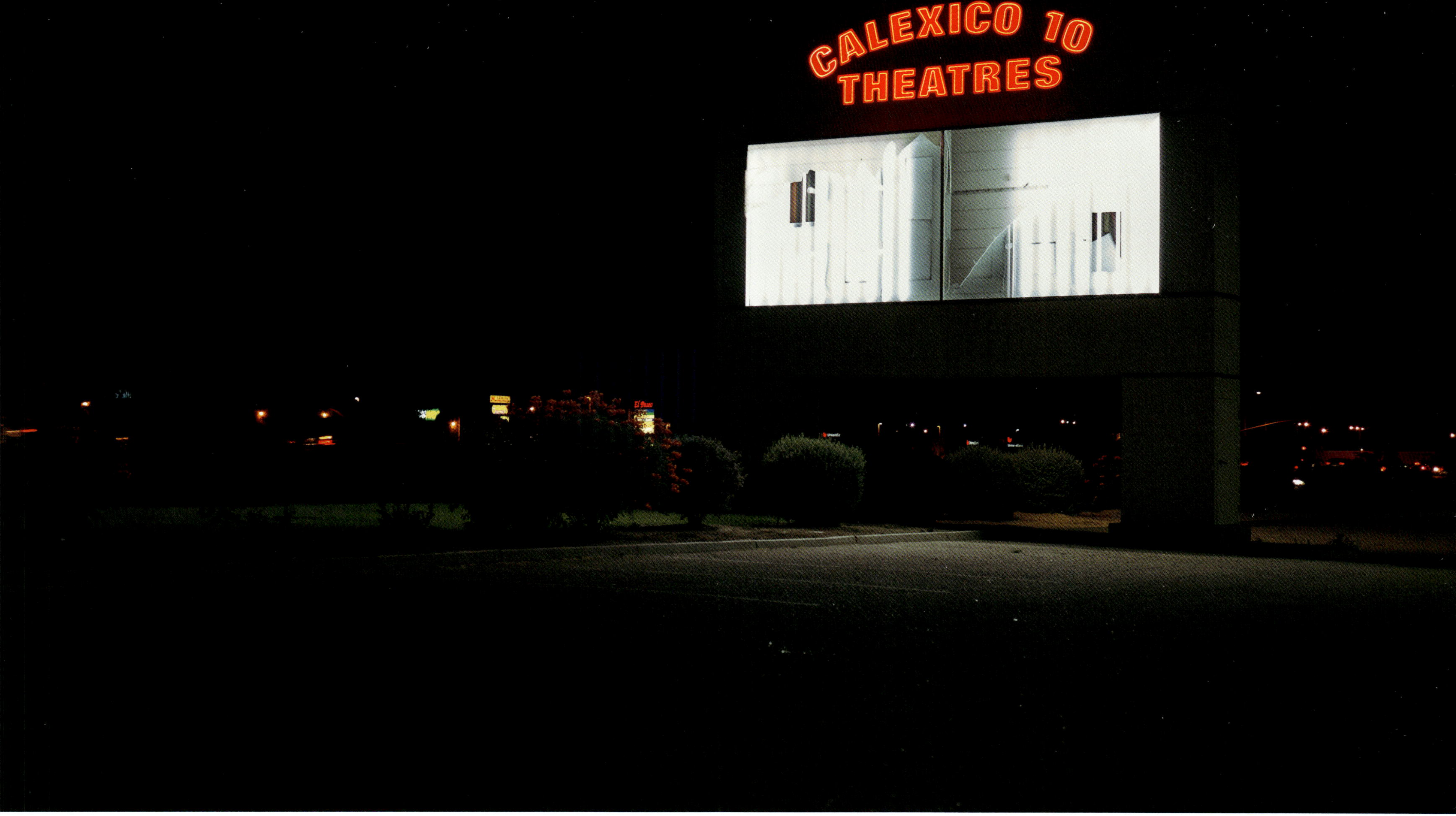

Cinema car park, El Centro

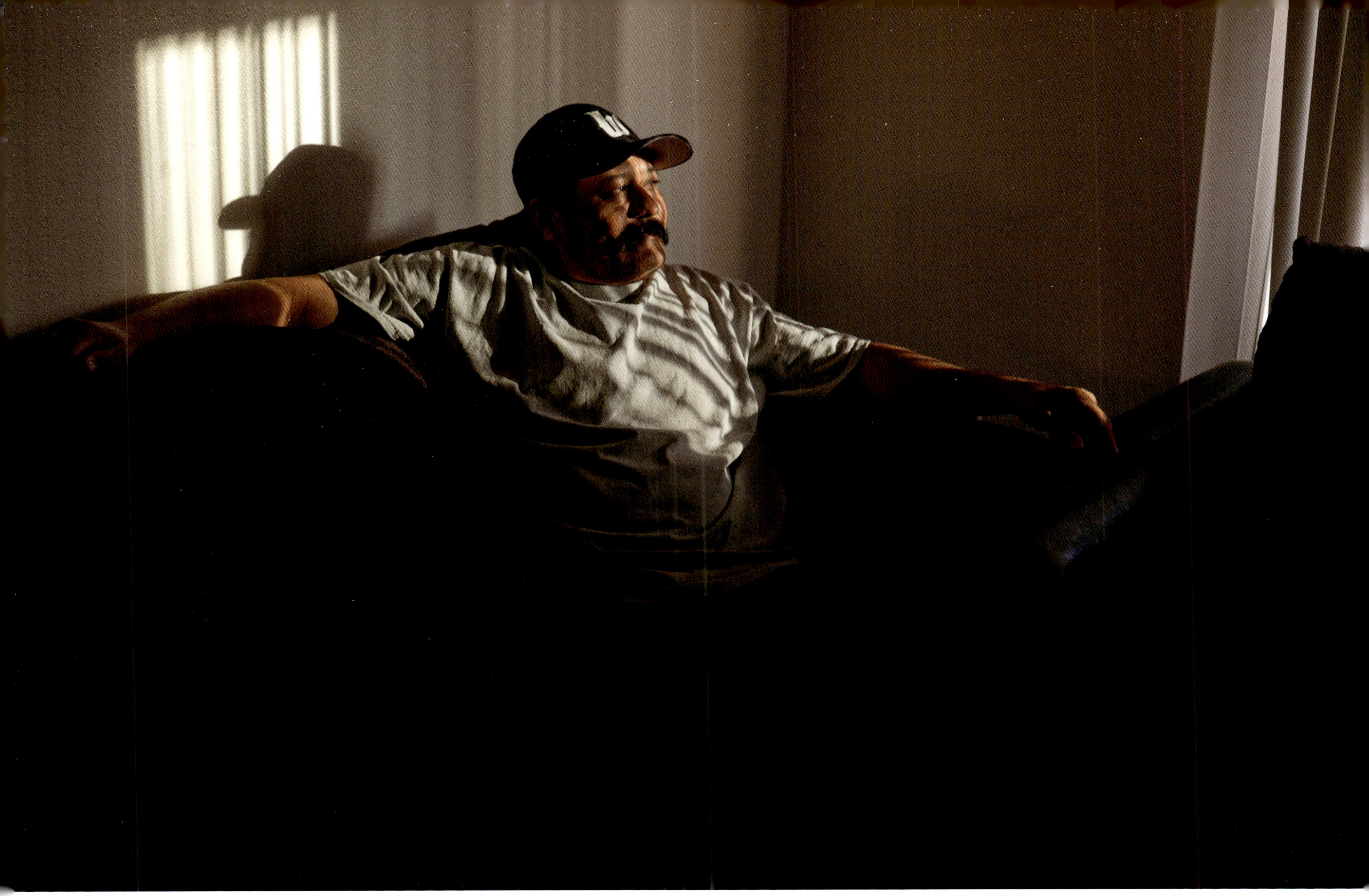

Hector senior, Calexico

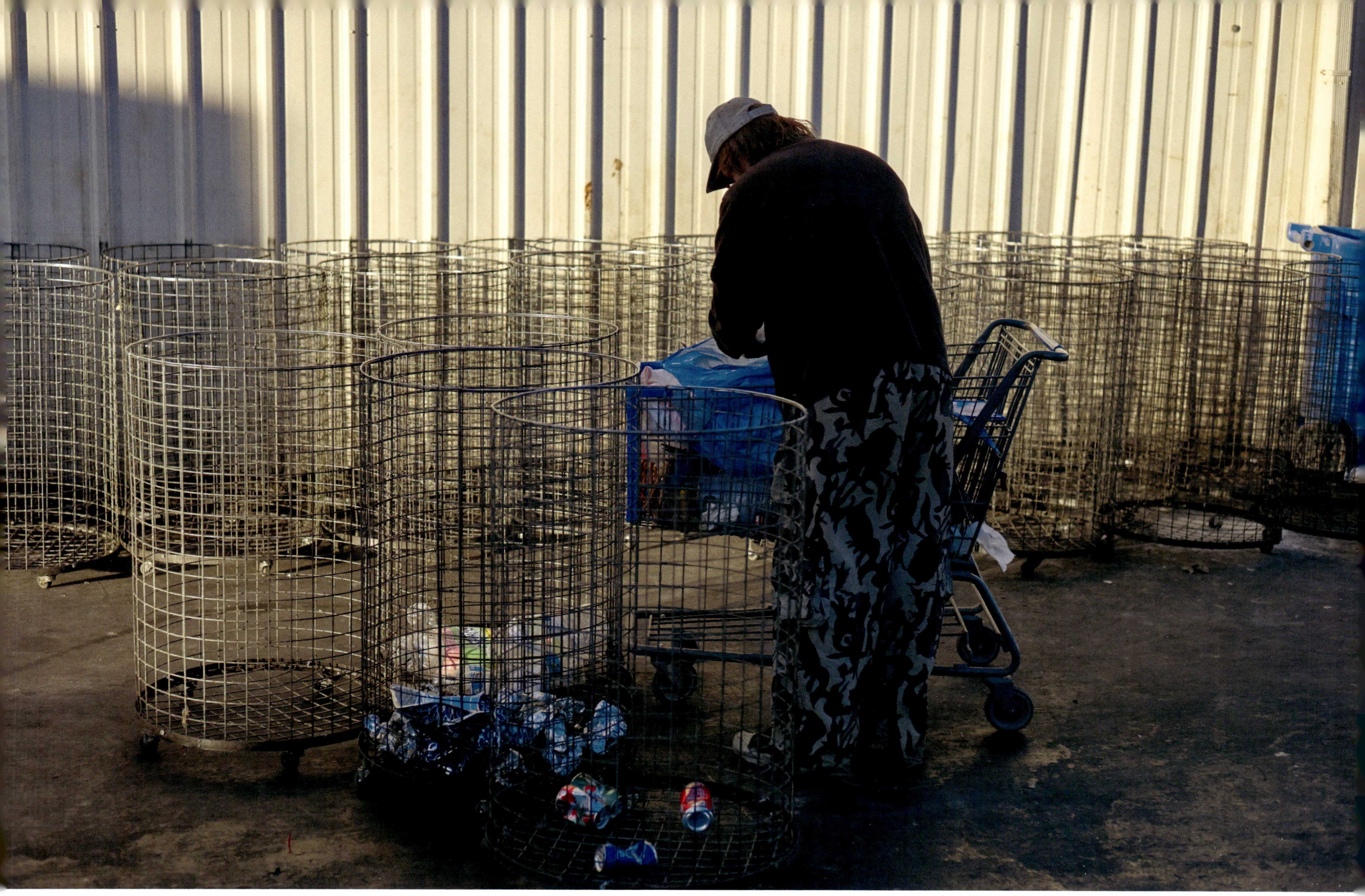

Chris at the Recycling Center, El Centro

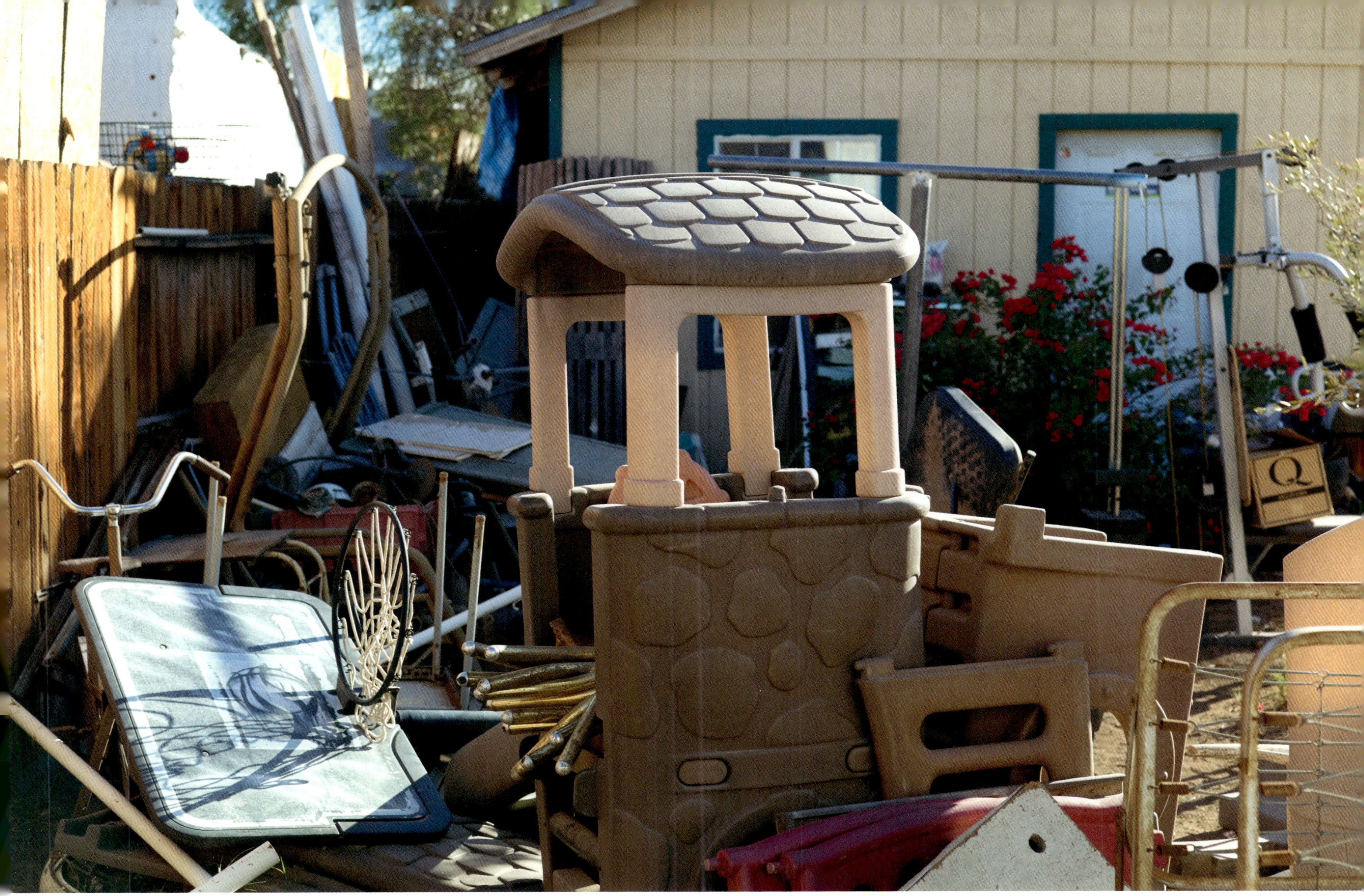

Yard, Calexico

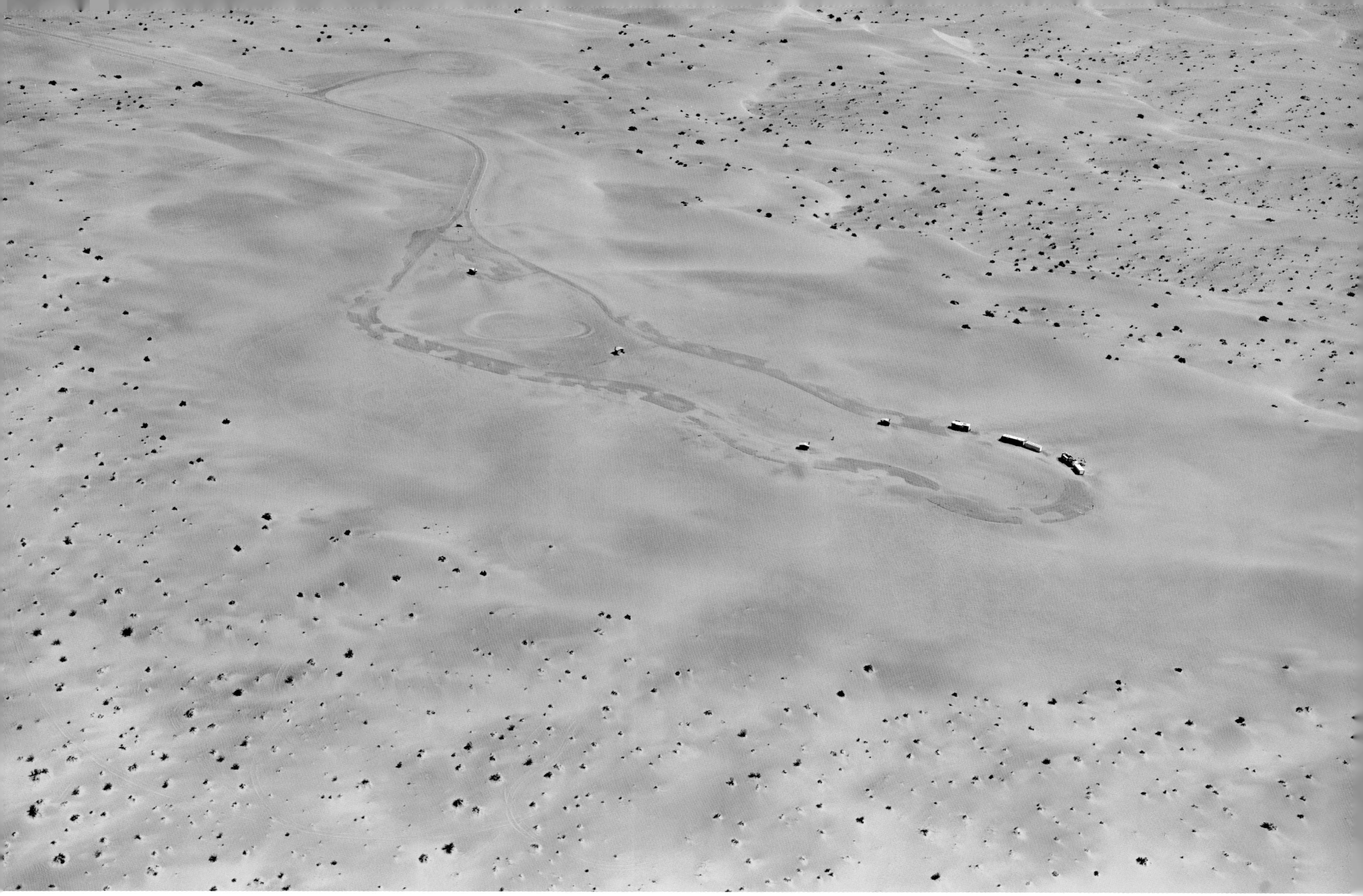

Imperial Sand Dunes Recreation Area, Glamis

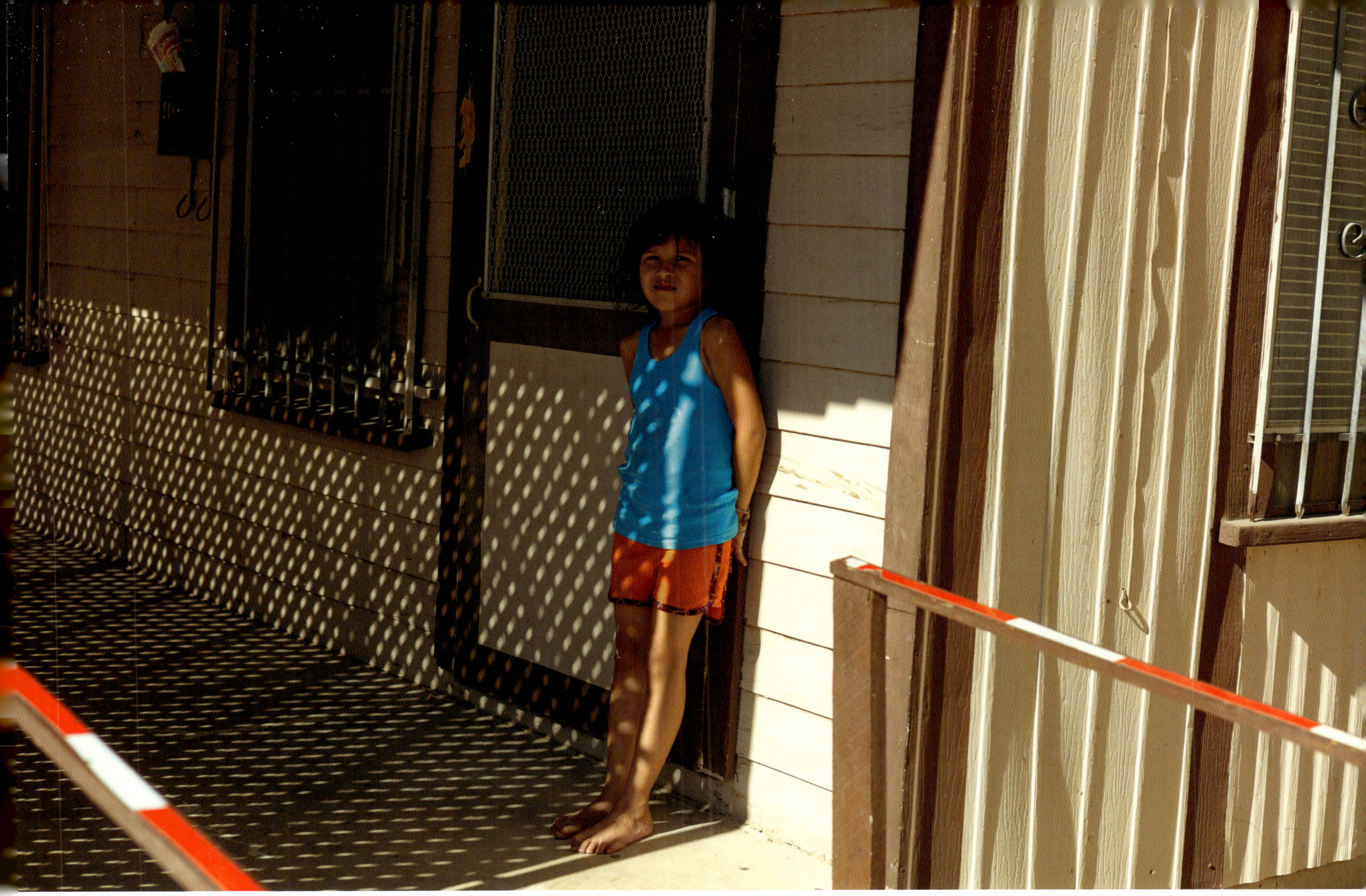

Boyd, Calexico

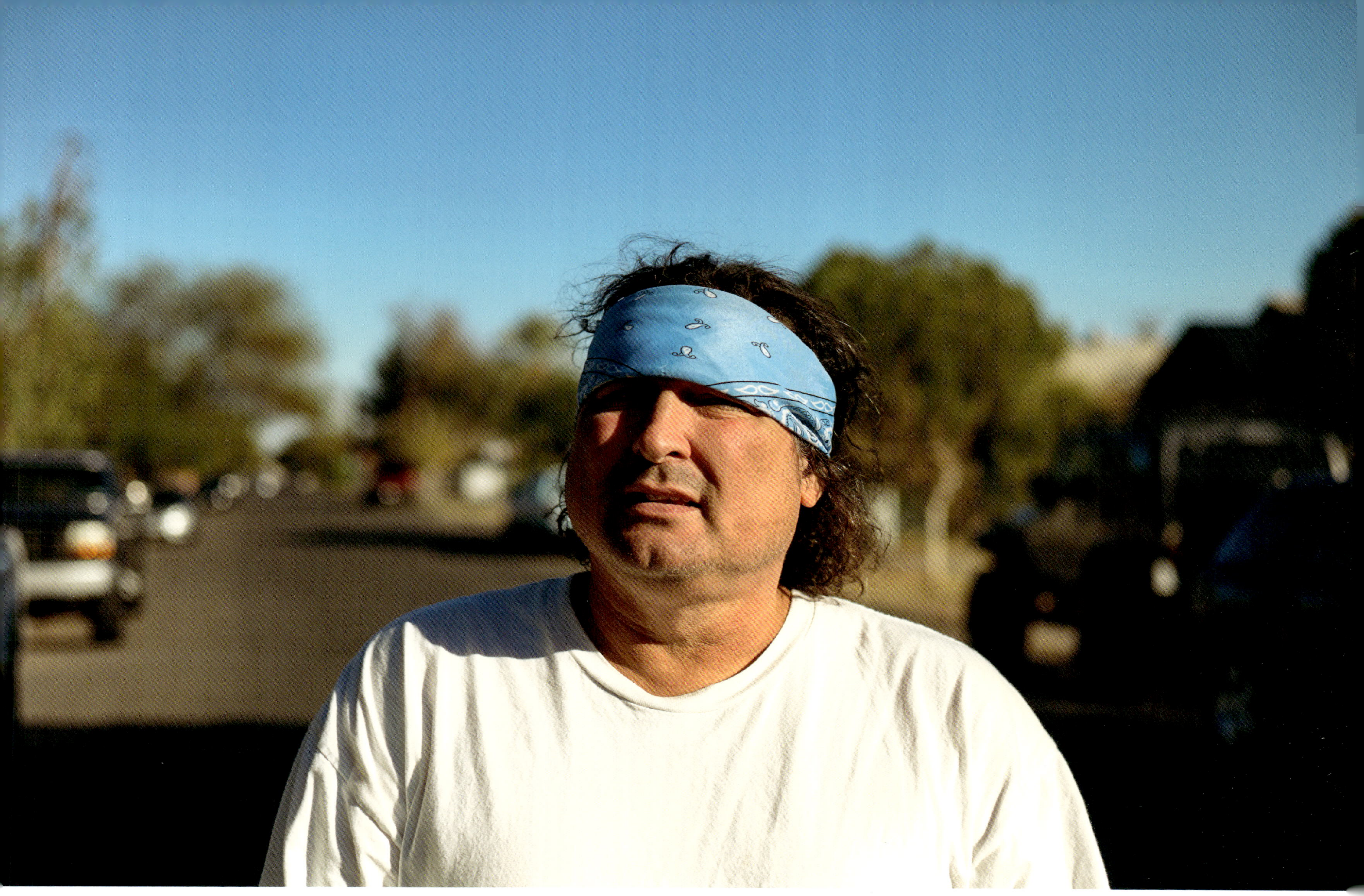

Moonie, El Centro

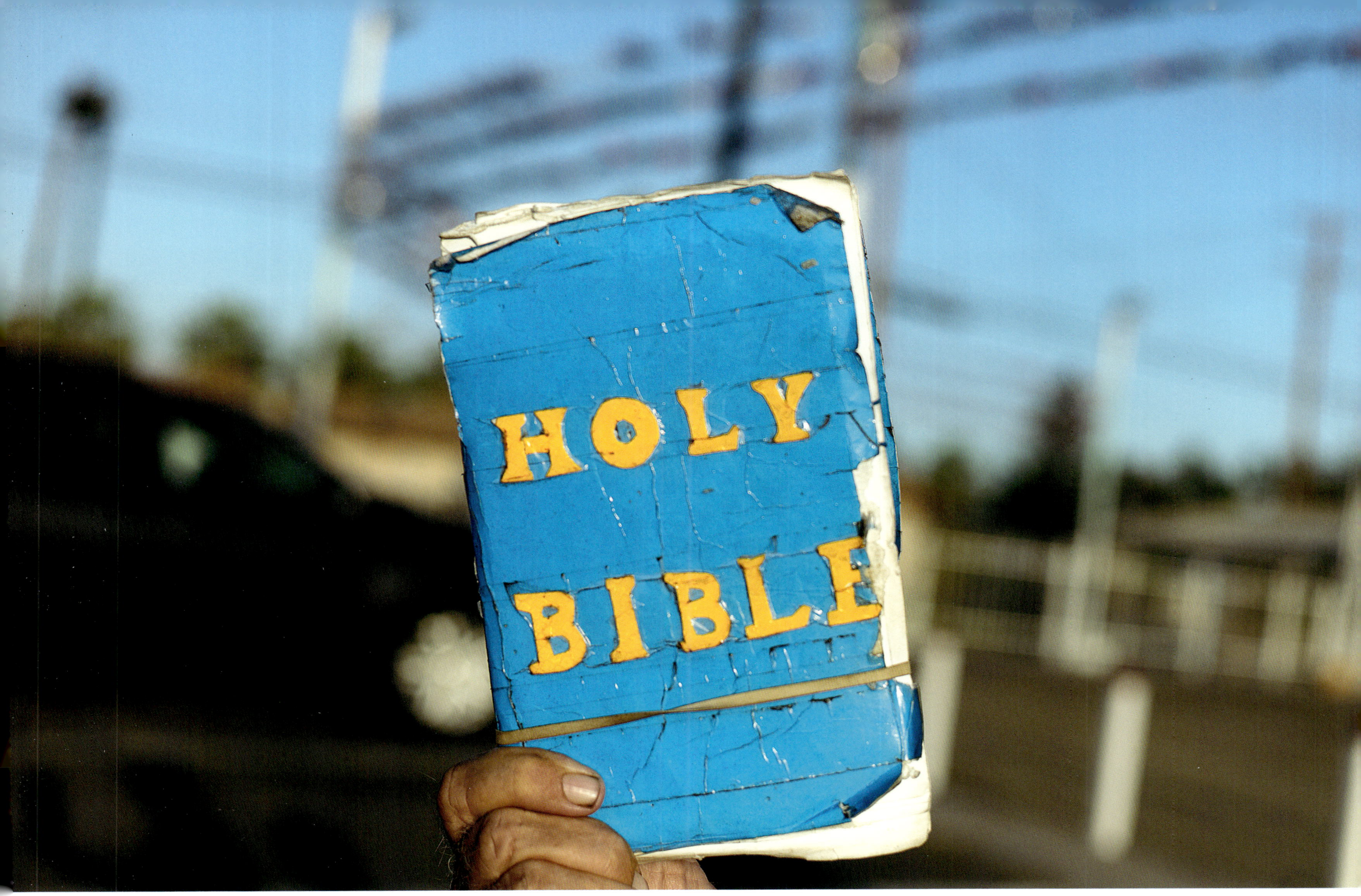

Missionary's Bible, Imperial

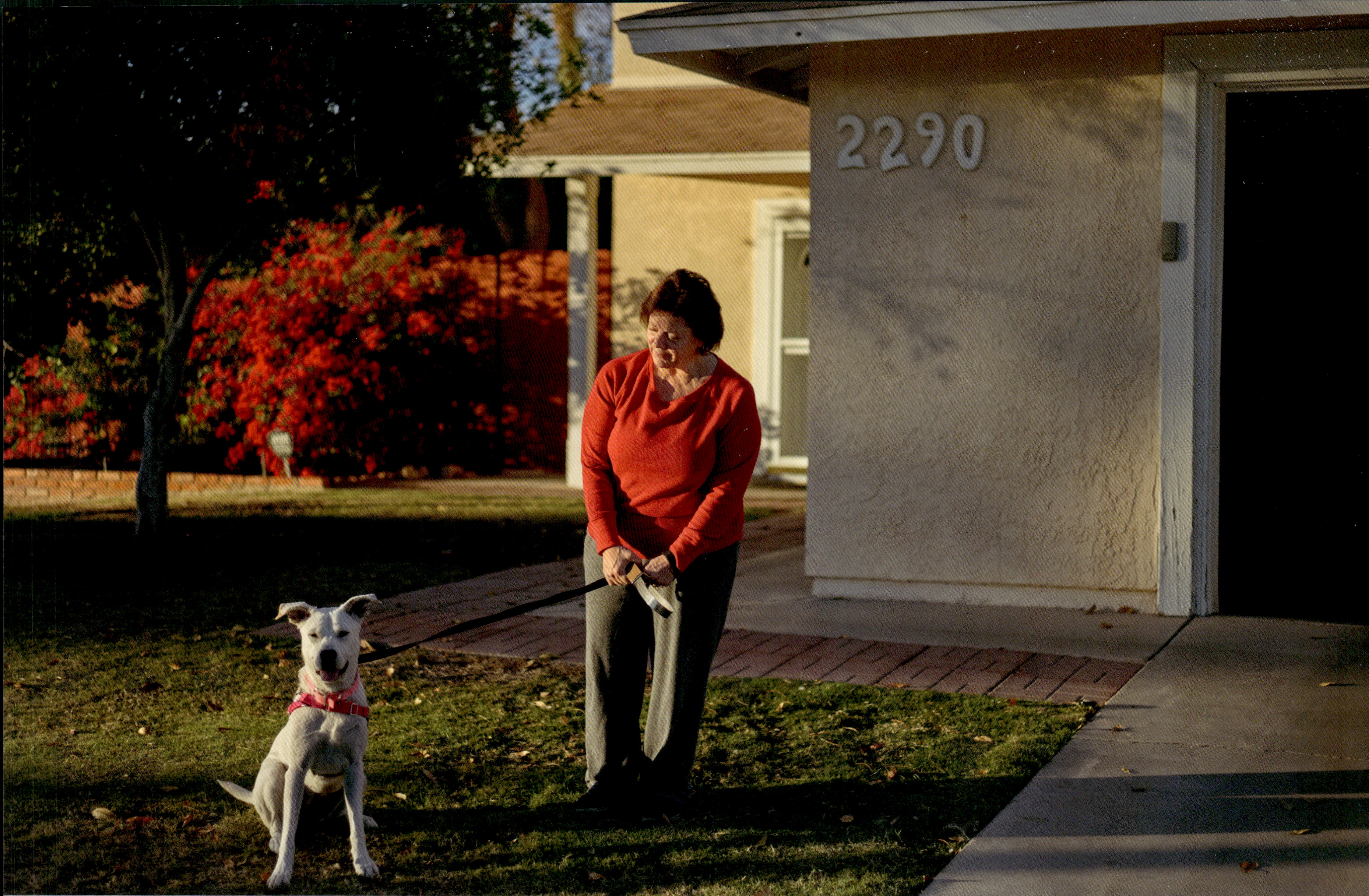

Stefanie and Brian, El Centro

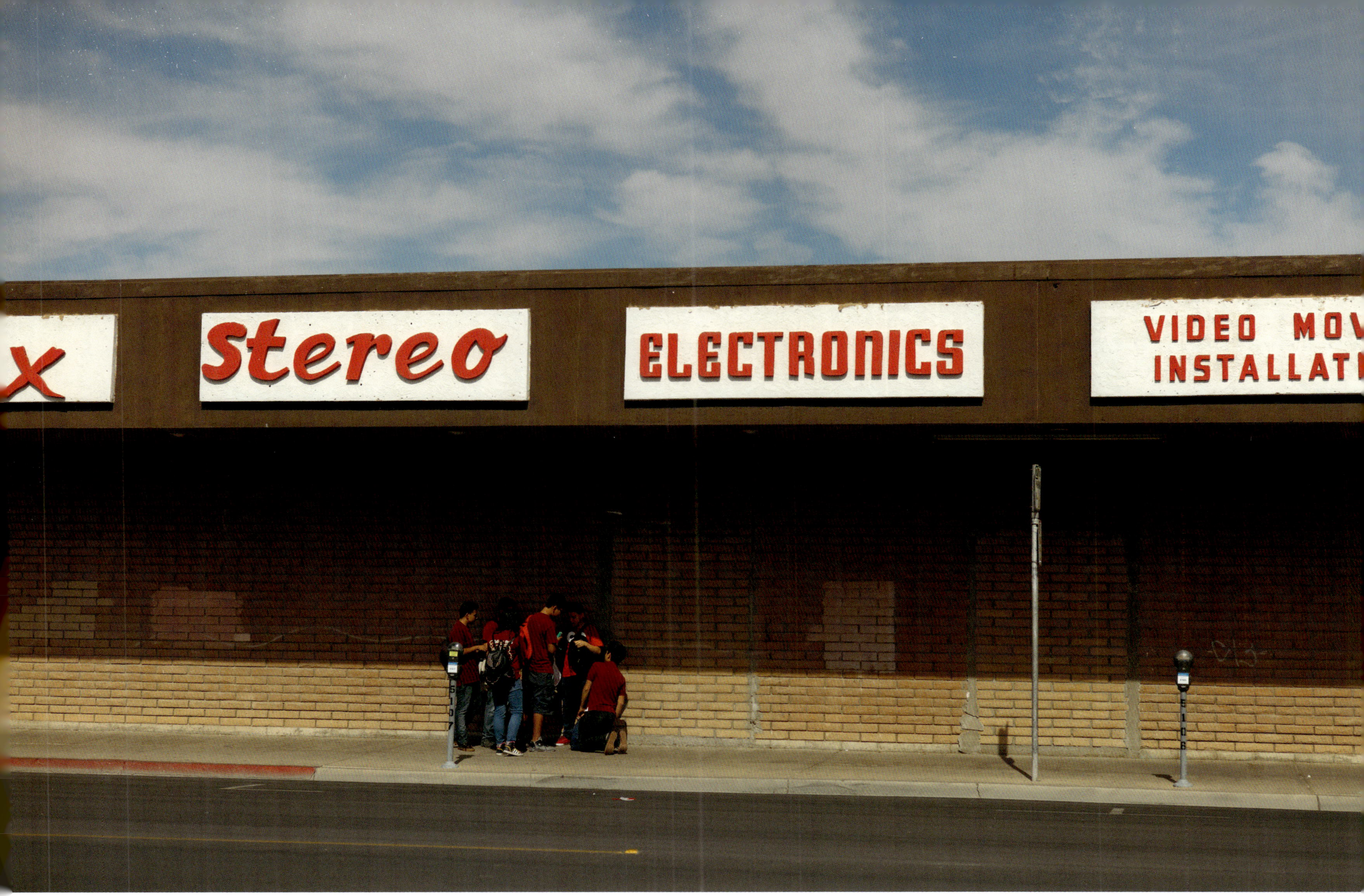

Closed down electronics store, Calexico

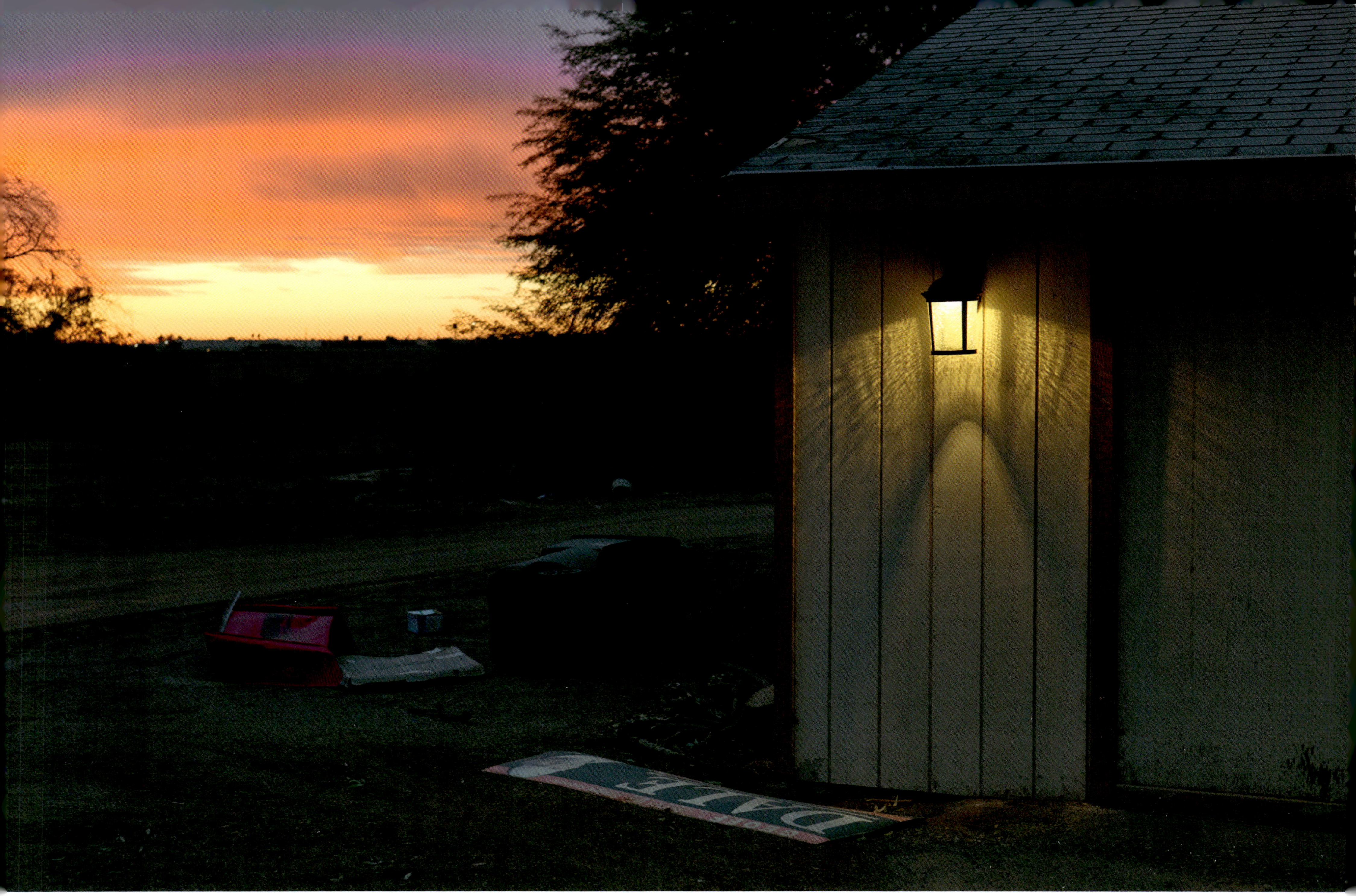

Barn, Imperial

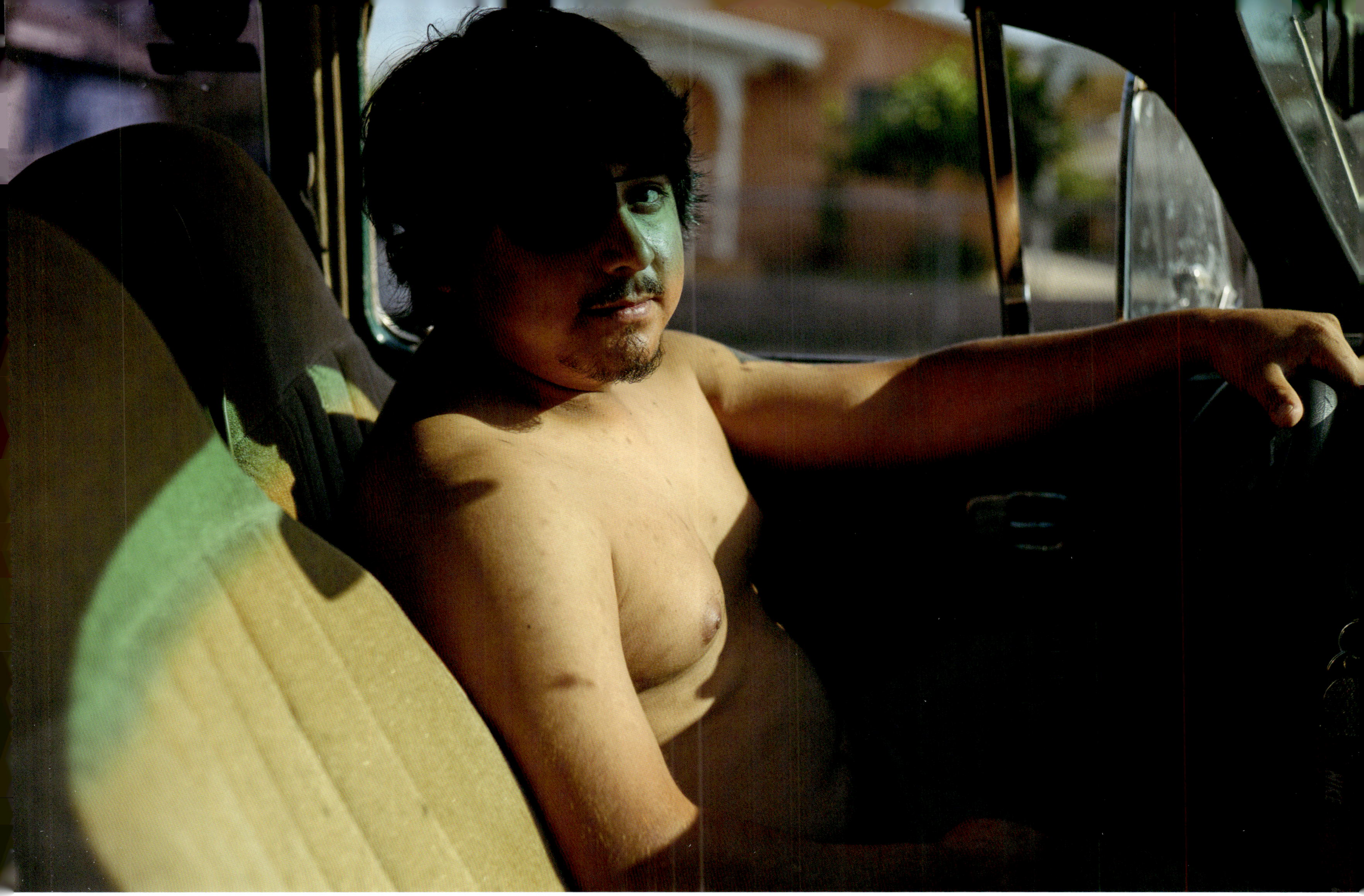

Chris in his Beetle, El Centro

Acknowledgment

A special thank you to Lisa and Levi, Dr. Enno Kaufhold, William T. Vollman, Klaus Kehrer, Hanne Reinhardt, Alexander Simon, Albert Valdez, Hector Arreola, Shedon Wyatt, Sherri Butler Dominick and her family, The Bujwah Tribe, Stefanie Williams, Simon Reinitzer, Strangers Bar, Prof. Manfred Paul, Niklas Goldbach, Edda Fahrenhorst, Steffen Lang, and Celeste Innocenti.

Dedicated to the people in the Imperial County, who allowed me into their lives to take theses photographs (and many more) or just shared their time, drinks, and wisdom with me.

Imprint

Texts
Enno Kaufhold, William T. Vollmann

Proofreading
Petra Joswig

Translations
Alisa Kotmaier (Enno Kaufhold), Claudia Kotte (William T. Vollmann)

Design
Studio Maven, Lisa Borges

Image Processing
Kehrer Design Heidelberg (Erik Clewe)

Production
Kehrer Design Heidelberg (Silke Küpperscheeg)

Bibliographic information published by the Deutsche Nationalbibliothek: The Deutsche Nationalbibliothek lists this publication in the Deutsche Nationalbibliografie; detailed bibliographic data is available on the Internet at http://dnb.dnb.de.

Printed and bound in Germany
ISBN 978-3-86828-781-3

Kehrer Heidelberg Berlin
www.kehrerverlag.com